Biomedical Signal Processing and Artificial Intelligence in Healthcare

Developments in Biomedical Engineering and Bioelectronics Series

Biomedical Signal Processing and Artificial Intelligence in Healthcare

Edited by

Dr. Walid Zgallai

Series Editor

Dr. Dennis Fitzpatrick

ELSEVIER

ACADEMIC PRESS

An imprint of Elsevier

Academic Press is an imprint of Elsevier
125 London Wall, London EC2Y 5AS, United Kingdom
525 B Street, Suite 1650, San Diego, CA 92101, United States
50 Hampshire Street, 5th Floor, Cambridge, MA 02139, United States
The Boulevard, Langford Lane, Kidlington, Oxford OX5 1GB, United Kingdom

Library of Congress Cataloging-in-Publication Data
A catalog record for this book is available from the Library of Congress

British Library Cataloguing-in-Publication Data
A catalogue record for this book is available from the British Library

ISBN 978-0-12-818946-7

For information on all Academic Press publications
visit our website at https://www.elsevier.com/books-and-journals

Publisher: Mara Conner
Acquisitions Editor: Fiona Geraghty
Editorial Project Manager: Joshua Mearns
Production Project Manager: Poulouse Joseph
Cover Designer: Matthew Limbert

My contribution is dedicated to my parents, Mr. Abdulhamid Zigalaie and Mrs. Amina Ibrahim.

Dr. Walid Zgalllai

Contents

Contributors

Dr. Noura AlHinai
Higher Colleges of Technology, Dubai, United Arab Emirates

Dr. J. Teye Brown
Faculty of Engineering Technology and Science, Higher Colleges of Technology, Dubai, United Arab Emirates

Christoph Janott
Munich School of BioEngineering, Technical University of Munich, Garching, Germany

Musa Sani Musa
Department of Biomedical Engineering, Faculty of Engineering, Near East University, Nicosia, Northern Cyprus, Turkey

Mubarak Taiwo Mustapha
Department of Biomedical Engineering, Faculty of Engineering; DESAM Institute, Near East University, Nicosia, Northern Cyprus, Turkey

Dr. Ilker Ozsahin
Department of Biomedical Engineering, Faculty of Engineering; DESAM Institute, Near East University, Nicosia, Northern Cyprus, Turkey

Dr. Dilber Uzun Ozsahin
Department of Biomedical Engineering, Faculty of Engineering; DESAM Institute, Near East University, Nicosia, Northern Cyprus, Turkey

Dr. Bashar Rajoub
Faculty of Engineering Technology and Science, Higher Colleges of Technology, Dubai, United Arab Emirates

Dr. Berna Uzun
DESAM Institute; Department of Mathematics, Near East University, Nicosia, Northern Cyprus, Turkey

Dr. Walid Zgallai
Faculty of Engineering Technology and Science, Higher Colleges of Technology, Dubai, United Arab Emirates

Foreword

This series on biomedical engineering provides an up-to-date and comprehensive review of the latest innovations within the field of biomedical engineering and bioelectronics. Each book in the series collectively brings together articles and supplementary learning materials to enhance or expand the reader's knowledge of that subject. Each subject is comprehensively introduced with in-depth articles by leading experts covering the latest technical innovations and biomedical engineering solutions.

The book series is aimed at anybody with an interest in biomedical engineering and bioelectronics whether it is on an academic or a professional level. Students studying undergraduate or postgraduate courses will find the subject introductions invaluable to enhance their academic studies and research projects. Professional biomedical and other engineers alike will find that they have access to the latest up to date articles and in-depth reviews in their subject field. The books will be supported by online media material to include online presentations, tutorials, application notes, algorithms, and working code examples.

Biomedical engineering encompasses engineering hardware and software for the diagnosis and remedy of medical conditions and diseases associated with the human body. The measurement and analysis of physiological signals inherent from the biological systems within the human body can help identify the cause and effect of medical conditions.

The first book in the series, Biomedical Signal Processing and Artificial Intelligence in Healthcare, provides an introduction to the foundation classes of biomedical signals based on the physiological recordings and measurements from the human body. The book then develops the different techniques used to capture and analyze these physiological signals using the latest artificial intelligence techniques such as machine learning algorithms that analyze the huge amount of data from biological systems and human traits to provide an understanding of the physiological parameters. The complex models that are developed ultimately lead to the development of therapeutic techniques and medical devices for the treatment and therapy of medical conditions.

The second book in the series, Drug Delivery Devices and Therapeutic Systems, introduces the technology behind the increasing number of biomedical devices that are used to deliver drug therapy in the treatment of various medical conditions and diseases. The book introduces the theory behind microfluidics and nanofluidics and the MEMS technology used to fabricate micropumps, reservoirs, and actuators in implantable drug delivery systems. The release of therapeutic drugs can be controlled using a variety of external physical stimuli, the medication being administered to specific localized tissue sites or direct into the bloodstream, the spinal canal, or the subarachnoid space. Using nanotechnology, nanoparticles can be used to carry anticancer drugs deep into tumors. The book also introduces drug-eluting stents; biodegradable hydrogels; and intranasal and transdermal drug delivery, with specific chapters on microneedles that pierce the skin using solid or hollow MEMS structures and the converse needle-free injectors. Finally the main therapeutic applications of drug delivery systems are presented, including cancer, diabetes, Parkinson's disease, and epilepsy.

The advancements in biomedical engineering provides not only more sophisticated diagnostic techniques but also more realistic technological solutions to the treatment and therapy of medical conditions and diseases. These biomedical engineering advancements will be covered in subsequent volumes in the book series with each book presenting the latest advances in biomedical engineering and bioelectronics.

Dr. Dennis Fitzpatrick

Preface

Book chapters

The human body consists of a complex network of subsystems that perform vital physiological processes. Biomedical signals acquired from organs using multiple sensors communicate information about the physiological processes and underlying pathologies. Such measurements can be plotted against time on a patient's chart. Analysis of these measurements provides useful information about the state of a patient's health.

Data modeling and analysis tools can be used to extract information from signals and reveal the underlying pathology that is reflected by the recorded signals. Typically the process starts with extracting meaningful features from the signal and subsequently using these features to learn a model that relates the extracted features to specific conditions. However, due to the vast amount of data recorded and the limited resources, physicians normally end up in actually making treatment decisions based on observing short isolated snapshots of biomedical signals. As such, providing physicians with reliable automated data analysis tools offers many potential benefits such as providing us with early warning signs of the onset of heart attacks, improve clinical diagnostic accuracy, and help clinicians make correct and timely medical interventions. Chapter 1, hence, introduces the basics of biomedical signal processing.

The main objective of Chapter 2 is to introduce the reader to the fundamentals of biomedical signal characterization. Feature engineering, feature extraction, generating alternative representations of biomedical signals form the main theme. We will first examine time-series data and how to represent them mathematically. We will discuss feature engineering from different perspectives: First, we begin by statistical feature generation using statistical moments. Next, we discuss transform-based feature extraction using the Fourier transform, time-frequency analysis, principal component analysis, independent component analysis, and factor analysis. The concepts of power spectrum, periodogram, and dimensionality reduction will be introduced, and examples of biomedical signals will be discussed. We will also discuss feature engineering using feature descriptor and conclude with a discussion of feature selection techniques.

Chapter 3 focuses on different supervised and unsupervised machine learning algorithms for biomedical signal analysis. Common algorithms in supervised learning include classification and regression, where different algorithms will be explained in details, permitting to effectively produce correct output data. Similarly, unsupervised learning algorithms such as clustering will be discussed. Performance of machine learning models will be illustrated using classification accuracy, region operating characteristics, and area under the curve. Finally, applications in biomedical signal processing will be presented in the form of a case study for automated detection of QRS complex in ECG signals based on temporal features.

Chapter 4 focuses on machine learning (ML) in biomedical signal processing with ECG applications and the advantages of machine learning to biomedical signal analysis. The tasks performed on ECG signals are commonly generated by the muscles of the heart resulting in an electrical signal. This is considered as one of the most important physiological parameters for feature extraction of ECG, and it is the most essential task in the manual and automated ECG analysis for use in instruments such as ECG monitors, Holter tape recorders and scanners, and ambulatory ECG recorders and analyzers. Machine learning applications apply artificial intelligent tools such as neural networks, genetic algorithms, fuzzy systems, and expert systems that are frequently used for detection and diagnostic tasks. This chapter will also address challenges associated with machine learning applications performed on ECG signals.

Chapter 5 will discuss how to apply deep learning, convolutional neural networks to process EEG signals in applications like controlling a robotic wheelchair. The process includes obtaining raw electroencephalogram (EEG) data in real time utilizing a brain-computer interface (BCI) device, providing a communication medium between brain activity signals and an external computer. These data are then processed using the fast Fourier transform algorithm (FFT). To convert these processed data into data conducive to processing with convolutional neural networks (CNNs), Python programming language and the NumPy and scikit-learn library are used. Finally, classification of the EEG data into four different commands is carried out using the popular TensorFlow and Keras machine learning libraries to train a convolutional neural network. The chapter presents deep convolutional neural networks. This is followed by explaining the deployment of Tensorflow and Keras in convolutional neural networks. A step by step explanation of acquiring EEG data with a BCI device is presented. Data processing and training utilizing Tensorflow and Keras is shown. Deployment and real time applications with embedded systems is introduced. The chapter offers also a tutorial on how to work with Pandas.

Fuzzy logic technique offers good solutions when it comes to vagueness in natural language and several other application domains. This is due to its characteristics to consider notions of truth and falsehood in a graded fashion when it comes to reasoning systems. Various diseases vary differently in behavior among patients. Also, similar symptoms can be caused by different diseases, leading to difficulty in diagnosis and as a result in medical treatment. Therefore the application of fuzzy logic in the medical field has gained popularity. For example, fuzzy expert systems were developed and tested in hospitals to diagnose diseases affecting the lungs, syndrome differentiation, and disease classification. Under vague conditions the physician requires assistance to make a diagnosis. Therefore fuzzy logic can be combined with other modeling approaches such as fuzzy linear programming where it aims to distribute several treatments to different disease population to minimize human productivity loss.

Fuzzy multiple-criteria decision analysis (MCDA) is another important aspect of operational research that has been employed in medicine because of its efficiency and effectiveness at evaluating alternatives with multiple conflicting criteria. In medicine and healthcare, there are various diagnostic and treatment devices that need evaluation according to their properties and needs of the hospital or patient. These methods support the decision-maker to obtain the best option among the alternatives. Chapter 6 introduces fuzzy logic and its application in medicine and healthcare systems. It discusses other fuzzy-based models such as fuzzy linear programming (FLP) and fuzzy multiple-criteria decision analysis (MCDA).

Factors associated with neurological and neuropsychiatric diseases can be caused by genetics, environment, and damage and degeneration of the nervous system. As a result, symptoms such as memory loss, mood swings, loss of bodily control, and behavioral changes arise, leading to more serious diseases. Examples of such disorders include Alzheimer's disease, Parkinson's disease, autism spectrum disorder, and attention deficit hyperactivity disorder. With early detection and diagnosis, these symptoms can be neutralized with the help of various treatments. However, with the limited current imaging techniques and variable human input, a patient can be misdiagnosed, and detection of the disease in its earlier stage can be inaccurate and challenging. Hence, it is of great importance to use automated detection methods for precise detection, classification, and prediction approaches. One form of artificial intelligence can be applied in these cases called artificial neural networks (ANNs). They are proven to perform better in extracting the biomarkers of heterogeneous data sets where the data volume and variety are great, hence providing early and more accurate diagnosis. In Chapter 7, we present an overview to the ANNs (shallow and deep neural network algorithms) and their applications in the classification and prediction of the neurological and neuropsychiatric diseases.

The interpretation of sleep data and support diagnosis can be time consuming for human experts; in recent years, machine learning methods for the interpretation and classification of sleep data have enhanced the ability of human experts to understand physiological information. The understanding of polysomnogram (PSG) data can be facilitated using the larger data sets of longer-term sleep monitoring obtained by the development of sophisticated machine learning models. These data sets include new findings in correlations between sleep structure and diseases as disturbing natural sleep is less, and novel combinations of sleep parameters are used. Chapter 8 will discuss methods of sleep signal processing and automated evaluation to support medical diagnosis and therapy decision-making.

Dr. Noura AlHinai

CHAPTER

Introduction to biomedical signal processing and artificial intelligence

1

Dr. Noura AlHinai

Higher Colleges of Technology, Dubai, United Arab Emirates

Abbreviations

1D	one-dimensional
AI	artificial intelligence
ASICs	application-specific integrated circuits
AV	atrioventricular
BPM	beats per minute
CAD	computer-aided diagnosis
DL	deep learning
ECG/EKG	electrocardiogram
EEG	electroencephalogram
EMF	electromagnetic field
FIR	finite impulse response
Hz	hertz
IIR	infinite impulse response
m-D	multidimensional
ML	machine learning
PLI	power-line interference
SA	sinoatrial

1.1 Introduction to signal processing

A signal is a mathematical function of one or more independent variables, representing a measureable quantity that can propagate in a certain medium [1]. Signals can be classified in many ways based on different parameters, such as time, periodicity of signal, nature of certainty, and causality. Subsequently signals can be classified as continuous time signals, discrete time signals, or digital signals as shown in Fig. 1.1 [2].

A continuous time signal is also known as an analog signal, where time and amplitude are continuous. Hence, time is an independent variable that belongs to real values. A discrete time signal is a signal that has been sampled at discrete intervals of

Biomedical Signal Processing and Artificial Intelligence in Healthcare. https://doi.org/10.1016/B978-0-12-818946-7.00001-9

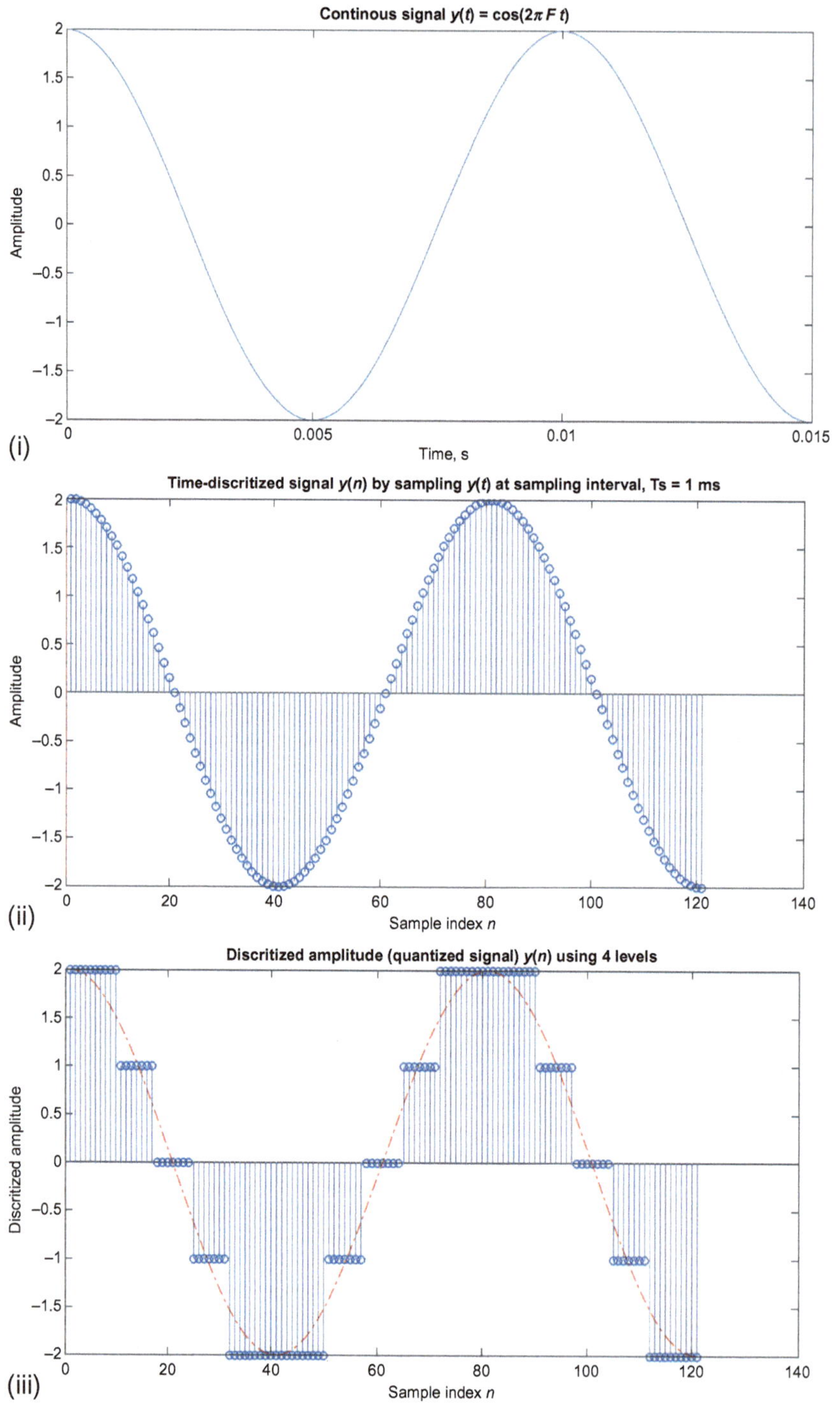

FIG. 1.1

Signal classification.

time. Hence, time is discrete, and amplitude is continuous. A digital signal is where both time and amplitude are quantized into discrete signal levels [2].

Signal processing involves manipulating a signal to change the basic characteristics of a signal or to extract some information from it. This is usually done by either using a computer program, application-specific integrated circuits (ASICs), or analog electrical circuit [3]. Software algorithms have advantage over analog electrical circuits in that they can be adapted for different scenarios and situations. The applications of signal processing are almost as diverse as the number of signals there are themselves. In the medical field, signal processing plays an important role in imaging, as well as monitoring, for example, the electrical activity in the heart and in the brain. There are three different classes of typical signal processing problems [4]:

(1) Eliminating *noise*: A noisy electrocardiograph can exhibit discontinuous behavior of the recorded signal. We know from the biology that the electrical activity of the heart should behave in a smooth fashion. Thus the goal of signal processing would be to eliminate or reduce noise and produce a clean signal that reflects the true underlying activity of the heart in a patient.

(2) Correction of distortion: Running a blurry image through a signal processing algorithm that can reconstruct a sharper, more focused image. Correcting distortion of images can be obvious; however, this can also be applied to signals being distorted in time.

(3) Extracting information embedded within the measured signals: For example, using a radar system to determine an aircraft position and velocity. Firstly, the position of the aircraft is governed by the time delay that it took for a pulse to travel from the radar to the airplane and back, and knowing the speed of light, we can figure out how far away it was. Secondly the relative velocity of the airplane with respect to the radar is embedded in the Doppler shift that can be seen in the received pulse.

In conclusion, signals and signal processing encompass every aspect of our lives. Signal processing is often used to address three different problems: (1) reduce noise in measured signals, (2) correct distortion, and (3) extract information from a signal. To do this, we rely on mathematical models, and it is the language of mathematics that is used to describe the field of signal processing.

1.2 Biomedical signals

The human body is made up of different systems that function in very unique ways, ensuring normal physiological processes, for example, the nervous system, the cardiovascular system, and the respiratory system. Abnormality in the physiological processes can alter the different physiological signals in the human body, which can cause diseases and lead to pathological processes. As a result the performance, health, and well-being of the human body will be affected. The nature of these physiological signals can be in the form of physical, electrical, or biochemical signals inherent within the human body [5].

A simple example of a biomedical signal is body temperature that can be easily detected in a qualitative manner via the palm of one hand or quantitatively measured using a thermometer. However, complicated diagnosis such as heart failure and epilepsy needs further signal analysis using different assessment methods, such as electrocardiogram (ECG/EKG) and electroencephalogram (EEG). The signals are small and reach the sensors attenuated and with noise; hence there is a need for amplifiers, which are used to amplify the signals and can be used for human computer interaction.

1.2.1 Electrocardiogram

The heart is a muscular organ that pumps blood around the body supplying the oxygen and nutrients the human body needs. It is divided into four chambers, namely, right atrium, left atrium, right ventricle, and left ventricle. The cardiac conduction system consists of the following components [6]:

- The sinoatrial node (SA node): This is located in the right atrium near the entrance of the superior vena cava. This is the natural pacemaker of the heart that initiates all heart beats and determines heart rate. Electrical impulses from the SA node spread throughout both atria and stimulate the muscles to contract. The SA node generates a heart rate of 60–100 BPM for adults and 100–150 BPM for babies and infants.
- The atrioventricular node (AV node): This is located on the other side of the right atrium near the AV valve. The AV node serves as an electrical gateway to the ventricles where it delays the passage of electrical impulses to the ventricles. This delay ensures that the atria have ejected all the blood into the ventricles before they contract. If the SA node fails, the AV node will "kick in" and generate its own series of impulses at a rate of 40–60 BPM.
- The AV node receives signals from the SA node and passes them into the atrioventricular bundle (bundle of His). This bundle is divided into right and left bundle branches, which conduct the impulses toward the apex of the heart. The signals are then passed onto Purkinje fibers turning upward and spreading throughout the ventricular myocardium. If the AV node and the bundle of His fails, the right and left bundle branches and the Purkinje fibers will generate their own impulses with a capacity to generate a heartbeat of 20–40 BPM.

The electrical activities of the heart can be recorded in the form of electrocardiogram (ECG/EKG). ECG or EKG measures the normal electrical signals of the heart to detect any heart problems such as heart attacks, irregular heartbeats, or heart failure [7]. Each wave or segments of the ECG correspond to a certain event of the cardiac electrical cycle. When the atria are full of blood, the SA node fires electrical signals to spread through the atria, causing the atria to depolarize. This is represented by the P wave on the ECG waveform. Atrial contraction starts about 100 ms after the

P wave begins. The P-Q segment represents the propagation time of the signal from the SA node to the AV node. The QRS complex marks the firing of the AV node and represents ventricular depolarization: (1) The Q wave corresponds to depolarization of the interventricular septum, (2) the R wave is produced by depolarization of the main mass of the ventricles, and (3) the S wave represents the last phase of ventricular depolarization at the base of the heart. The S-T segment reflects the plateau in the myocardial action potential. This is when the ventricles contract and pump blood. The T wave represents ventricular repolarization immediately before ventricular relaxation. The cycle repeats itself with every heartbeat [8]. Fig. 1.2 shows segments of the ECG waveform corresponding to events of the cardiac electrical cycle.

1.2.2 Electroencephalogram

The brain is the command center for the entire body. It receives information from our senses and controls our thoughts and movement. To better explore this complex organ, scientists have divided the brain into parts and regions [9]. The largest part is the cerebrum, which is divided into two hemispheres. The outer layer is called the cortex, which is a Latin term for bark and is only 1/8 inch thick. The cortex is divided into four regions: (1) the frontal lobe is for personality and emotions; (2) the temporal lobe helps process your hearing and other senses and helps with language and reading; (3) the parietal lobe is involved with your senses, attention, and language; and (4) the occipital lobe helps your eyes see, including recognition of shapes and colors. The thalamus in the center of the brain relays sensory and motor information into the cortex and helps with consciousness, sleep, and alertness. Twelve pairs of cranial nerves carry information from your senses to and from the brain and body. The cerebellum is found in the lower part of the brain, which plays a key role in motor control, coordination, and spatial navigation. Below the cerebellum is the brain stem, which connects the brain to the spinal cord, a nerve

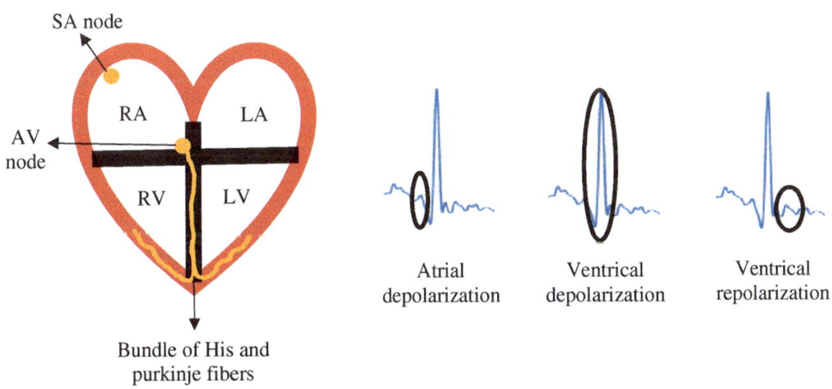

FIG. 1.2

Segments of the ECG corresponding to a certain event of the cardiac electric cycle.

pathway that runs all the way down the spine sending and receiving information from your senses. The brain stem includes (1) pons, which helps control breathing, and (2) medulla oblongata, which regulates our heart and other body reflexes such as vomiting, coughing, sneezing, and swallowing.

The electroencephalogram (EEG) measures the summation of electrical activity recorded on the scalp, primarily derived from neurons and the cortex [10]. Neurons communicate by passing electrical current that travels along dendrites or axons due to ions moving through voltage-gated channels in the neuron's plasma membrane. Voltage-gated channels open and close in response to an electrical voltage, so they are affected by changes in electrical charge around them. When a neuron is at rest, a charged difference is maintained between the inside and outside of the cell [11]. The system by which EEG electrodes are applied to the head and then displayed on EEG recordings is called "the international 10–20 system." The international 10–20 system is a standard method of measuring the head for electrode placement. It depends on four main positions on the head that are easily transferrable between patients: (1) the nasion at the bridge of the nose; (2) the inion, the bony part at the back of the head; and (3) two preauricular points just interior to each ear [12]. Fig. 1.3 is a schematic illustration using the 10–20 system of electrode placement for EEG recording.

1.3 Noise

Most biomedical signals are weak in amplitude and can easily be distorted especially in an environment with a multitude of other signals from various sources. Undesired signals that do not carry information are called interference, artifacts, or simply noise. The nature of artifacts that are encountered in biomedical signals varies and in return degrade the performance of signal processing. The physiological, instrumentational, or experimental environment could be potential sources of noise. In this section the various types of artifacts that could potentially corrupt biomedical signals and filtering techniques will be explored [13].

A patient undergoing an ECG test may not be able to control all physiological processes and systems. It is even more challenging when dealing with infants as the maternal ECG gets added to the fetal ECG of interest, and external control is not desirable. Coughing and breathing are some of the examples of physiological interference or motion artifacts and can vary with the level of the activity of relevance. In the case of normal breathing, the associated EMG of the chest muscles can cause interference with the desired ECG signal. Recording of the signal with the patient holding their breath for a few seconds can be an effective solution. However, it is not applicable if the patient is critically ill or during the recording of the ECG of infants. Factors such as electrode properties, electrolyte properties, skin impedance, and the movement of the patient affect the peak amplitude and duration of the artifact. Hence the physician is forced to develop solutions that are effective in removing or reducing physiological interference [4].

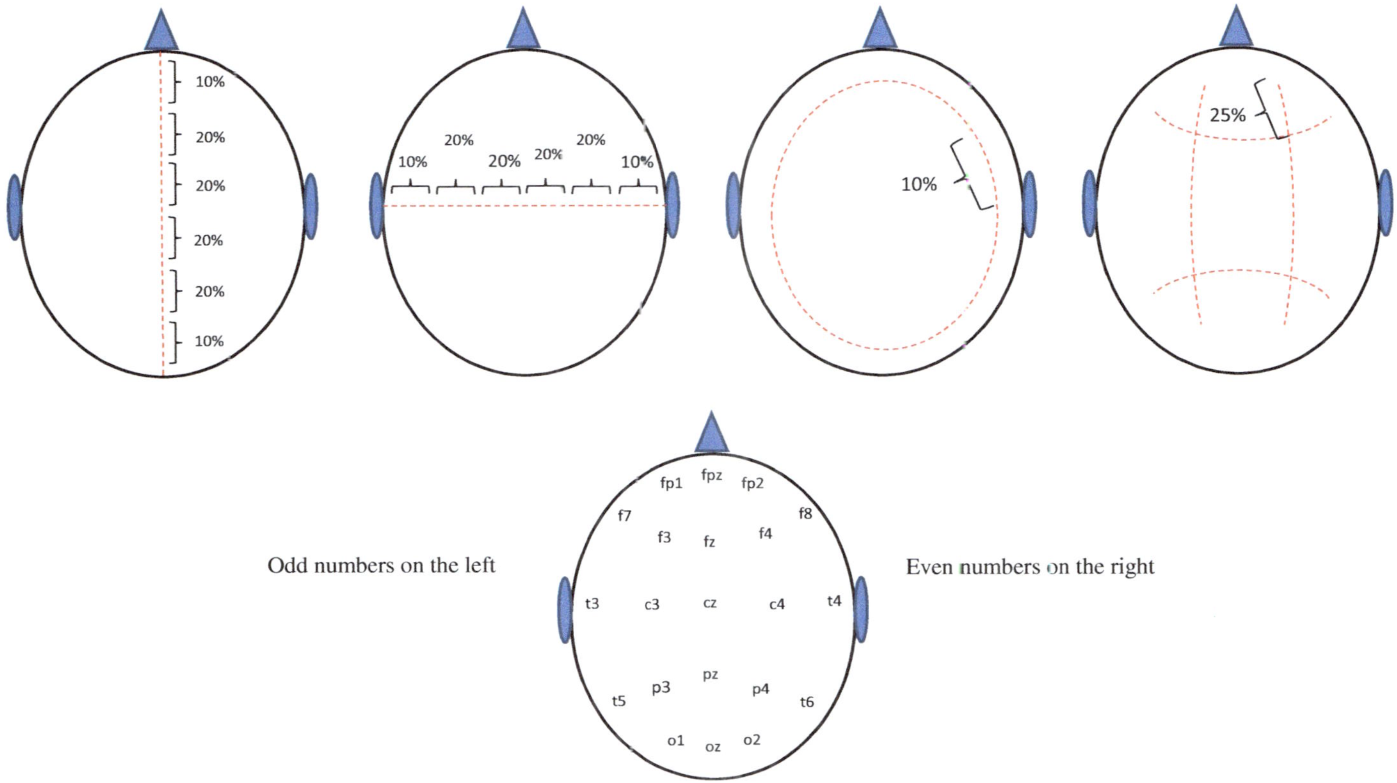

FIG. 1.3

The 10–20 system of electrode placement for EEG recording. Labels: *fp*, prefrontal; *f*, frontal; *p*, partial; *c*, central; *o*, occipital; *t*, temporal; *z*, midline.

1.3.1 Thermal noise

Thermal noise is always present in the electrical equipment used and is one of the major sources of noise that can affect the weak levels of biomedical signals at their source. Thermal noise was first detected and measured by John B. Johnson in 1926 and later explained by Harry Nyquist [14]. Hence, thermal noise is also known as Johnson-Nyquist noise, Johnson noise, or Nyquist noise. Thermal noise occurs due to the vibration of charge carriers within an electrical conductor and is directly proportional to the temperature, regardless of the applied voltage. Elimination of thermal noise is impossible; however, it can be reduced by reducing the temperature of operation or reducing the value of the resistance in electrical circuits. The thermal noise power is proportional to the bandwidth and is effectively white noise. However, the power spectrum equation suggests that at frequencies higher than 100 Hz, the level of thermal noise starts to drop off. The power spectrum equation is defined as [14]

$$V_n^2 = 4kTR \tag{1.1}$$

where k is the Boltzmann's constant, T is the temperature, and R is the resistance. Another type of instrumentational noise is called flicker noise.

1.3.2 Flicker noise

In contrast to thermal noise, flicker noise or $1/f$ noise is a function of frequency, and its effects are usually observed at low frequencies in electronic components. Flicker noise can be expressed in the form [15].

$$S(f) = \frac{K}{f} \tag{1.2}$$

Flicker noise is believed to be caused by charge carriers that are randomly trapped and released between the interfaces of two materials. This phenomenon typically occurs in semiconductors that are used in instrumentation amplifiers to record electrical signals. Flicker noise can be effectively reduced by a technique called chopper stabilization or chopper, where the amplifier offset voltage is reduced. In reality the input terminals are at slightly different DC potentials. The offset voltage is the differential voltage that must be applied to the input of an op-amp to produce zero output. Chopper stabilization technique is equivalent to modulation using a square wave, where the signal is alternated and gets chopped twice, first at the input stage and secondly at the output stage [16].

1.3.3 Power-line interference

Power-line interference (PLI) introduces 50–60 Hz frequency and is present in cables carrying signals from the examination room to the monitoring equipment. PLI can totally dominate physiological measurements like ECG or EEG due to the presence of electromagnetic interference or electromagnetic field (EMF) radiation from electrical machinery, computers, or other electrical equipment placed nearby. Other factors that dominate noise interference include stray currents caused by impedance mismatching of electrodes and cables and improper grounding of the ECG machine or even the patient [17]. Fig. 1.4 shows an ECG signal distorted with PLI, degrading the signal quality and potentially masking any significant small level signal features that may be crucial for monitoring and diagnosis.

1.4 Filters

Different filtering techniques can be used to reduce the effect of PLI corrupting a biomedical signal. The simplest filter design is a digital filter using the infinite impulse response (IIR) algorithm to remove the stationary power-line interference. However, since ECG signals corrupted with power-line interference is nonstationary in nature (i.e., its amplitude, frequency, and phase vary over time), an IIR notch filter practically fails to eliminate the line interference at frequencies other than the power-line frequency, 50 Hz in the United Kingdom and 60 Hz in the United States. Therefore other filtering techniques are used that will be explained later in this chapter.

1.4.1 FIR filters

A finite impulse response (FIR) filter is one of the categories of discrete time filters. The output of an FIR filter is expressed simply as the sum of the weighted values of the past input. This is also sometimes known as a moving average filter [18]. Thus the output of an FIR filter is given as

$$y[n] = \sum_{k=0}^{M} b_k x[n-k] \tag{1.3}$$

The FIR system function can be described as

$$H(z) = \sum_{k=0}^{M} b_k z^{-k} \tag{1.4}$$

So if we take the inverse of the z-transform to find the impulse response, we find that it is given by

$$h[n] = \left\{ \begin{array}{ll} b_n & ,0 \le n \le M \\ 0 & ,\text{otherwise} \end{array} \right\} \tag{1.5}$$

hence the term finite impulse response because this impulse response dies out after M turns. Fig. 1.5 shows the block diagram representing the FIR filter. The z^{-1} block represents a unit delay, so another way to think about the z^{-1} block in terms of actually implementing it in a computer is that each of these blocks represents a memory storage locations [19].

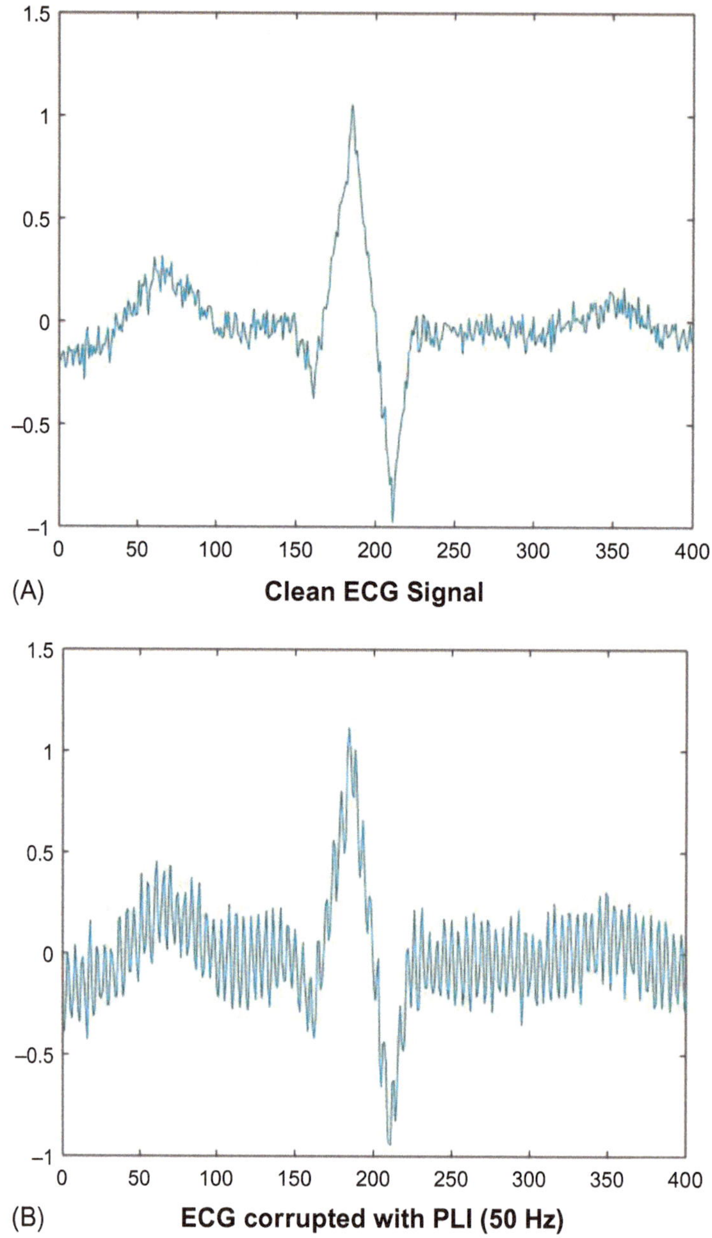

FIG. 1.4

An ECG signal distorted with PLI, degrading the signal quality and disturbs the significant features that may be crucial for monitoring and diagnosis. (A) Clean ECG signal; (B) ECG corrupted with PLI (50 Hz).

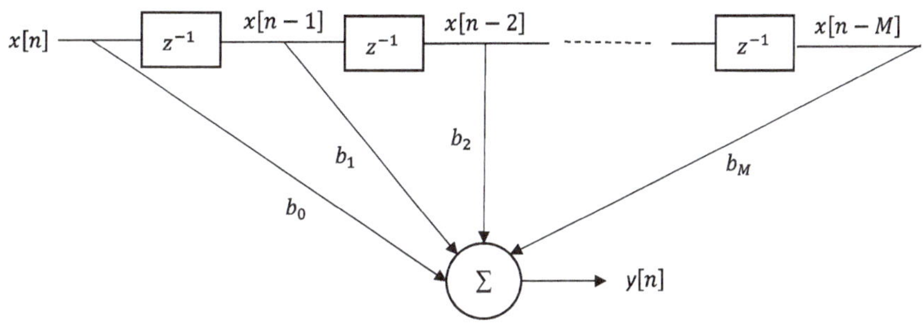

FIG. 1.5

FIR filter block diagram.

Assuming that we have a desired frequency response $H_d(e^{j\omega})$, our goal is to design a filter that approximate this desired frequency response. So in FIR design filter, we get to choose the coefficients b_k [18, 19]. Therefore the equation is given by

$$H\left(e^{j\omega}\right) = \sum_{k=0}^{M} b_k e^{-jk\omega} \tag{1.6}$$

It turns out that because of the simplicity of the form of the FIR filter, namely, that all the coefficients are in the numerator, you can develop optimization-based designs for choosing b_k so that $H(e^{j\omega})$ approximates $H_d(e^{j\omega})$. This means optimization can be achieved by minimizing the mean square error between H and H_d. You can set up the design problem in an optimization framework and then use numerical optimization to find the coefficients b_k. Another consequence in the FIR filter is that because we can formulate optimization based designs strategies, we can find FIR filters that have arbitrary magnitude/phase response. Hence, we approximate arbitrary magnitudes and phase responses, and then the question is how big M needs to be to achieve the desired level of approximation? In addition, with FIR filter, you can obtain exactly linear phase, so that these filters can be designed to have zero-phase distortion. Finally, to get an acceptable FIR filter design requires very large values of M. This is because the FIR filter only has zeroes available for placement in the z-plane and thus does not have much flexibility in terms of the types of frequency responses that can be easily designed [18, 19].

An application of an FIR filter to remove artifacts from an ECG signal at a cutoff frequency of 36 Hz and filter order $n=20$ is illustrated in Fig. 1.6.

```
close all
clear all
fs = 360; % sampling frequency
shift = 500 % plot offset
fc = 0.2; % fc normalized
wn = 20 % filter order
% ecg = load('sample.txt');
v = load('100m (0).mat')
ecg = v.val;
```

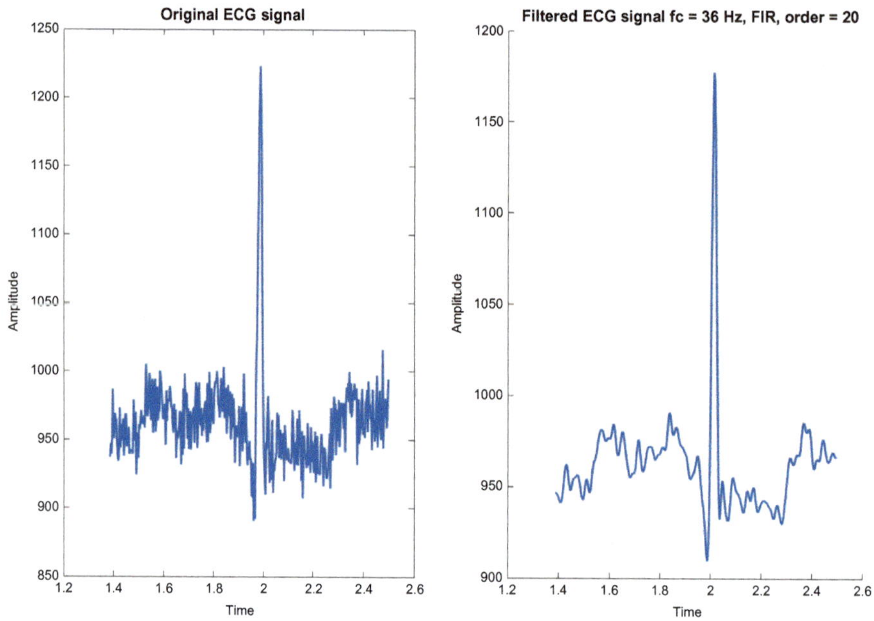

FIG. 1.6

Application of FIR filter to remove artifacts from an ECG signal.

```
K = fix(length(ecg)/4)
ecg = ecg(1:K)';
ecg = ecg+randn(K,1)*15; % add Gaussian noise
N = length(ecg);
t = [0:N-1]/fs;
[b,a] = butter(wn, fc);
[h,w] = freqz(b,a)
ecg_out = filter(b,a,ecg);
h = fir1(wn,fc)
y = filter(h,1,ecg);
figure
subplot 121
plot(t(shift:end),ecg(shift:end),'linewidth',1.5);
xlabel('time')
ylabel('amplitude')
title("original ECG signal")
subplot(122)
hold on,
plot(t(shift:end),y(shift:end),'linewidth',1.5);
title(['filtered ECG signal fc = ' num2str(fc*fs/2) ' Hz, FIR,
order = ' num2str(wn)])
xlabel('time')
ylabel('amplitude')
```

1.4.2 Frequency domain filters

A Butterworth filter, also called a maximally flat filter, is one of the most commonly used frequency domain filters. This is due to the filter having a sharp frequency roll-off characteristic, a monotonically changing magnitude function with frequency, ω, and a more linear phase response in the passband compared with the other traditional Chebyshev Type I/Type II and elliptic filters [20]. Therefore the Butterworth filter can be defined with an amplitude response of

$$|H(j\omega)| = \frac{1}{\sqrt{1+\left(\frac{\omega}{\omega_C}\right)^{2n}}} \tag{1.7}$$

where ω_c is the filter cutoff frequency and n is the filter order. At low frequencies, we can obtain a gain closer to one, and as the frequency increases, the gain decreases. The way this transition occurs is highly dependent on the filter order; with low filter order a smooth roll-off is attained; however, as the filter order increases, the curve can look more like a step function with very sharp transition and at higher frequencies will have very low gain [21]. Fig. 1.7 shows the Butterworth low pass filter response with different filter order.

```
% cutoff frequency fc
% sampling frequency fs
% filter order wn
close all
wn1 = 2
wn2 = 10
wn3 = 20
fc = 1000
fs = 5000
[b,a] = butter(wn1, fc/(fs/2));
[h1,w1]=freqz(b,a)
[b,a] = butter(wn2, fc/(fs/2));
[h2,w2] = freqz(b,a)
[b,a] = butter(wn3, fc/(fs/2));
[h3,w3] = freqz(b,a)
figure,
plot(w1/pi,20*log10(abs(h1)),'k','linewidth',2)
hold on
plot(w2/pi,20*log10(abs(h2)),'b','linewidth',2)
plot(w3/pi,20*log10(abs(h3)),'r','linewidth',2)
xlabel('normalized frequency')
grid on
ylabel('magnitude response, dB')
legend(num2str(wn1),num2str(wn2),num2str(wn3))
title('low pass Butterworth filter (different filter orders)')
```

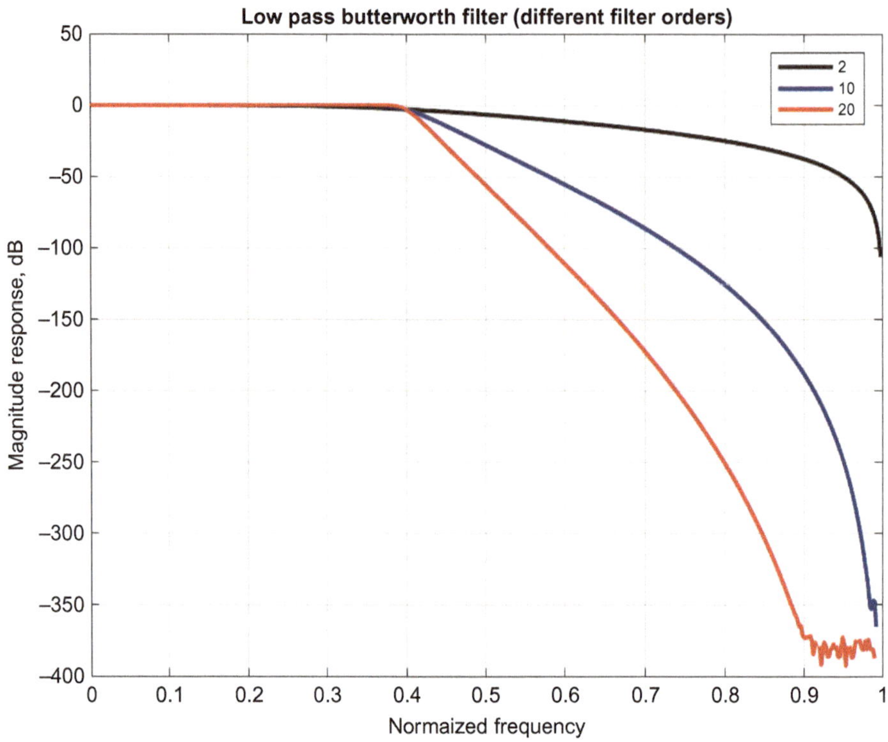

FIG. 1.7

Butterworth low pass filter with different filter order.

To design a normalized filter, the filter cutoff frequency is basically set to 1 (i.e., $\omega_c = 1$) [20]. Thus the normalized amplitude response can be expressed as follows:

$$|H_n(j\omega)| = \frac{1}{\sqrt{1+\omega^{2n}}} \tag{1.8}$$

Now let's look into the transfer function of a Butterworth filter, where a transfer function of a filter is denoted as $H(s)$ and s in general is a complex number written as $s = \sigma + j\omega$. The frequency response $H(j\omega)$ can be obtained from the transfer function by evaluating the transfer function along a certain set of points, mainly the imaginary axis. So, substituting $s = j\omega$ (i.e., $\sigma = 0$), the amplitude response can also be expressed as follows [20]:

$$|H_n(j\omega)|^2 = \frac{1}{1+\left(\frac{s}{j}\right)^{2n}} \tag{1.9}$$

Analyzing the equation further, this quantity has a total of $2n$ poles; they are actually $2n$ places in complex plane where this quantity $\frac{1}{1+\left(\frac{s}{j}\right)^{2n}}$ goes to infinity. This occurs at any time when $\left({}^{s}/_{j}\right)^{2n} = -1$, yielding to

$$s^{2n} = -(j)^{2n} \tag{1.10}$$

To find the poles the earlier equation is expanded by substituting $-1 = e^{j\pi(2k-1)}$ and $j = e^{j\pi}/2$; the equation is given as follows, which is a complex number on the unit circle [20]:

$$s_k = \cos\left(\frac{\pi}{2n}(2k+n-1)\right) + j\sin\left(\frac{\pi}{2n}(2k+n-1)\right) \quad \text{where } k = 1,2,\ldots,2n \tag{1.11}$$

The poles on the left hand plane correspond to $H_n(s)$, while the poles on the right hand plane correspond to $H_n(-s)$. The left hand plane poles are the ones that we care about because they correspond to a causal and stable filter. Finally the transfer function of the normalized Butterworth filter is given as [20, 22]

$$H_n(s) = \frac{1}{B_n(s)} \tag{1.12}$$

where $B_n(s)$ is the nth order Butterworth polynomial and can be looked up in table [20].

How to design a Butterworth filter with a cutoff frequency other than $\omega_c = 1$? [22] This is done by scaling the normalized filter up to the desired cutoff frequency, simply by replacing ω with ω/ω_c in $H_n(\omega)$. Equivalently, we can scale our filter in the s domain by replacing s with s/ω_c in $H_n(s)$. Another parameter that we want to control is the gain; this is the amount the frequency is changed in amplitude at a given frequency. Hence, typically it is specified using a passband gain and a stopband gain. Normally for a low pass filter, we have a gain of approximately 1 at low frequencies, and then it starts falling off, and ω_p is the passband frequency. At the passband frequency, we usually specify exactly how much gain we should have. Thus, when designing a filter, there are four parameters: ω_p, ω_s, and their corresponding gains G_p and G_s. From these filter specifications, we can figure out the filter order that we need. The gain is measured in dB given by [23]

$$G_x = -10\log_{10}\left[1 + \left(\frac{\omega_x}{\omega_c}\right)^{2n}\right] \tag{1.13}$$

Evaluating the earlier equation at ω_p and ω_s, the gain will be expressed as follows:

$$G_{p,dB} = -10\log_{10}\left[1 + \left(\frac{\omega_p}{\omega_c}\right)^{2n}\right] \rightarrow \left(\frac{\omega_p}{\omega_c}\right)^{2n} = 10^{-G_{p,dB}/10} - 1 \tag{1.14}$$

$$G_{s,dB} = -10\log_{10}\left[1 + \left(\frac{\omega_s}{\omega_c}\right)^{2n}\right] \rightarrow \left(\frac{\omega_s}{\omega_c}\right)^{2n} = 10^{-G_{s,dB}/10} - 1 \tag{1.15}$$

By dividing passband gain and the stopband gain, the equation can then be solved for the filter order n yielding to the following equation:

$$n = \frac{10\log_{10}\left[\left(10^{-G_{s,dB}/10} - 1\right)\left(10^{-G_{p,dB}/10} - 1\right)\right]}{2\log_{10}\left(\omega_s/\omega_p\right)} \tag{1.16}$$

In summary, by defining the filter specifications ω_p, ω_s, and their corresponding gains G_p and G_s, the needed filter order can be found to design the required filter [24]. A Butterworth low pass filters with order $n = 20$ and $\omega_c = 36$ Hz and with order $n = 3$ and $\omega_c = 2$ Hz were applied in series to the ECG signal. Fig. 1.8 shows the application of Butterworth low pass filter to remove artifacts from an ECG signal.

```
close all
clear all
fs = 360; % sampling frequency
shift = 500 % plot offset
fc = 0.2; % fc normalized
wn = 20 % filter order
% ecg = load('sample.txt');
v = load('100m (0).mat')
ecg = v.val;
K = fix(length(ecg)/4)
ecg = ecg(1:K)';
ecg = ecg+randn(K,1)*15; % add Gaussian noise
N = length(ecg);
t = [0:N-1]/fs;
[b,a] = butter(wn, fc);
[h,w] = freqz(b,a)
ecg_out = filter(b,a,ecg);
figure
subplot 121
plot(t(shift:end),ecg(shift:end),'linewidth',1.5);
xlabel('time')
ylabel('amplitude')
title("original ECG signal")
subplot(122)
hold on,
plot(t(shift:end),ecg_out(shift:end),'linewidth',1.5);
title(['filtered ECG signal fc = ' num2str(fc*fs/2) 'Hz,
Butterworth, order = ' num2str(wn)])
xlabel('time')
ylabel('amplitude')
```

1.5 Computer-aided diagnosis (CAD): Why?

One of the branches of signal processing is multidimensional (mD) signal processing. It is utilized when specific data need to be detailed and sampled using more than one-dimension (1D). As a result, images are formed based on the manipulation of multiple signals. Compared with 1D, proceeding in mD requires more complex algorithms and is directly associated with digital signal processing. Hence the actual computations grow with the number of dimensions, and the use of computer modeling is needed.

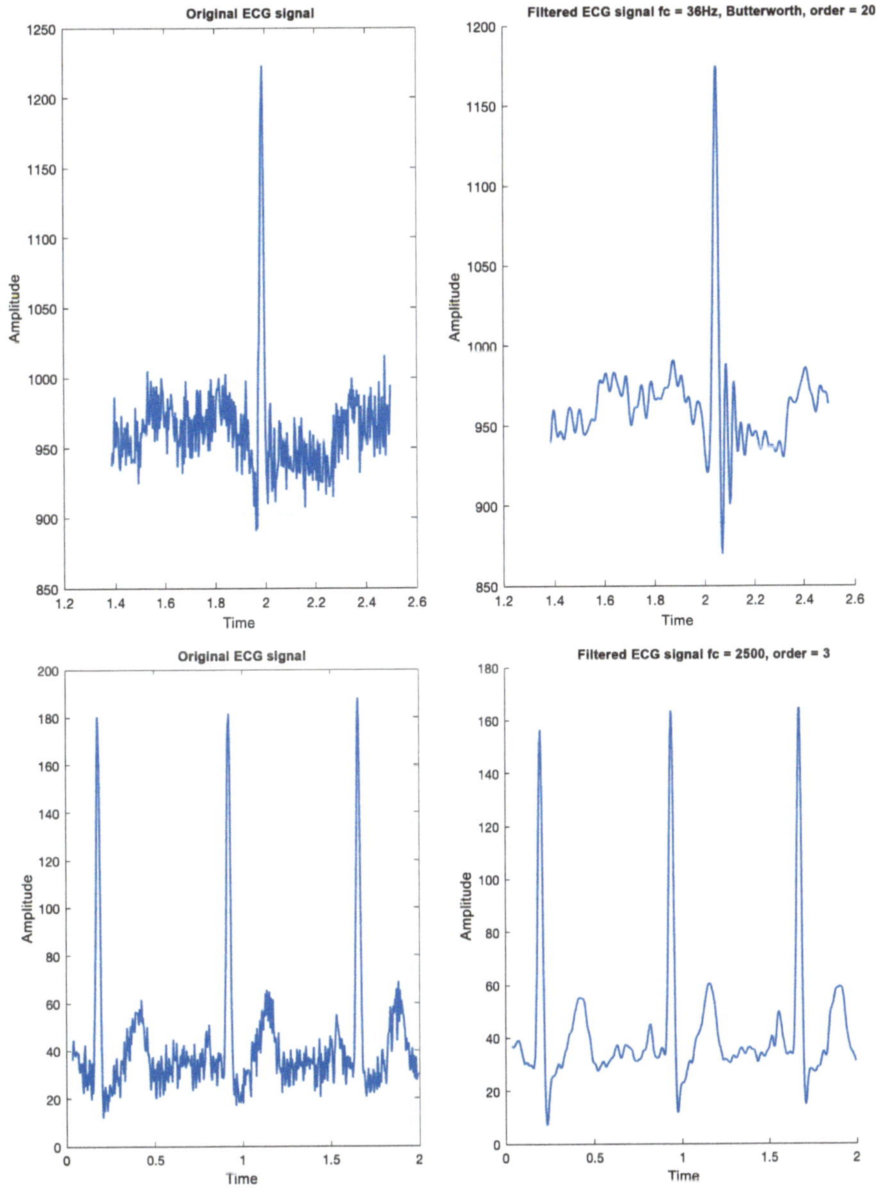

FIG. 1.8

Application of Butterworth filter to remove artifacts from an ECG signal.

The concept of CAD was first reported by Fred Winsberg in 1967. Winsberg and his team examined the use of computers to analyze the detection of abnormalities on mammograms [25]. In 1972 the concept of CAD was expanded by classifying four properties a computer could use to detect lesions on mammograms, namely, (1) calcification, (2) speculation, (3) roughness, and (4) shape. Many other features have been defined since this initial classification [26]. Today, computer-aided diagnosis is helping physicians to make diagnoses, in particular acting as second readers, which means a physician will make their first attempt at diagnosing a disease in a patient and then the computer will come in as a backup to confirm that diagnosis. The main objective of CAD is to decrease the rate of false diagnosis by assisting physicians with a second opinion.

In this age of technology, artificial intelligence (AI) knows no bounds; once thought a futuristic threat to human kind, AI is changing and saving lives. Not intended to replace clinicians or clinical judgments, AI serves the purpose to enhance and compliment the very human interaction of provider and patient. In healthcare, AI is changing the game with its applications in decision support, image analysis, and patient triage. With their ability to reduce variation and duplicate testing, decision support systems quickly decipher large amounts of data within the electronic medical record. AI technology is also taking the uncertainty out of viewing patients' scans by highlighting problem areas on images, aiding in the screening and diagnosis process. Artificial intelligence helps with the issue of physician burnout by collecting patient data via an app or text messaging. Chatbox will ask patients a series of questions regarding their symptoms, taking the guesswork out of self-diagnosis and saving both the patient and provider time and money [27].

CAD uses a pattern recognition software that detects unusual patterns on the image for the physician to take into consideration when making a diagnosis. There are typically four general schemes for a computer-aided diagnosis system [28]:

1. Preprocessing: The data are being processed into a sufficient enough quality so that the computer is able to recognize the image. Filters, as well as window level adjustment techniques, are applied for image contrast. The main objective of this step is to reduce noise and artifacts.
2. Segmentation: In this step the body is segmented into regions. The computer uses data from an anatomical databank to identify whether the region of interest on the image represents mass, micro calcification, or tissue.
3. Feature extraction: The region of interest is analyzed for special characteristics, such as morphological features, gray level features, and texture features.
4. Feature classification: The goal is to apply various algorithms to classify: (a) whether the identified structure is benign or malignant and (b) differentiate true lesions from normal anatomical structures.

The effects of CAD on quality and efficiency of services are as follows [4]:

1. CAD can improve the time efficiency as it can help reduce times for image diagnosis for certain cases. Signal processing is used to remove noise or extract parameters using complicated mathematical procedures that humans cannot perform.

2. Human observers are prone to commit errors when monitoring a patient's status for prolonged periods due to factors such as fatigue, boredom, and environmental factors. However, computers can be designed to record all episodes or transients in the signal in a mathematical and consistent manner.
3. CAD can help increase the accuracy in image diagnosis as it may be able to detect diseases if they are too small or in early stages and cannot be seen by human eyes. This allows for early diagnosis that can be beneficial for a better patient outcome.
4. CAD can help reduce the workload for a highly experienced radiologist as the system can help improve the accuracy and interpretation time for less experienced physicians. This will allow for less stress and demand for highly experienced radiologists and therefore increase productivity [4].

In conclusion, CAD only provides quantitative analysis and is consistently applied in routine or repetitive tasks [4]. Signal analysis alone is not enough to make a diagnosis and needs to be integrated with other information that a physician can include such as the general physical appearance and mental state of the patient and family history. Accordingly, it is further emphasized that computer-aided diagnosis is used as a secondary source of diagnosis. The physicians are still the primary source of diagnosis. The CAD system will be used to provide a second opinion [4].

1.6 Artificial intelligence (AI): An overview

The history of artificial intelligence (AI) goes back to the early 1920s when Karel Čapek's play, "Rossum's Universal Robots" (RUR), opened in London and first used the word "robot" in English. In 1956 John McCarthy coined the term *artificial intelligence* a demonstration of the first running AI program at Carnegie Mellon University, and in 1958 John McCarthy invented the LISP programming language for AI. Major advances occurred in 1990s in different areas of AI, such as machine learning, reasoning, problem solving, natural language, and perception [29]. Although AI was born some time ago, today's artificial intelligence is receiving a lot of attention from different sectrs, such as transportation, education, and health. So the question is what is different this time?

The definition of artificial intelligence has evolved in different eras based upon the goals intended to be achieved by different industries using AI. It first started with a neutral definition, introduced by John McCarthy when he invited a group of researchers to develop the concepts around "thinking machines" that included cybernetics, automata theory, and complex information processing. At the Dartmouth Summer Research Project on Artificial Intelligence conference, John McCarthy proposed [30], "Every aspect of learning or any other feature of intelligence can in principle be so precisely described that a machine can be made to simulate it. An attempt will be made to find how to make machines use language, form abstractions and concepts, solve kinds of problems now reserved for humans, and improve themselves." The modern definition of artificial intelligence in the English Oxford Living

Dictionary is [31] "The theory and development of computer systems able to perform tasks normally requiring human intelligence, such as visual perception, speech recognition, decision-making, and translation between languages." Thus investing in AI became a priority to many industry leaders to solve problems defined in the field and to use the unique capabilities of AI to enhance services or products offered, rather than replicating the human brain [32].

The fear of the future driven by AI has been overwhelming on the society, although we use AI almost every day in our lives without even knowing it. As a matter of fact, many of us mistakenly use the word "robot" as a synonym to AI. Hence, it is very important to understand the various types of AI, before making assumptions on what the future holds. There are two types of artificial intelligence, namely, "weak" AI and "strong" AI [33].

The key feature that makes us humans different to a machine is the brain, which enables us to make decisions, be sentient, creative, and emotionally driven when responding to situations. Weak AI, also known as artificial narrow intelligence (ANI), lacks the ability to perform human-like tasks that require self-awareness and emotions. ANI as the name implies can only perform specific real-time tasks by retrieving information from specific data sets that is within a predetermined and predefined range. A good example of "weak" AI is Siri. When we ask Siri a question about the weather, we get an accurate response. However, if Siri was asked a question on its opinion about a personal problem, we receive a vague response. This is because Siri was designed to process the human language, enter it into a search engine (Google), and return to us with results. However, the benefit of "weak" AI cannot be denied as it has made tasks such as ordering a pizza online a lot easier [33].

In contrast to "weak" AI, "strong" AI, also known as artificial general intelligence (AGI), are machines that are able to operate without outside intervention and act independently when dealing with different situations. The ultimate goal of "strong" AI is to develop artificial intelligence machines to mimic the human brain and function just like humans. As mentioned earlier, industry leaders are making rapid progress to achieve this goal, and as such, there are no proper existing examples [34].

There is a lot of data today generated not only by humans but also by computers, phones, and other devices. This will only continue to grow in the years to come; as the volume of data surpasses the ability for humans to make sense of it and manually write those rules, efficient training of large complex model is required. This will in turn allow machines to learn from the data and more importantly the changes in the data. Hence, machine learning and deep learning were introduced. Often, both terms are used interchangeably and have caused confusion. For simplification purposes, artificial intelligence, machine learning, and deep learning are subsets of one another [35].

Machine learning (ML) is a technique that uses statistical methods, enabling machines to learn from their past data or experience. Machine learning has gained popularity in areas where (a) equations are complex, for example, face recognition; (b) tasks are constantly changing, for example, fraud detection; and (c) the nature of

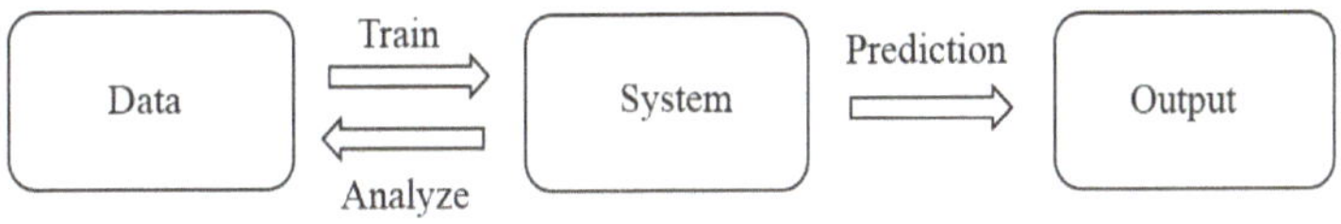

FIG. 1.9

Simplified machine learning workflow.

the data keeps changing and the program needs to adapt, for example, energy production, for price and load forecasting [36]. When the data come in, machines immediately start analyzing the data and eventually get "trained up" and learn from the data. When a new data point comes in, machines accurately make prediction and decisions based on the past data. Fig. 1.9 demonstrates the machine learning workflow.

Machine learning can be divided into two branches, namely, (a) supervised learning and (b) unsupervised learning [36]. Supervised learning has several data points or samples, described using predictor variables or features and a target variable. The data are commonly represented in a table structure, where there are rows for each data point and columns for each feature. The aim of supervised learning is to build the model to be able to predict the target variable, given the predictor variables. In supervised learning, we have machine learning algorithms for (a) classification that is the organization of labeled data and (b) regression that is the prediction of trends in labeled data to determine future outcomes. On the other hand, unsupervised learning is a machine learning task uncovering hidden patterns and structures from unlabeled data. One branch of unsupervised learning is clustering, which is the analysis of patterns and groupings of unlabeled data [37]. Fig. 1.10 summarizes the difference between supervised learning and unsupervised learning.

Deep learning is a subfield of machine learning and uses neural network architectures to emulate human brain abilities such as observing, analyzing, learning, and making decisions [38]. So far, no one really understands what happens inside a neural network and why it works so well, so currently, it is called a black box. To understand deep learning better, let us consider a simple example and see how it works on a conceptual level such as how to recognize a square from other shapes [39]. So the first thing you do is check the following: (a) whether there are four lines associated with the figure or not. If yes, (b) we further check if they are connected and closed. If yes, (c) we finally check whether it is perpendicular and all its sides are equal. If everything fulfills, then it is a square. Thus what we did is we took a complex task of identifying a square and broke it into simpler tasks. Now deep learning does the same thing but at a larger scale. Fig. 1.11 illustrates a classic example of utilizing deep learning to recognize whether a given image is of a cat or a dog. Similarly the first thing is to define the feature of the animal such as whether it has whiskers or not or check whether it has pointed ears or not. The system will then define which features are more important in classifying a particular animal [40].

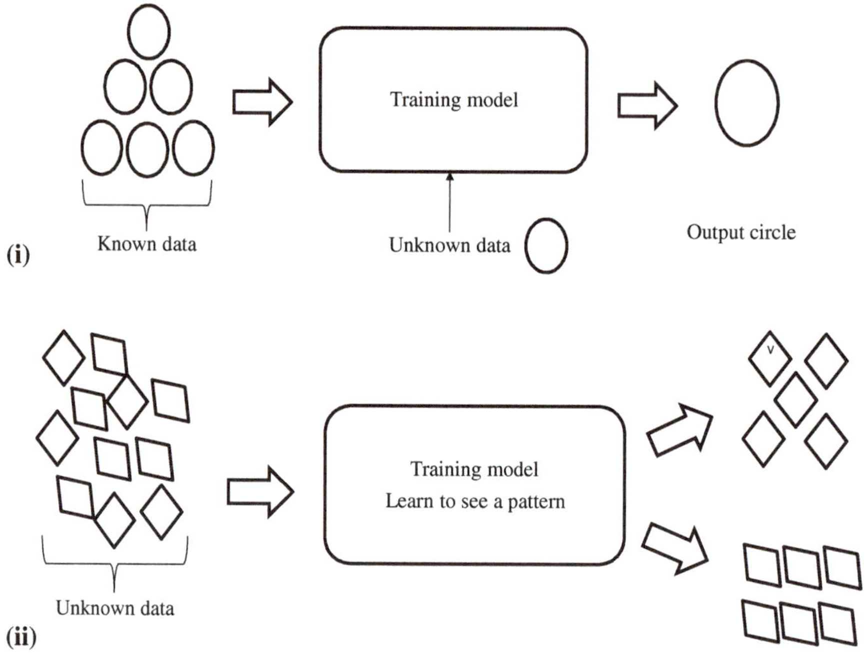

FIG. 1.10

The difference between (i) supervised learning and (ii) unsupervised learning.

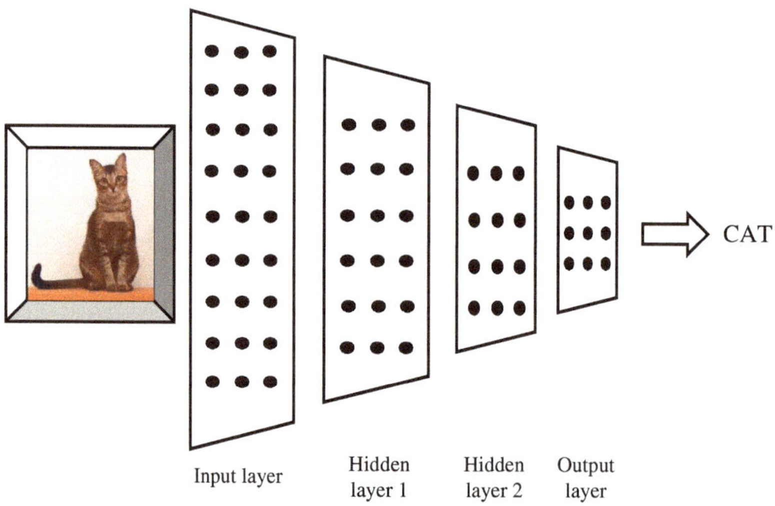

FIG. 1.11

A classic example of utilizing deep learning to recognize whether a given image is of a cat or a dog.

1.7 Fuzzy logic in artificial intelligence

In 1965 Lotfi A. Zadeh introduced the concept of fuzzy logic. As the name implies, the output of any event, process, or function that is changing continuously needs to be defined in a fuzzy manner, taking into consideration inaccuracies and uncertainties. In simple terms, fuzzy logic takes the ambiguity of a human input and transforms it into a degree of membership; memberships make up a fuzzy set that is used to evaluate a number of rules [41]. Fig. 1.12 shows the difference between traditional logic and fuzzy logic using tap water temperature as an example. In traditional logic the temperature is either represented as hot or cold, representing 0 or 1 respectively, while in fuzzy logic, there is a gradient from hot to cold.

Real-world applications of fuzzy logic are numerous and are gaining more popularity over the course of time, for example, weather forecasting, business decision-making, and neural networks in artificial intelligence. The reason why fuzzy logic applies so well in most real-world scenarios is because most of the scenarios do not have a distinct value but based on approximations [42]. For example, the number of red cells in your blood cannot be accurately counted, but we can always have an estimated value. Another example is the growth of bacteria in an environment, which

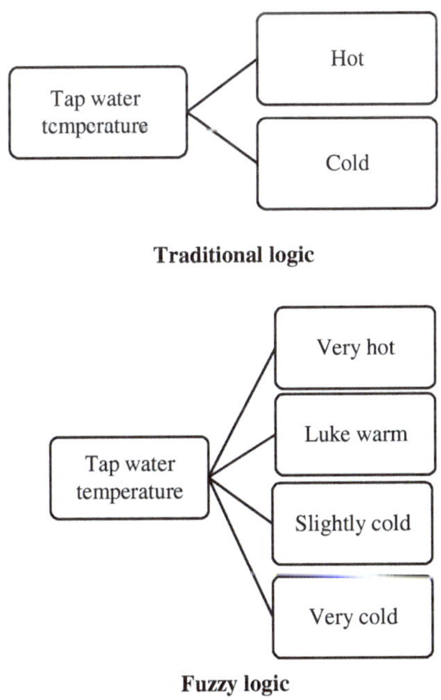

FIG. 1.12

The difference between traditional logic and fuzzy logic using tap water temperature as an example.

can only be predicted. As mentioned earlier, fuzzy logic operates under the concept of membership and degree of membership, which ranges from 0 to 1. So, depending on a membership function, as in the example of tap water temperature, the member function can be considered as "what is the tap water temperature?" The gradient outputs are the membership values. To understand the concept better, we need to understand the difference between crisp set and fuzzy set. Crisp sets are usually classical sets that have distinct objects, for example, where A is a set of even numbers and can be represented as follows: $A = \{2, 4, 6, 8, \ldots\}$. Each individual number is called an entity or a member of the set. Fuzzy set is where the degree of membership concept is applied and can be represented as follows: $A = \{\frac{0.9}{\text{Car}}, \frac{0.6}{\text{Train}}, \frac{0.1}{\text{Cycle}}\}$, where the numerator is called the membership degree to which the denominator is associated with set A. So, we can say that "train" has a degree of membership of 0.6 associated with fuzzy set A. As a result the highest value of membership degree is 1, and the lowest value of membership degree is 0. In this representation the element "cycle" is least associated with set A, and "car" is strongly associated with set A [43].

The initial concept of crisp sets was used by system experts to introduce fuzzy set theory, in imprecisions and vague situations. The significance of fuzzy set theory has increased in the attempt to imitate the human brain in artificial intelligence.

In conclusion, studies revealed the importance of integrating artificial intelligence systems in biomedical signal processing applications that provides an insight into solutions to minimize the challenges faced by physicians when making a diagnosis. The concept of fuzzy logic has common features with neural networks when it comes to mimicking human psychology; it is a mathematical representation near to the human thinking and natural activities. Therefore fuzzy logic can be considered a branch of artificial intelligence, especially in situations of vagueness. Reduction of noise using different filtering techniques produces improved readings for disease detection, which assists physicians to better diagnose.

Questions and answers

Describe other types of biomedical signals such as EMG and ERG

Electromyography (EMG) is a diagnostic procedure to measure the electrical activities between the muscles and nerves. The test is ordered by a physician if the patient shows symptoms of numbness, tingling, or weakness in the limbs. An EMG procedure takes about 30–60 min to complete, in which the electrodes will deliver tiny electrical signals to the nerves. It is composed of two procedures:

1. Nerve conduction: Several electrodes are placed on the surface of the skin, usually in the area where the symptoms are experienced, to evaluate how well nerve cells communicate with the muscles. The electrodes are removed once the test is completed.
2. Needle EMG: Needle electrodes are inserted into the muscle to evaluate the electrical activity of the muscle when it contracts and relax.

Electroretinogram (ERG) is an eye test that evaluates the function of the retina, which is a film that outlines the inside of the eye. The idea of the ERG test is that when flashes of light comes to the eye, the rods and the cones in the inner cells of the retina produce tiny amounts of electricity. Some retinal abnormalities that an ERG can detect include Leber congenital amaurosis, achromatopsia, and choroideremia. ERG is performed by the following steps:

- Your doctor will ask you to lie down or sit in a comfortable position.
- They will dilate your eyes with eye drops in preparation for the test.
- Your doctor will place anesthetic drops in your eyes, which will make them numb.
- They will use a device known as a retractor to hold open your eyelids. This will enable them to carefully place a small electrode on each eye. The electrodes are about the size of a contact lens.
- Your doctor will attach another electrode to your skin so that it functions as a ground for the faint electrical signals made by the retina.
- You will then watch a flashing light. Your doctor will conduct the test in normal light and in a darkened room. The electrode enables the doctor to measure your retina's electrical response to light. The responses recorded in a light room will mainly be from your retina's cones. The responses recorded in a darkened room will mainly be from your retina's rods.
- The information from the electrodes transfers to a monitor. The monitor displays and records the information. It appears as a-waves and b-waves. The a-wave is a positive wave that originates mainly from your eye's cornea. It represents the initial negative deflection of a flash of light. The b-wave, or positive deflection, follows. The plot of the b-wave's amplitude reveals how well your eye reacts to light.

State any two difficulties encountered in biomedical signal acquisition and analysis

- Inadequate data acquisition to different variables due to the location of organs within the body.
- Biomedical signals are generally weak at the source. Therefore transducers with integrated amplifiers are required with low noise levels.
- Patients' protection as the risks involved when conducting a procedure needs to thoroughly assessed to avoid electrical shocks or radiation hazards.
- Movement of the subject, such as coughing, can cause undesirable artifact such as EMG.

Provide a comparison between stationary and nonstationary processes. Are biosignals such EEG and ECG stationary or nonstationary and why?

A signal is nonstationary when the statistics of the signal (mean, variance, and higher-order statistics) change with time. A signal that is independent of time is called stationary signal.

The ECG represents the electrical activity of the heart. The heart has its own oscillator that is modulated by signals from the brain at every heartbeat. Therefore, since the process changes with time (i.e., the way that the heart beats changes at each heartbeat), then it is considered nonstationary. The same applies for the EEG. The EEG represents a sum of localized electrical activity of neurons in the brain. The brain cannot be considered stationary in time since a human being performs different activities. Conversely, if we were to fix the observation window, we could claim some form of stationarity, and the signal can be referred to as quasi-stationary. One of the techniques that is used for time-frequency representations is short-time Fourier transform (STFT); the short time-duration window is subsequently slid along the time axis to cover the entire duration of the signal and to obtain an estimate of the spectral content of the signal at every time instant.

References

[1] L. Van Biesen, Signals and information and classification of signals, in: Signal Theory, Vrije Universiteit Brussel, 2012, pp. 1–18.

[2] tutorialspoint.com, Signals & Systems—Classification of Signals, TutorialsPoint, 2019. Available: https://www.tutorialspoint.com/signals_and_systems/signals_and_systems_classification_of_signals.asp. (Accessed 1 July 2019).

[3] D.C.B. Chan, P.J.W. Rayner, S.J. Godsill, Multi-channel signal separation, in: 1996 IEEE International Conference on Acoustics, Speech, and Signal Processing Conference Proceedings, vol. 2, 1996, pp. 649–652.

[4] R.M. Rangayyan, Biomedical Signal Analysis, John Wiley & Sons, 2015.

[5] C. Singh, J. Singh, Biomedical signal processing, artificial neural network: a review, Indian J. Sci. Technol. 9 (47) (2016).

[6] T. Newman, The Heart: Anatomy, Physiology, and Function, Medical News Today, 2019. Available: https://www.medicalnewstoday.com/articles/320565.php. (Accessed 30 June 2019).

[7] WebMD, 2019. "Heart Disease and Electrocardiograms, Available: https://www.webmd.com/heart-disease/electrocardiogram-ekgs (Accessed 30 June 2019).

[8] R. Klabunde, Cardiovascular Physiology Concepts, Lippincott Williams & Wilkins, 2011.

[9] R. Carter, The Human Brain Book: An Illustrated Guide to Its Structure, Function, and Disorders, Penguin, 2014.

[10] Healthline, EEG (Electroencephalogram): Purpose, Procedure, and Risks, Available: https://www.healthline.com/health/eeg, 2019. (Accessed 30 June 2019).

[11] imotions, What Is EEG (Electroencephalography) and How Does It Work?, Available: https://imotions.com/blog/what-is-eeg/, 2019. (Accessed 30 June 2019).

[12] 10–20 system (EEG), *Wikipedia*. 20-Jun-2019.

[13] M.H. Limaye, M.V.V. Deshmukh, ECG noise sources and various noise removal techniques: a survey, Int. J. Appl. Innov. Eng. Manag. 5 (2) (2016).

[14] Electronics Notes, RF Thermal Noise | Johnson-Nyquist Noise, Available: https://www.electronics-notes.com/articles/basic_concepts/electronic-rf-noise/thermal-johnson-nyquist-basics.php, 2019. (Accessed 30 June 2019).

[15] Electronics Notes, What Is Flicker Noise | 1/f Noise, Available: https://www.electronics-notes.com/articles/basic_concepts/electronic-rf-noise/flicker-noise-1-f-what-is.php, 2019. (Accessed 30 June 2019).
[16] Analog Devices, Understanding and Eliminating 1/f Noise, Available: https://www.analog.com/en/analog-dialogue/articles/understanding-and-eliminating-1-f-noise.html, 2019. (Accessed 30 June 2019).
[17] S.G. Thalkar, D. Upasani, Various techniques for removal of power line interference from ECG signal, Int. J. Sci. Eng. Res. 4 (2013) 12–23.
[18] ElProCus—Electronic Projects for Engineering Students, What Is FIR Filter?—FIR Filters for Digital Signal Processing, Available: https://www.elprocus.com/fir-filter-for-digital-signal-processing/, 2015. (Accessed 30 June 2019).
[19] ScienceDirect Topics, Finite Impulse Response Filter—An Overview, Available: https://www.sciencedirect.com/topics/computer-science/finite-impulse-response-filter, 2019. (Accessed 30 June 2019).
[20] ScienceDirect Topics, Butterworth Filters—An Overview, Available: https://www.sciencedirect.com/topics/engineering/butterworth-filters, 2019. (Accessed 30 June 2019).
[21] Butterworth Filter Design and Low Pass Butterworth Filters, Basic Electronics Tutorials, 14-Aug-2013.
[22] Butterworth Filters [Online]. Available: https://tttapa.github.io/Pages/Mathematics/Systems-and-Control-Theory/Analog-Filters/Butterworth-Filters.html (Accessed 30 June 2019).
[23] Active Low Pass Filter—Op-amp Low Pass Filter, Basic Electronics Tutorials, 14-Aug-2013.
[24] Mateo Aboy, Butterworth Filter design: Finding "n".
[25] F. Winsberg, M. Elkin, J. Macy, V. Bordaz, W. Weymouth, Detection of radiographic abnormalities in mammograms by means of optical scanning and computer analysis, Radiology 89 (2) (1967) 211–215.
[26] U. Bick, F. Diekmann, Digital Mammography, Springer Science & Business Media, 2010.
[27] Artificial Intelligence in Healthcare, *Wikipedia*, 03-Oct-2019.
[28] B. Halalli, A. Makandar, Computer aided diagnosis—medical image analysis techniques, Breast Imag. 10 (2018).
[29] tutorialspoint.com, Artificial Intelligence Overview, Available: https://www.tutorialspoint.com/artificial_intelligence/artificial_intelligence_overview.htm, 2019. (Accessed 30 June 2019).
[30] A Proposal for the Dartmouth Summer Research Project on Artificial Intelligence [Online]. Available: http://www-formal.stanford.edu/jmc/history/dartmouth/dartmouth.html (Accessed 30 June 2019).
[31] Lexico Dictionaries, Artificial Intelligence | Definition of Artificial Intelligence in English by Lexico Dictionaries, Available: https://www.lexico.com/en/definition/artificial_intelligence, 2019. (Accessed 30 June 2019).
[32] B. Marr, The Key Definitions of Artificial Intelligence (AI) That Explain Its Importance, Forbes, 2018. Available: https://www.forbes.com/sites/bernardmarr/2018/02/14/the-key-definitions-of-artificial-intelligence-ai-that-explain-its-importance/. (Accessed 30 June 2019).
[33] T.D. Jajal, Distinguishing between Narrow AI, General AI and Super AI, Medium, 2018. Available: https://medium.com/@tjajal/distinguishing-between-narrow-ai-general-ai-and-super-ai-a4bc44172e22. (Accessed 30 June 2019).

[34] Machine Design, What's the Difference Between Weak and Strong AI?, Available: https://www.machinedesign.com/robotics/what-s-difference-between-weak-and-strong-ai, 2017. (Accessed 2 July 2019).
[35] sas, Machine Learning: What It Is and Why It Matters, Available: https://www.sas.com/en_ae/insights/analytics/machine-learning.html, 2019. (Accessed 30 June 2019).
[36] MathWorks, What Is Machine Learning? | How It Works, Techniques & Applications, Available: https://www.mathworks.com/discovery/machine-learning.html, 2019. (Accessed 30 June 2019).
[37] M. Colins, Machine Learning: An Introduction to Supervised and Unsupervised Learning Algorithms, CreateSpace Independent Publishing Platform, 2017.
[38] J. Brownlee, What Is Deep Learning? Machine Learning Mastery, 2016.
[39] Y. Bengio, Deep learning of representations for unsupervised and transfer learning, in: Proceedings of ICML Workshop on Unsupervised and Transfer Learning, 2012, pp. 17–36.
[40] I. Goodfellow, Y. Bengio, A. Courville, Deep Learning, MIT Press, 2016.
[41] tutorialspoint.com, Fuzzy Logic Introduction, Available: https://www.tutorialspoint.com/fuzzy_logic/fuzzy_logic_introduction.htm, 2019. (Accessed 30 June 2019).
[42] O. Terrada, A. Raihani, O. Bouattane, B. Cherradi, Fuzzy cardiovascular diagnosis system using clinical data, in: 2018 4th International Conference on Optimization and Applications (ICOA), 2018, pp. 1–4.
[43] Difference Between Fuzzy Set and Crisp Set (With Comparison Chart), Tech Differences, 02-Nov-2018.

CHAPTER

Characterization of biomedical signals: Feature engineering and extraction

2

Dr. Bashar Rajoub

Faculty of Engineering Technology and Science, Higher Colleges of Technology, Dubai, United Arab Emirates

2.1 Introduction

Generating alternative representations of biomedical signals define the identity of this chapter. Fig. 2.1 shows a block diagram of a typical pattern recognition system. The pipeline comprises a sensor that captures data from the "real world" and presents these data as raw data objects. It requires a preprocessing mechanism to prepare the data for the following stages, such as removing artifacts and unwanted noise, transformation of the data to get alternative modalities, adjusting of average intensity/amplitude levels, and downsampling (decimation) or upsampling (interpolation). Feature generation and engineering require expert domain knowledge to extract important features from the signal (e.g., segment specific regions of interest and calculate feature descriptors).

We expect the generated features to have strong correlations with the latent structure we are trying to model in the data. However, the number of generated features can be very high; therefore we need a feature selection step. Feature selection aims to produce a new feature space that comprises a subset of the original features, weighted combinations of best features, or extracted features obtained by projective or nonlinear embedding. Finally, we train a predictive model on the new feature space to learn a mapping that relates the extracted features to the clinical information we are trying to predict, for example, the presence or absence of a disease given measurements of several biomarkers in the blood (e.g., features such as sugar levels, white blood cell count, proteins, lipids, or metabolites).

2.2 Feature engineering

Characterization of biomedical signals is challenging because of noise, stochastic nature of the signals, and the large variability both within and between individuals. A *feature* is a measurable quantity obtained from the patterns present in the signal. Raw features obtained from sensors are fed to a feature engineering step. Feature engineering extracts essential features that can be used to detect different patterns.

Biomedical Signal Processing and Artificial Intelligence in Healthcare. https://doi.org/10.1016/B978-0-12-818946-7.00002-0

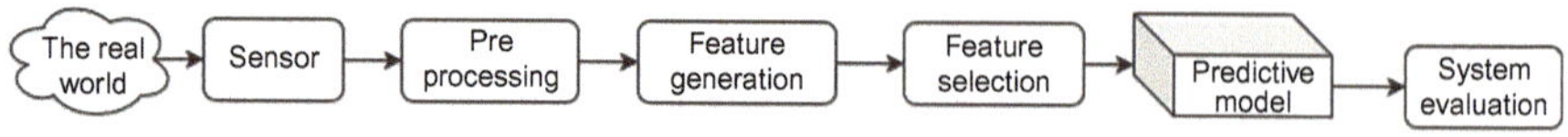

FIG. 2.1

Typical pattern recognition system.

Good feature representations allow us to build robust models that learn the salient structures in the data. For example, to obtain new representations of the data, we can apply sliding filtering operations, Fourier transform, and extract descriptive statistical measures from local regions in the data.

We can express a signal $f(t)$ in terms of a d-dimensional feature space $\mathbf{x}$, using a finite set of d measurements $x_1, \ldots, x_d$, where d is the total number of features.

We can now discard the raw signal and replace it with the new feature vector $\mathbf{x}$

$$\mathbf{x} = [x_1, \ldots, x_d]^{\mathrm{T}} \in R^d \tag{2.1}$$

when repeated for every signal f_i, $i = 1, 2, \ldots, N$ in the dataset, we get a feature matrix $\mathbf{X} \in R^{N \times d}$ where each row represents a data instance and each column represents a feature.

In this section, we will utilize feature engineering to generate frequency-based features using Fourier analysis, time-frequency features using the short-time Fourier transform and the wavelet transform, statistical features using moments and correlation analysis, and generating local features using local binary patterns.

2.2.1 Discrete Fourier transform

Fourier analysis is useful in gaining insight into the frequency content of the signal. The discrete Fourier transform (DFT) $\mathbf{X}$ of a discrete signal $\mathbf{x} \in R^N$ is defined as a linear projection of $\mathbf{x}$ onto a unitary symmetric matrix $\mathbf{W}$ with fixed basis functions $W_N \equiv \exp\left(-j\frac{2\pi}{N}\right)$ as

$$\mathbf{X} = \widetilde{\mathbf{W}}\mathrm{x} \tag{2.2}$$

where

$$\widetilde{\mathbf{W}} = \mathbf{W}^{-1} = \mathbf{W}^* \tag{2.3}$$

$$\widetilde{\mathbf{W}} = \frac{1}{\sqrt{N}} \begin{bmatrix} 1 & 1 & 1 & \ldots & 1 \\ 1 & W_N & W_N^2 & \ldots & W_N^{N-1} \\ \vdots & \vdots & \vdots & \ldots & \vdots \\ 1 & W_N^{N-1} & W_N^{2(N-1)} & \ldots & W_N^{(N-1)(N-1)} \end{bmatrix} \tag{2.4}$$

The DFT $\mathbf{X}$ is a complex quantity that encodes the magnitude and phase information of the frequencies in the signal. It is a symmetric and periodic function with a period

2π. The magnitude of **X** is plotted in the range $[0, \pi]$ or $[0, F_s/2]$ where F_s is the sampling frequency.

The resolution of the DFT depends on the number of samples in the signal as **x**. It is therefore advised to use all the samples of the original signal to avoid loss of information.

The DFT is invertible; we can reconstruct the original signal using the inverse DFT, also expressed as a projection:

$$\mathbf{x} = \mathbf{W}\mathbf{X} \tag{2.5}$$

Naive computation of the DFT requires N^2 operations; however, thanks to the Fast Fourier Transform, the computational complexity becomes $N \log N$. To compute the DFT, we can use the fast Fourier transform algorithm (FFT), but one needs to first zero pad the signal to make the number of samples a power of two (e.g., see Cooley-Tukey FFT algorithm, Wikipedia).

One aspect of Fourier analysis is to identity frequency bands that compact most of the signal's energy. Parseval's theorem states that the total energy is the same in both the time domain and the frequency domain:

$$\sum_{n=0}^{N-1} |x(n)|^2 = \frac{1}{N} \sum_{k=0}^{N-1} |X(k)|^2 \tag{2.6}$$

$|X(k)|^2$ represents the spread of power spectral density (PSD) in the signal over frequency.

Fourier features preserve the correlation between neighboring data points. However, the temporal structures are lost in the frequency domain. This makes it possible that different signals produce very similar magnitude representations under Fourier mappings.

2.2.2 Time-frequency analysis

The short-time Fourier transform (STFT) allows us to perform time-frequency analysis. It is used to generate representations that capture both the local time and frequency content in the signal. Similar to the Fourier transform, the STFT still relies on fixed basis functions; however, it uses fixed-size time-shifted window functions $w(n)$ to get a transformation of the signal and can be expressed as

$$X(k, m) = \sum_{n=0}^{N-1} x(n+m) w(n) W_N^{nk};\ k, m = 0, 1, \ldots, N-1 \tag{2.7}$$

where m is the amount of shift.

However, the STFT has better temporal and frequency localization properties compared with the Fourier transform. However, since the product of temporal and frequency resolution is constant (because of the classical Heisenberg's uncertainty principle), the generated features cannot achieve instantaneous localization of both time and frequency. In addition, due to using a fixed window length and fixed basis functions, the STFT still cannot capture events with different durations or when the signal contains fast (sharp) events.

The wavelet transform is among the widely used techniques for extracting features from biomedical signals. The wavelet transform tries to mitigate the limitations of the STFT and do a better job. It starts by defining special basis functions called "mother wavelets." Mother wavelets are not restricted to a single family of functions (e.g., periodic functions as the case in the FT). In addition, the basic functions have both temporal and frequency components. This allows us to generate a series of variable-sized wavelet functions; each has a share of the time-frequency spectrum. Fig. 2.2 shows the difference between the STFT and wavelet transform. The STFT divides the time-frequency space into equally sized grid, while for the wavelet transform, we see a coarse-to-fine (i.e., nonuniform) representation of the signal.

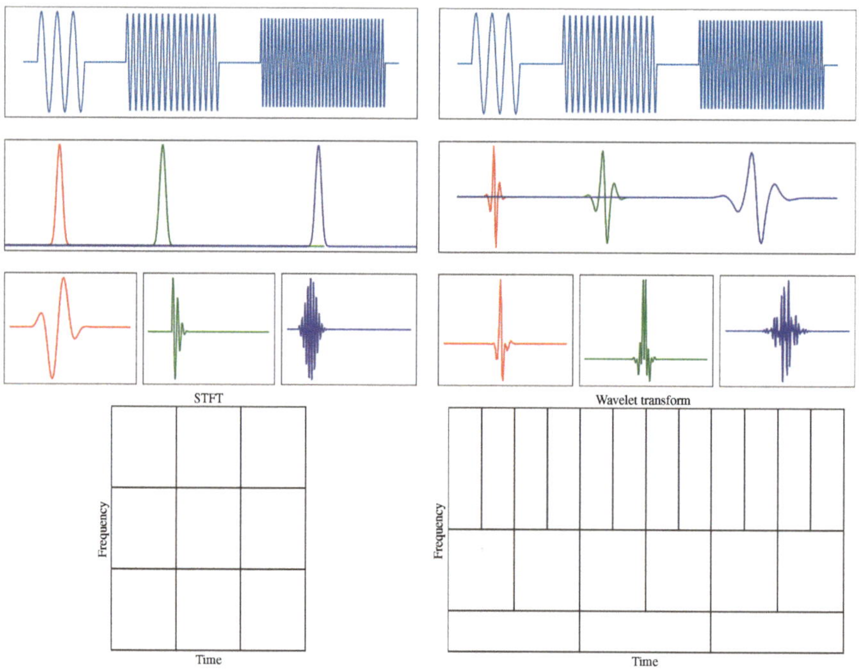

FIG. 2.2

Comparison between the STFT and wavelet transforms. In the STFT (left panel), a fixed-size sliding window is used to compute the Fourier transform of the signal. This results in uniform time/frequency representation of the signal. However, computing the WT (right panel) involves one time application of a filter bank on the overall signal. As such, we end up with time/frequency representation that is nonuniform (i.e., coarse-to-fine resolution).

2.2.3 Statistical features

Statistical features have been used in various intelligent signal processing applications. Statistical features consider modeling the data in terms of statistical traits—such as maximum, minimum, range, interquartile range, median, mode, and statistical moments such as the mean, variance, kurtosis, and skewness—besides other measures such as information-based metrics.

Statistical moments can capture information about the properties of the distribution on the features. Given samples from a random variable X, we can define statistical moments about the origin of any order p using the geometric series:

$$m_p = E[X^{\mathrm{p}}] = \frac{\sum_{n=1}^{N} x_n^p}{N} \tag{2.8}$$

where N is the number of samples generated from a random variable, X, x_n is the nth sample, and $E[.]$ is the expectation operator. The pth moment about the mean of X is

$$\nu_p = E\left[(X - E[\mathrm{X}])^p\right] \tag{2.9}$$

The first moment (i.e., $p = 1$) represents the empirical *mean* (*i.e., arithmetic mean*) of the data and is given by

$$\mu = \frac{1}{N}\sum_{n=1}^{N} x_n \tag{2.10}$$

The *mean* is a measure of central tendency. Using the mean to measure central tendency can sometimes mislead since it is sensitive to outliers. Alternative measures such as the mode (most frequent data value) or the median (middle data point when data are sorted) are more robust to outliers. One way to test for outliers for unimodal random variables is to compare the values of mean and the median: if the difference between the mean and median is large, then probably outliers are present in the data.

The second moment around the mean is called the *variance*; σ^2 is obtained from Eq. (2.8) by subtracting the mean of the data from each data point, that is, $x_n - \mu$ and setting $p = 2$. The square root of the variance is called the standard deviation; σ indicates the spread (concentration) of the data around the mean. A small standard deviation means the values are very similar to the mean of the data:

$$\sigma = \sqrt{\frac{1}{N}\sum_{n=1}^{N}(x_n - \mu)^2} \tag{2.11}$$

A related measure, the root mean square of the signal, is defined as

$$RMS = \sqrt{\frac{\sum_{n=1}^{N} x_n^2}{N}} \tag{2.12}$$

The third and fourth moments are standardized measures (i.e., normalized by the standard deviation). The third moment is called *skewness* and is obtained from Eq. (2.8) by substituting $p = 3$:

$$\text{Skewness} = \frac{\sum_{n=1}^{N} (x(n) - \mu)^3}{N\sigma^3} = \frac{E\left[(X-\mu)^3\right]}{\sigma^3} \tag{2.13}$$

Skewness describes the shape of the distribution by quantifying its asymmetry about the mode. It is used to measure the distance of the data distribution from a normal distribution of the same variance: a skewness of zero indicates a symmetric distribution, while a positive skew indicates a long tail in the positive direction. Skewness can be approximated by $(\mu - \text{median})/\sigma$. Fig. 2.3 shows a right-skewed distribution where the mean is larger than the median. The fourth moment ($p = 4$) is called the *kurtosis*:

$$\text{kurtosis} = \frac{\sum_{n=1}^{N} (x(n) - \mu)^4}{N\sigma^4} - 3 \tag{2.14}$$

where -3 in the definition is included to ensure we get zero kurtosis for normal distributions.

The kurtosis can also describe the shape of the distribution; it shows the extent of flatness of the distribution. Positive kurtosis indicates that the distribution has a pointed (peaked) shape, while negative kurtosis indicates a broad flat distribution (see Fig. 2.4.)

The fifth moment is a measure that is entirely determined by the tails of the distribution. It is a quantitative representation of tail skewness (i.e., the asymmetry of the tails of a univariate distribution). It also quantifies the relative importance of the tails versus the mode in causing skew. We rarely use higher moments for data analysis since they are difficult to approximate and describe in layman's terms.

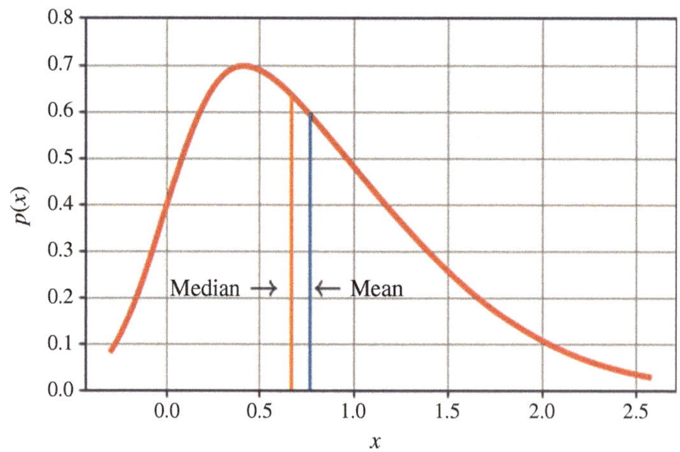

FIG. 2.3

Right-skewed distribution: Mean is to the right of the median.

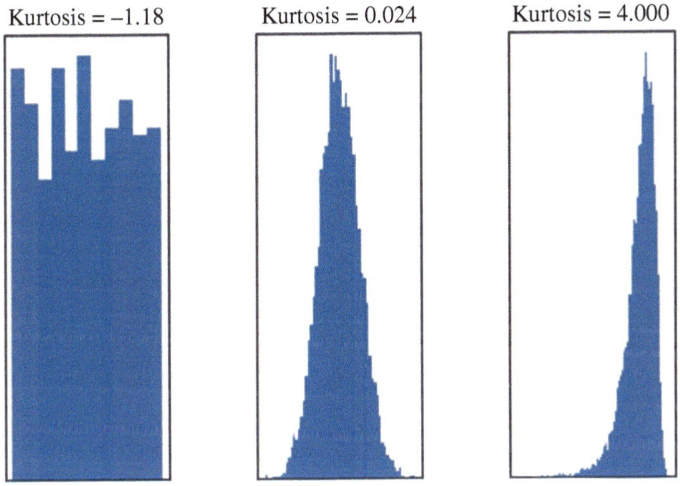

FIG. 2.4

Positive kurtosis (right) indicates that the distribution has a pointed or peaked shape, while negative kurtosis (left) indicates a broad flat distribution; a normal distribution (middle) has zero kurtosis.

2.2.4 Local binary patterns

Local binary patterns (LBP), first originated by computer vision research, have been adapted to 1-D biomedical signals such as EEG and ECG signals. LBP compare each sample in a neighborhood window to the middle sample and generate a binary code that encodes the local behavior of the signal. Characterizing the signal, therefore, is done by analyzing the patterns produced for all the neighborhoods scanned by the sliding window.

For example, an LBP can be generated by applying a binary neighborhood operation $G(.)$ over signal regions R_i, each having a width of k samples. The function $G(.)$ compares the samples in the neighborhood to a reference sample, the first or the middle sample, and produces a k-bit binary number, where 1 means that the kth sample in the window is greater than the reference sample. A signal with N regions will produce N, k-bit binary patterns. We convert each binary pattern to decimal representation to produce a feature vector $\in R^k$. We then compute a histogram on the resulting patterns using p-bins. The histogram, therefore, becomes the new feature vector describing the signal in terms of the distribution of its local binary patterns.

2.3 Feature ranking

Feature ranking is ordering the features based on their relevancy. We can obtain feature relevancy using scoring functions that measure feature relevance based on specific criteria, such as variance, correlations, independence, and mutual information.

2.3.1 Variance threshold

We can rank features by their variance; the more the variance, the more relevant is the feature (or feature subset), while we can assume low variance features do not provide much information. The extreme case is constant features where the variance is zero. We can deem low variance features irrelevant and therefore removed from the dataset. This can be done by computing the variance of each feature and finding a variance threshold to eliminate unimportant features (e.g., keeping the top p-features with the largest variance.)

Using a variance threshold to rank individual features does not consider the correlation between other features. This can result in selecting redundant features. As such, we need a subsequent stage to remove highly correlated features. In addition, we can have a selected feature that is uncorrelated with the response variable; here, we need to drop that feature as well.

2.3.2 Correlation measures

Correlation is a bivariate measure that examines the linear relationship between two random variables. Correlation analysis is concerned with testing the statistical dependence between two random variables and can be expressed in terms of their inner product:

$$p=\sum^{N} xy \tag{2.15}$$

The correlation coefficient R is large if there is a sizable collinear similarity between two signals.

Univariate ranking methods can generate redundant features because they do not take into account the correlation between other features; they could generate irrelevant features because they do not consider correlations with the response variable. However, relying on the correlation coefficient in its basic form can still fail. For example, signals that are shifted versions of each other can have a low correlation, yet they are similar! If we incorporate the sample shift, k, we get the cross-correlation as a function of k:

$$\rho_{x,y}(k)=\sum^{N} x(n)y(n+k) \tag{2.16}$$

The cross-correlation function can be used to obtain the maximum similarity between two signals. A similar measure can be obtained if we further subtract the means from the signals before computing the sum; in this case, we get the covariance function:

$$C_{xy}(k)=\sum^{N}(x(n)-\mu_x)(y(n+k)-\mu_y) \tag{2.17}$$

If we further normalize the covariance function by the product of the standard deviations of the random variables, we now get the Pearson's correlation coefficient:

$$p_{xy}(k) = \frac{C_{x,y}(k)}{\sigma_x \sigma_y} \quad (2.18)$$

Pearson correlation coefficient measures the linear correlation between two variables and produces values between [−1; 1], with ±1 meaning perfect positive/negative correlation, and 0 meaning no linear correlation between the two variables.

2.3.3 Information measures

One obvious drawback of correlation for feature ranking is that it does not capture nonlinear relationships between variables; it only measures the strength of linear relationships. Alternative measures that are more suited for nonlinear relationships include mutual information (MI) and maximal information coefficient (MIC). Information-based metrics can capture any kind of statistical dependency but require more data samples for accurate estimation.

Mutual information measures mutual dependence between variables. It is a more robust measure for correlation. MI quantifies the amount of information obtained about one feature (random variable X), through the other feature (random variable, Y):

$$I(X, Y) = \sum_{y \in Y} \sum_{x \in X} p(x, y) \log \frac{p(x, y)}{p(x)p(y)} \quad (2.19)$$

where $p(x, y)$ is the joint probability density and $p(x)$, $p(y)$ are the marginal density functions. From the equation, if X and Y are unrelated, then $p(x, y)$ factors as $p(x)p(y)$, and the sum would be zero.

Given N subsets of candidate features of size k, S_n; $n = 1, 2, \ldots, N$; feature selection is achieved by choosing the subset that maximizes the joint mutual information between S_n and the response variable y, $I(\mathbf{X}_{Sn}; y)$. The complexity of computing $I(\mathbf{X}_{Sn}; y)$ can be high if k, that is, the number of features in a subset S_n is large since this requires the sum over a k-dimensional space that becomes quickly intractable.

Unlike Pearson's correlation coefficient, MI is not a normalized measure and is not a valid distance metric, that is, $I(X, Y) \neq I(Y, X)$. For continuous variables, integrals replace the sums and the MI can become inconvenient to compute. Maximal information coefficient (MIC) resolves these problems and turns mutual information score into a metric that lies between 0 and 1. In addition, MIC does not make any assumptions about the distribution of the variables nor requires that we know the distribution of the data. MIC assigns the same score to equally noisy relationships and works well regardless of the structural relationships between variables.

MIC is the mutual information between random variables X and Y normalized by their minimum joint entropy:

$$\text{MIC}(x, y) = \max\left\{I(x, y)/\log_2 \min\left\{n_x, n_y\right\}\right\} \quad (2.20)$$

where $I(x,y)$ is the mutual information between variables x and y and n_x and n_y are the number of bins into which x and y are partitioned.

2.3.4 Class separability measures

Class separability, for example, based on distance measures, is another metric that can be used to rank features. The intuition for adopting distance metrics is that we expect good features to embed objects of the same class close together for all classes in the dataset (i.e., small interclass distance); in addition, good features also embed objects of different classes far away from each other (i.e., large intraclass distance). This can measure the discriminative power of a feature. Figs. 2.5 and 2.6 show examples of good and bad features for a single feature and two-dimensional class distributions.

To estimate the interclass distance, we need to find the center of mass for the class, for example, using the mean, median, or mode of **x**, then compute the average distance between all class objects and the class center. This can be done based on the absolute, Euclidean, Mahalanobis or nearest-neighbor distances, etc. The intraclass distances can be estimated by computing the average of absolute distances between the means of the class-conditional densities.

We can also formulate a distance metric in terms of the spread and the means of the classes. Let μ_i and σ_i be the mean and standard deviation of the ith class, and μ and σ be the mean and standard deviation of the whole dataset for a specific feature, x_r. The Fisher score (also called Fisher discriminant ratio, FDR) for feature selection computes an independent score for each feature using the Fisher ratio:

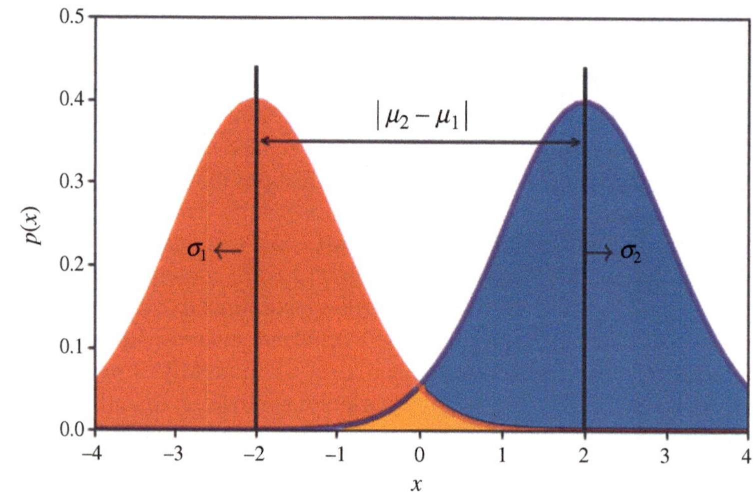

FIG. 2.5

Distance metric for measuring class separability: here, we have two class-conditional densities for two equiprobable classes. Notice that the classes can be partially separated based on the information about the class means. Classification errors are expected for features, *x*, that lie within the orange region.

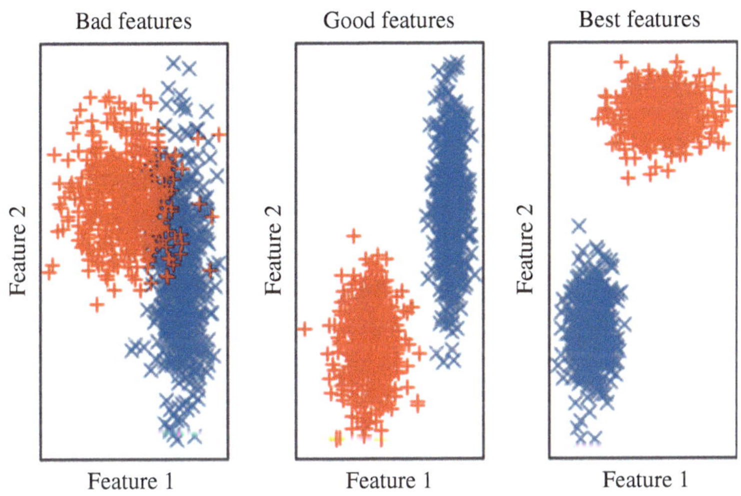

FIG. 2.6

Scatter plots showing class separability of two-dimensional datasets. Notice that higher separability can be achieved by selecting those features that have large interclass means yet small within class variance.

$$F_r = \frac{\sum_{i=1}^{C} n_i(\mu_i - \mu)^2}{\sum_{i=1}^{C} n_i \sigma_i^2} \tag{2.21}$$

In one dimension and for two equiprobable classes, the ratio reduces to

$$F_r = \frac{\mu_1^2 - \mu_2^2}{\sigma_1^2 + \sigma_2^2} \tag{2.22}$$

where n_i is the number of patterns of class C_i.

We can use the trace of the within scatter matrix S_w as a measure of the average class compactness and use the spread of the between-scatter matrix S_b as a measure of the scatter of class means about the overall mean. This allows us to write the Fisher feature ranking metric as

$$J = \text{trace}\left(S_w^{-1} S_b\right) \tag{2.23}$$

2.4 Feature selection

Finding the optimal feature subset relies on scoring functions for assessing the goodness of a subset. Feature selection is concerned with selecting the top-ranked features that contribute most to the predictive performance. Feature selection offers several advantages: it reduces the dimensionality of data allowing us to build models that are more efficient and less prone to overfitting. In addition, feature selection produces an ensemble of features that have higher explainability; this helps us build interpretable models that we can use to extract meaningful rules and gain new domain knowledge from the data. Last but not least, in some applications, features can be expensive to obtain or measure; here, feature selection proves useful, especially if a hard-to-measure feature is irrelevant.

Feature subset selection methods are classified into three broad categories: filter methods, wrapper methods, and embedded methods.

2.4.1 Filter methods for feature selection

Filter methods test the goodness of features independently of any modeling assumptions and are not optimized to a specific model. Filter methods are efficient as the model is not part of the process; that is, there is no need to train and cross-validate the test performance. Filter methods rank features only, based on their intrinsic properties of the features and the response variable. Standard measures for ranking features include information value (information gain), correlation coefficient, mutual information, variance ranking, inter-/intraclass distance (Fisher score), and the scores of significance tests such as chi-squared test, t-test, F-test, and ANOVA. Features with high relevance scores are deemed important and kept, while those having low scores are removed. It is also possible to add the selected features and discarded features to different pools to allow for reconsidering previous decisions, for example, reconsider a previously discarded feature.

For example, correlation analysis is considered a filter method for feature selection. Here the feature relevance is tested based on the mutual relationships between the feature and (a) the response variable (supervised feature selection) and/or (b) with another feature. The generated features are agnostic about any modeling assumptions and are not optimized to a specific model. A good feature subset contains features that are correlated with the response variable and uncorrelated with each other (i.e., not predictive of each other). For example, if the correlation between feature x_1 and the response variable is larger than the correlation between feature x_2 and the response variable, we can claim that feature x_1 is more important than feature x_2. In addition, if feature x_1 is also correlated with feature x_3, then we can claim that x_3 is redundant and can be removed from the dataset.

Let $Y_p = [x_1 x_2, \ldots, x_p]$ denote a feature subset, and let ρ_{ic} denote the correlation coefficient between feature i and the class label c. Let ρ_{ij} denote the correlation coefficient between features i and j. Now a good feature subset is expected to have features that are correlated with the response variable; hence, we would expect the sum of individual correlations between the features and class label, that is, $\sum_{i=1}^{m} \rho_{iC}$ to be large. We would also expect that the sum of all possible between-feature correlations in the subset, that is, $\sum_{i=1}^{m} \sum_{j=i+1}^{m} \rho_{ij}$ be as small as possible. This allows us to formulate the following objective function:

$$J(Y_p) = \frac{\sum_{i=1}^{m} \rho_{iC}}{1 + \sum_{i=1}^{m} \sum_{j=i+1}^{m} \rho_{ij}} \tag{2.24}$$

Another example of filter methods is selecting features based on class separability. Class separability is classified as a filter method since the goodness of a feature is not evaluated directly in terms of the model output: instead, it is evaluated in terms of the model objective function.

2.4.2 Wrapper methods: Feature subset search

Wrapper methods attempt to find those features that are best tuned for a specific model. Feature selection using wrapper methods use model-based ranking metrics. Such methods guarantee to select the combination of features that produces the best performance and hence are prone to overfitting. Wrapper methods are computationally expensive due to a large number of possible feature subsets and also because we need to train and test the model for each subset. Therefore, to reduce the number of candidate features, we can use filter methods as a preprocessing step for wrapper methods.

Feature subset search makes up two main components: a search strategy and feature ranking mechanism. Search strategies propose candidate feature subsets, while feature ranking utilizes specific criterion function J to evaluate the goodness of the proposed subsets. The model is trained and tested for each candidate subset. We then assign a ranking score based on the predictive performance of the model to each subset.

Feature subset search is a combinatorial problem and can be expensive. For example, exhaustive search (ES) considers all feature subsets, including individual features. A feature vector of m features produces 2^m feature subsets that reduce to $\binom{m}{p}$ if we restrict the subset size to p-features. Exhaustive search is feasible for a small number of features and achieves a global best feature subset. However, if the feature vector is large, ES becomes NP-hard and infeasible. As such, we need a good search strategy to make the process of feature selection computationally feasible.

Greedy search algorithms such as sequential forward and sequential backward selection are used to search through the space of all feature combinations. Sequential forward selection (SFS) attempts to reduce the number of trained models by building the "optimal" feature subset iteratively. SFS starts with an empty feature subset and a list of all individual candidate features. A predictive model is trained from scratch based on each feature; then a ranking score for the features is estimated on a holdout test set (or by using statistical resampling or cross-validation). We select the best feature; then the first feature is tried in combination with all the other features in the candidates' list, thus incrementally building the optimal feature subset by adding the feature that has the best model performance at every step. This process is repeated until a specified number of features are selected. Assume we have $m = 20$ and $p = 5$, and we want to build a model using the best two features. The number of possible feature combinations of size 2 is $\binom{20}{5} = 15504$. However, using forward feature selection reduces this number to $20 + 19 + 18 + 17 + 16 = 90$, which is quite a significant saving! The general formula for the number of trained models is $pm - \frac{p(p-1)}{2}$.

The algorithm for SFS is summarized in Algorithm 2.1.

Algorithm 2.1 Sequential forward selection.

1. Start with the empty set $Y_0 = \Phi$.
2. Select the next best feature $x^+ = \arg\max_{x/\in Yk} J(Y_k + x)$.
3. Update $Y_{k+1} = Yk + x^+$; $k = k + 1$.
4. Go to 2.

Sequential backward selection (SBS) performs a greedy search to find the best performing feature subset. The first step of the backwards feature selection is to initialize the feature subset to all features in the original set. We train the model using all features and estimate model performance. Then, we iteratively create models and determine the best or the worst performing feature at each iteration. The number of feature subsets created is

$$1+\frac{1}{2}((m+1)m-p(p+1))$$

For $m = 20$ and $p = 5$, we need to train 196 models, which is more than the 90 required for SFS.

The algorithm for SBS is summarized in Algorithm 2.2.

Algorithm 2.2 Sequential backward selection.

1. Train m models with only one feature removed from the feature set at a time and evaluate the model performance.
2. The feature set that yields the best performance is then set as the new feature subset.
3. Again, one feature is removed from the new subset to train $m - 1$ models, and we select the combination that has the best performance.
4. This process continues until the specified number of features has been selected for the dataset.

Sometimes a wrong choice is made while running SFS or SBS, for example, discarding an important feature that appeared irrelevant or accepting a bad feature that was judged as good. Once a choice is made during SFS/SBS, there is no way to reconsider it in the following steps. This is called the nesting effect. Therefore the algorithm should reconsider a previously discarded feature or discard a feature that was previously chosen. This is called floating search.

2.4.3 Embedded methods

Embedded methods consider feature selection as part of the model construction process; that is, we learn both the model parameters and features relevance scores, while the model is being created. Embedded methods have moderate computational complexity and offer the advantages of both filter and wrapper methods. Examples of embedded methods include decision trees, LASSO (or L1) regression, ridge regression, and elastic nets (add both L1 and L2 penalties).

We particularly need regularization when the number of features is high compared with the number of training samples. Regularization reduces overfitting and improves generalization. For example, we can write the cost function for linear regression with L1 regularization as

$$J_{reg}(\mathbf{w}, \mathbf{D}) = J(\mathbf{w}, \mathbf{D}) + \lambda \|\mathbf{w}\|_1 \tag{2.25}$$

where $\mathbf{w}$ is a p-dimensional weight vector and λ is a hyperparameter that controls regularization strength. Regularization adds a penalty that only depends on the model, not the data, and hence penalizes model complexity.

The $L1$ norm induces sparsity in the solution $\mathbf{w}$, which forces a certain number of model coefficients to zero. Features with zero weights can be treated as irrelevant and do not contribute to the model. Automatic feature selection is achieved by adding $L1$ regularization as part of the model. The nonzero coefficients are treated as associated with the "selected features" by the LASSO algorithm.

2.5 Feature extraction

Feature extraction aims to extract informative features by transforming the original signal into new feature spaces and extract new features with a high information density and low redundancy. Feature extraction offers several advantages: it can help in getting better data visualizations, reduce the dimensionality of the data, and build more accurate and efficient models. We can consider both feature selection and feature extraction as a form of dimensionality reduction techniques.

Feature selection differs from feature extraction in the following way: Feature selection optimizes over the features directly based on their intrinsic properties (filter methods) or predictive performance (wrapper methods), discarding irrelevant features and keeping only the best $p \ll m$ features. On the other hand, feature extraction optimizes for the best mapping/transformation that maximizes intrinsic criterion (unsupervised: keeping only those $p \ll m$ directions that keep most of the variance as in PCA) or by maximizing a separability criterion (supervised: such as Fisher ratio for LDA).

2.5.1 Principal component analysis

Principal component analysis (PCA)—also referred to as Karhunen-Loeve transform or the Hotelling transform—is a basic technique that has many applications in pattern recognition, signal processing, dimensionality reduction, and data visualization. Unlike the Fourier and wavelet transforms, which rely on fixed basis functions, the Karhunen-Loeve transform utilizes data-dependent and optimal basis functions. As a result, PCA is more expensive to compute; however, while Fourier/wavelet transforms produce features that have some correlations and redundancy, the transformation produced by PCA provides us with uncorrelated features (i.e., the redundancy in the data is removed automatically). In addition, if the original features are correlated, then a large reduction in dimensionality can be achieved.

PCA assumes that the data can be embedded in a lower-dimensional linear subspace $R^p \ll R^m$. The new representation tries to account for the variations in the data by finding directions with high variance. Although there are as many directions as the number of features m in the data; however, in practice, we only use the first $p \ll m$ directions (principal components or eigenvectors), while we can ignore the rest of the components. This is because they retain most of the variance of the original data in these p directions.

To perform PCA analysis, we first identify the projection that accounts for as much of the variability in the data as possible; that is, the direction that has the highest variance. The second direction is constrained to be orthogonal to the first and must account for as much of the remaining variability in the data that are not modeled by the first principal component (PC). We can repeat these steps until we obtain all m PCs. PCA solution can be achieved by expressing the extracted features $\mathbf{y} \in R^p$ as a linear projection of the original features $\mathbf{x}$ using the projection matrix $\mathbf{A}$:

$$\mathbf{y} = \mathbf{A}^{\mathrm{T}}\mathbf{x} \tag{2.26}$$

We constrain the projection matrix $\mathbf{A}$ to be orthogonal so that the elements of $\mathbf{x}$ are optimally mutually uncorrelated (i.e., we remove the redundancy in the data), that is,

$$E[y(i)y(j)] = 0, i \neq j \tag{2.27}$$

Besides the requirement that projection $\mathbf{A}$ is orthogonal, we also want projections that retain the largest variance. The variation in the projected features, $\mathbf{y}$, is, therefore,

$$\mathrm{R}_y = E\left[\mathbf{y}\mathbf{y}^{\mathrm{T}}\right] = E\left[\mathrm{A}^{\mathrm{T}}\mathbf{x}\mathbf{x}^{\mathrm{T}}\mathrm{A}\right] = \mathrm{A}^{\mathrm{T}}\mathrm{R}_x\mathrm{A} \tag{2.28}$$

where we assumed zero-mean random variables, so we can write the covariance Σ as the autocorrelation matrix $\mathbf{R}$.

PCA solution is achieved by choosing a projection matrix $\mathbf{A}$ such that its columns $\mathbf{a}_i$ are the orthogonal eigenvectors of $\mathbf{R}_x$. This will make $\mathbf{R}_y$ in diagonal form, that is,

$$\mathbf{R}_y = \mathbf{A}^{\mathrm{T}}\mathbf{R}_x\mathbf{A} = \lambda \tag{2.29}$$

The eigenvalues λ_i will then become the diagonal elements of λ.

We can recover our original features from the projected ones if we use all m principal components:

$$\mathbf{x} = \sum_{i=1}^{m} y(i)\mathbf{a}_{\mathrm{i}}, y(i) = \mathbf{a}_i^{\mathrm{T}}\mathbf{x} \tag{2.30}$$

However, if we project $\mathbf{x}$ into the subspace spanned by the first (largest) p principal eigenvectors, then our reconstructed original features becomes

$$\hat{\mathbf{x}} = \sum_{i=1}^{p} y(i)\mathbf{a}_{\mathrm{i}} \tag{2.31}$$

The errors however are as small as possible since PCA solution is also the solution that minimizes the mean squared reconstruction error:

$$E\left[\|\mathbf{x}-\hat{\mathbf{x}}\|^2\right] = E\left[\left\|\sum_{i=l}^{m} y(i)\mathrm{a}_i\right\|^2\right] \tag{2.32}$$

PCA is considered an unsupervised technique, that is, it treats all data points as belonging to one class. Pattern classification using PCA will fail if the directions with maximum variance do not separate the classes. Hence, we need to use alternative methods if our interest is in finding the direction of maximum class separation rather than largest variance as shown in Fig. 2.7.

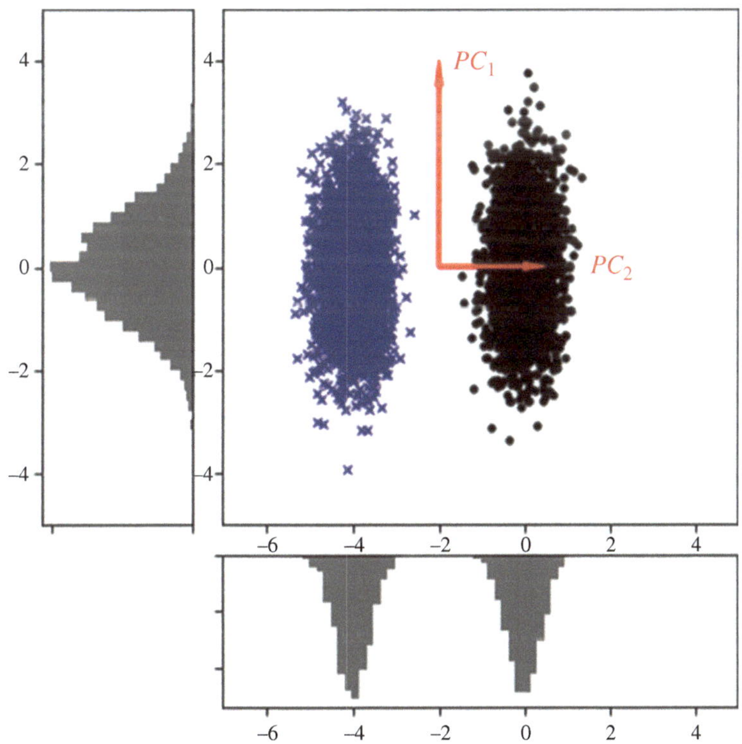

FIG. 2.7

PCA captures the direction that retains maximum variance, i.e., PC1. Here PCA fails because the class information is stored in the means not the variance.

2.5.2 Fisher linear discriminant

PCA finds the best linear subspace lower-dimensional representation of the data. The representation aims to capture the largest modes of variation in the data and is agnostic to class information. The principal components are best for data representation but not for data discrimination since directions of maximum variance are not always best for discriminating between classes. The Fisher's ratio, introduced as a separability measure for ranking features, can be used as the optimization criterion to find projections that maximize class separability. Fisher's linear discriminant analysis (LDA) aims to find a linear subspace projection that has the most discriminative power. Fig. 2.8 shows an example of different projections and their ability to separate classes. LDA transforms the original features $\mathbf{x} \in R^m$ using a linear projection $\mathbf{A}$. This results in new features $\mathbf{y} \in R^p$:

$$\mathbf{y} = \mathbf{A}^{\mathrm{T}}\mathbf{x} \tag{2.33}$$

Unlike projections obtained using PCA, LDA finds the best projection that maximizes class separation taking class information into account as shown in Fig. 2.9. Specifically, LDA formulates the problem in terms of scatter matrices (scatter and variance both measure the spread of data around the mean; however, scatter is just on a different scale than variance). The assumption is that class separability is higher if the "projected" class means are far from each other while same-class examples cluster around the projected mean for all classes, which is exactly what Fisher ratio measures:

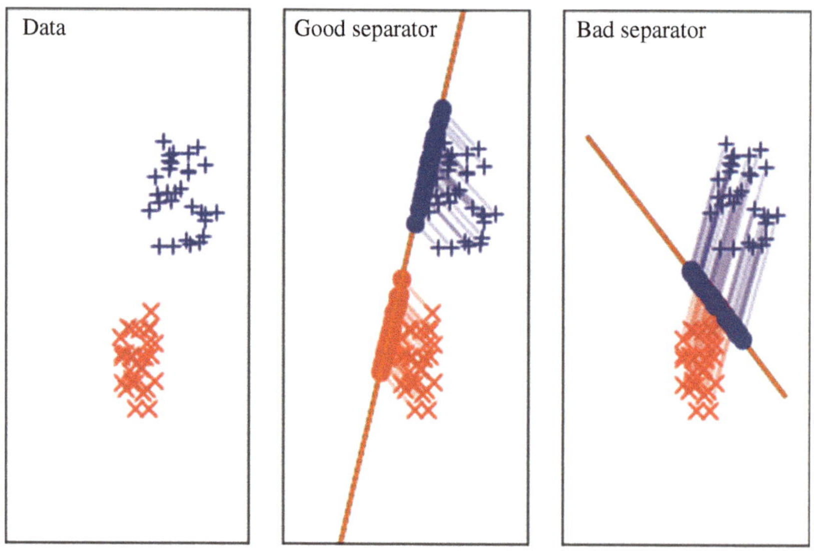

FIG. 2.8

Separability measures can be used as the optimization criterion for finding projections that maximize class separability.

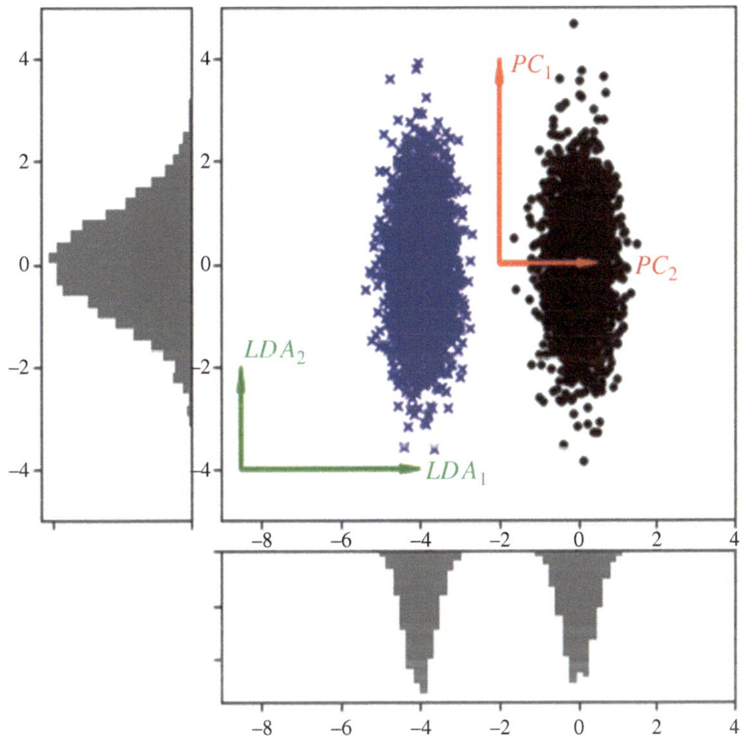

FIG. 2.9

PCA versus LDA: PCA fails to separate the classes since the projection is agnostic about class information. LDA on the other hand finds the best projection that can discriminate between the two classes (i.e., the x axis).

$$J = \text{trace}\left(S_w^{-1} S_b\right) \tag{2.34}$$

Assume a single projection direction **v**, and let us define the projected mean for class C_i as

$$\widetilde{\mu}_i = \mathbf{v}^{\mathrm{T}} \mu_i \tag{2.35}$$

the scatter for projected samples for class C_i is

$$\widetilde{s_i^2} = \sum_{y_k \in C_i} (y_k - \widetilde{\mu}_i)^2 = \mathbf{v}^{\mathrm{T}} S_i \mathbf{v} \tag{2.36}$$

for two classes, the within and between-class scatter are

$$\widetilde{S_W} = \widetilde{s_1^2} + \widetilde{s_2^2} = \mathbf{v} S_W \mathbf{v} \tag{2.37}$$

where S_W is a full rank invertible matrix, which is obtained using $S_W = S_1 + S_2$, that is, the sum of scatters based on original features. The between-class scatter matrix for the projected features measures the separation between the projected class means:

$$(\tilde{\mu}_1 - \tilde{\mu}_2)^2 = \mathbf{v} S_B \mathbf{v} \tag{2.38}$$

where $S_B = (\mu_1 - \mu_2)(\mu_1 - \mu_2)^{\mathrm{T}}$. The Fisher ratio now becomes

$$J(\mathbf{v}) = \frac{(\tilde{\mu}_1 - \tilde{\mu}_2)^2}{\tilde{S}_1^2 + \tilde{S}_2^2} = \frac{\mathrm{v}^{\mathrm{T}} S_B \mathbf{v}}{\mathrm{v}^{\mathrm{T}} S_W \mathbf{v}} \tag{2.39}$$

This expression can be differentiated with respect to $\mathbf{v}$ and solve for the direction with maximum discriminative power. It can be shown that the result will be a generalized eigenvalue problem:

$$S_B \mathbf{v} = \lambda S_W \mathbf{v} \tag{2.40}$$

for which the solution for the optimal direction $\mathbf{v}$ is given by

$$\mathrm{v} = S_W^{-1}(\boldsymbol{\mu}_1 - \boldsymbol{\mu}_2) \tag{2.41}$$

In case of c classes, we can use LDA to find $c - 1$ directions, that is, the dimensionality of the data is reduced to $c - 1$ dimensions.

$$J(\mathrm{A}) = \frac{\mathrm{A}^{\mathrm{T}} S_B \mathbf{A}}{\mathrm{A}^{\mathrm{T}} S_W \mathbf{A}} \tag{2.42}$$

The optimal projection, $\mathbf{A}$, will have $c - 1$ dimensions, that is, spanned by the eigenvectors $\mathbf{v}_1, \ldots, \mathbf{v}_{c-1}$, and hence, there is a loss of information.

2.6 Summary

This chapter gives an overview of feature engineering, feature extraction and feature selection techniques. Characterization of biomedical signals involves the use of domain knowledge and mathematical tools to extract informative features from the raw data. Feature selection further selects a subset of the generated features by identifying the most informative feature subset. The resulting features are expected to separate the underlying phenomena in the signals from noise and other irrelevant structures. It also makes machine learning computationally more efficient and enhances the predictive performance of the model.

Further reading

H. Abdi, L.J. Williams, Principal component analysis, WIREs Comput. Stat. 2 (4) (2010) 433–459.

D.W. Aha, R.L. Bankert, A comparative evaluation of sequential feature selection algorithms, in: D. Fisher, H.-J. Lenz (Eds.), Learning from Data: Artificial Intelligence and Statistics V, Springer, New York, NY, 1996, pp. 199–206. Lecture Notes in Statistics.

SpringerLink A Review of Feature Selection Methods Based on Mutual Information — SpringerLink (n.d.), https://link.springer.com/article/10.1007/s00521-013-1368-0.
R. Bala, Survey on Texture Feature Extraction Methods, (2017)p. 3.
A. Bansal, R. Agarwal, R.K. Sharma, Statistical feature extraction based iris recognition system, Sadhana 41 (5) (2016) 507–518.
M.R. Canal, Comparison of wavelet and short time Fourier transform methods in the analysis of EMG signals, J. Med. Syst. 34 (1) (2010) 91–94.
G. Chandrashekar, F. Sahin, A survey on feature selection methods, Comput. Electr. Eng. 40 (1) (2014) 16–28.
K. Chomboon, P. Chujai, P. Teerarassammee, K. Kerdprasop, N. Kerdprasop, An empirical study of distance metrics for k-nearest neighbor algorithm, in: The 3rd International Conference on Industrial Application Engineering 2015 (ICIAE2015), 2015.
IEEE Comparison Between Short Time Fourier and Wavelet Transform for Feature Extraction of Heart Sound—IEEE Conference Publication (n.d.), https://ieeexplore.ieee.org/abstract/document/818731.
K. Delac, M. Grgic, S. Grgic, Independent comparative study of PCA, ICA, and LDA on the FERET data set, Int. J. Imaging Syst. Technol. 15 (5) (2005) 252–260.
S.M.P. Dinakarrao, A. Jantsch, M. Shafique, Computer-aided Arrhythmia diagnosis with bio-signal processing: a survey of trends and techniques, ACM Comput. Surv. 52 (2) (2019) 23: 1–23: 37.
ScienceDirect EEG Signal Classification Using PCA, ICA, LDA and Support Vector Machines—ScienceDirect (n.d.), https://www.sciencedirect.com/science/article/pii/S0957417410005695.
P.A. Estevez, M. Tesmer, C.A. Perez, J.M. Zurada, Normalized mutual information feature selection, IEEE Trans. Neural Netw. 20 (2) (2009) 189–201.
Wikipedia, Euclidean Distance, 2020. Wikipedia. Page Version ID: 940470023.
I. Guyon, A. Elisseeff, An introduction to variable and feature selection, J. Mach. Learn. Res. 3 (2003) 1157–1182.
T. Hastie, R. Tibshirani, Discriminant adaptive nearest neighbor classification and regression, in: D.S. Touretzky, M.C. Mozer, M.E. Hasselmo (Eds.), Advances in Neural Information Processing Systems 8, MIT Press, 1996, pp. 409–415.
L.-Y. Hu, M.-W. Huang, S.-W. Ke, C.-F. Tsai, The distance function effect on k-nearest neighbor classification for medical datasets, Springerplus 5 (1) (2016).
Wikipedia, *K*-Nearest Neighbors Algorithm, 2020. Wikipedia. Page Version ID: 938393063.
M. Llamedo, Mart´ınez, J., Heartbeat classification using feature selection driven by database generalization criteria, IEEE Trans. Biomed. Eng. 58 (3) (2011) 616–625.
ScienceDirect Local Pattern Transformation Based Feature Extraction Techniques for Classification of Epileptic EEG Signals—ScienceDirect (n.d.), https://www.sciencedirect.com/science/article/abs/pii/S174680941730006X.
V.B.S. Prasath, H.A.A. Alfeilat, A.B.A. Hassanat, O. Lasassmeh, A.S. Tarawneh, M.B. Alhasanat, H.S.E. Salman, Distance and similarity measures effect on the perfor mance of K-nearest neighbor classifier—a review, Big Data 7 (4) (2019) 221–248.
A. Puglisi, A. Sarracino, A. Vulpiani, Thermodynamics and Statistical Mechanics of Small Systems, MDPI, 2018.
V. Rangappa, L. Vidyapeeth, S. Prasad and A.C. Agarwal, Classification of cardiac arrhythmia stages using hybrid features extraction with K-nearest neighbour classifier of ECG signals. Int. J. Int. Eng. Syst. 11(6), 21–32, doi: 10.22266/ijies2018.1231.03

T. Rückstieß, C. Osendorfer, P. van der Smagt, Sequential Feature Selection for Classification, in: D. Wang, M. Reynolds (Eds.), AI 2011: Advances in Artificial Intelligence, Springer, Berlin, Heidelberg, 2011, pp. 132–141. Lecture Notes in Computer Science.

M.S. Sainin, R. Alfred, Nearest neighbour distance matrix classification, in: L. Cao, Y. Feng, J. Zhong (Eds.), Advanced Data Mining and Applications, Springer, Berlin, Heidelberg, 2010, pp. 114–124. Lecture Notes in Computer Science.

P. Schober, C. Boer, L.A. Schwarte, Correlation coefficients: appropriate use and interpretation, Anesth. Analg. 126 (5) (2018) 1763–1768.

P.P.M. Shanir, K.A. Khan, Y.U. Khan, O. Farooq, H. Adeli, Automatic seizure detection based on morphological features using one dimensional local binary pattern on long-term EEG, Clin. EEG Neurosci. 49 (5) (2018) 351–362.

P. Sharma, M. Kaur, Classification in Pattern Recognition: A Review, 2013.

S. Theodoridis, Classifiers based on Bayes decision theory, in: Matlab Introduction to Pattern Recognition, Elsevier, 2010, pp. 1–27.

J. Walters-Williams, Y. Li, Comparative study of distance functions for nearest neighbors, in: K. Elleithy (Ed.), Advanced Techniques in Computing Sciences and Software Engineering, Springer Netherlands, Dordrecht, 2010, pp. 79–84.

S. Wold, K. Esbensen, P. Geladi, Principal component analysis, Chemom. Intell. Lab. Syst. 2 (1) (1987) 37–52.

CHAPTER

Supervised and unsupervised learning

3

Dr. Bashar Rajoub

Faculty of Engineering Technology and Science, Higher Colleges of Technology, Dubai, United Arab Emirates

3.1 Introduction

Two major directions of pattern recognition are supervised and unsupervised learning. Supervised pattern recognition relies on labeled data to learn a mapping function that maps input features (i.e., measurements) $\mathbf{x}$ to the output variable y; that is, $y = f(\boldsymbol{X}, \boldsymbol{\theta})$. Unsupervised learning tries to discover patterns and structure of unlabeled data. Sometimes, unsupervised learning strategies are used before proceeding with building a supervised model. Some applications of unsupervised learning techniques include clustering, anomaly detection, and latent variable mixture models. Regression and classification are examples of supervised machine learning. In classification the goal is to train a model to predict a discrete or categorical output variables y, for example, determine for a given observation which of k classes $\{C_1, C_2, \ldots C_k\}$ it belongs to. Regression on the other hand deals with the problem of predicting a continuous response variable, for example, predict CO_2 emissions on a specific date.

3.2 Density estimation

3.2.1 Maximum likelihood, maximum a posteriori, and Bayesian parameter estimation

Let $\mathbf{X} = \{\mathbf{x_1}, \mathbf{x_2}, \ldots, \mathbf{x_N}\}$ be independent samples generated from a probability density function $p(\mathbf{X}; \boldsymbol{\theta})$ with a known functional form but unknown parameters $\boldsymbol{\theta}$. We wish to estimate the unknown parameters such that the joint probability of observing the data under the model is high, that is,

$$p(\boldsymbol{X}; \boldsymbol{\theta}) \equiv p(\mathbf{x_1}, \mathbf{x_2}, \ldots, \mathbf{x_N}; \boldsymbol{\theta}) \tag{3.1}$$

If we assume independent data samples (i.e., choosing the next sample is not influenced by the previous samples), then the joint probability can be written in factored form as

$$p(\mathbf{X}; \boldsymbol{\theta}) = \prod_{k=1}^{N} p(\mathbf{x_k}; \boldsymbol{\theta}) \tag{3.2}$$

Biomedical Signal Processing and Artificial Intelligence in Healthcare. https://doi.org/10.1016/B978-0-12-818946-7.00003-2

When viewed as a function of $\boldsymbol{\theta}$ (i.e., *with respect to* fixed data $\mathbf{X}$), this equation becomes the likelihood function of $\boldsymbol{\theta}$. Fig. 3.1 shows an example of maximum likelihood function. The parameter $\hat{\boldsymbol{\theta}}_{ML}$ that maximizes the likelihood function can be written as

$$\hat{\boldsymbol{\theta}}_{ML} = \arg\max_{\boldsymbol{\theta}} \prod_{k=1}^{N} p(\mathbf{x_k}; \boldsymbol{\theta}) \tag{3.3}$$

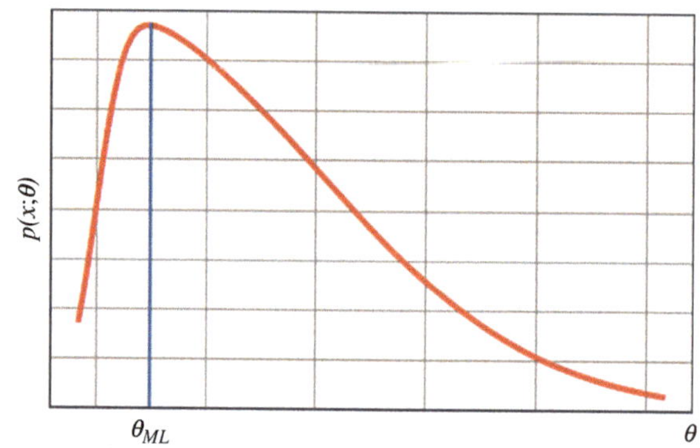

FIG. 3.1

The maximum likelihood estimator chooses the parameter that makes the observed data under the most probable model.

Applying the logarithm gives

$$\mathcal{L}(\boldsymbol{\theta}) = \ln p(\mathbf{X}; \boldsymbol{\theta}) = \sum_{k=1}^{N} \ln p(\mathbf{x_k}; \boldsymbol{\theta}) \tag{3.4}$$

Maximizing the likelihood function can be achieved analytically by differentiating $\mathcal{L}(\boldsymbol{\theta})$ with respect to the parameters and setting the gradients to zero:

$$\hat{\boldsymbol{\theta}}_{ML} = \frac{\partial \mathcal{L}(\boldsymbol{\theta})}{\partial \boldsymbol{\theta}} = \frac{1}{p(\mathbf{x_k}; \boldsymbol{\theta})} \frac{\partial p(\mathbf{x_k}; \boldsymbol{\theta})}{\partial \boldsymbol{\theta}} = 0 \tag{3.5}$$

Maximum likelihood estimators are asymptotically unbiased and consistent in the sense that it always converges to the true parameters as N approaches infinity:

$$\lim_{N \to \infty} E[\boldsymbol{\theta}_{ML}] = \boldsymbol{\theta}_{true} \tag{3.6}$$

or

$$\lim_{N \to \infty} E\left\| \hat{\boldsymbol{\theta}}_{ML} - \boldsymbol{\theta}_{true} \right\|^2 = 0 \tag{3.7}$$

Notice that maximum likelihood estimation provides us with the single best estimate of the parameter, $\hat{\boldsymbol{\theta}}_{ML}$, which makes seeing the observations $\mathbf{X}$ most likely under the model. This, however, turns out to be a bad choice, especially if the number of data samples is very small compared with the number of parameters of the model. This is because point estimates of the parameters could easily overfit the data and hence the resulting model fails to generalize.

To reduce the problem of overfitting, maximum a posteriori probability density estimation (MAP) can be used. MAP estimation is still optimizing for the single best settings (i.e., point estimate) of the parameters, $\hat{\boldsymbol{\theta}}_{MAP}$. Unlike maximum likelihood, MAP estimation views the parameters θ as a random variable with a known form of prior, that is, a probability density function over the parameters $p(\boldsymbol{\theta})$. Maximum a posteriori estimation considers the data as given (or known) and uses Bayes rule to get a posterior probability density over the estimated parameter given the data, that is, $p(\boldsymbol{\theta}|\mathbf{X})$.

We start by expressing the joint distribution (using Bayes theorem) of the data and the parameters

$$
\begin{aligned}
p(\boldsymbol{\theta})p(\mathbf{X}|\boldsymbol{\theta}) &= p(\mathbf{X})p(\boldsymbol{\theta}|\mathbf{X}) \\
\Rightarrow p(\boldsymbol{\theta}|\mathbf{X}) &= \frac{p(\mathbf{X}|\boldsymbol{\theta})p(\boldsymbol{\theta})}{p(\mathbf{X})}
\end{aligned}
\tag{3.8}
$$

We obtain the MAP estimate by computing the maximum of $p(\boldsymbol{\theta}|\mathbf{X})$:

$$
\begin{aligned}
\hat{\boldsymbol{\theta}}_{MAP} &= \arg\max_{\boldsymbol{\theta}} p(\boldsymbol{\theta}|\mathbf{X}) \\
&= \arg\max_{\boldsymbol{\theta}} p(\mathbf{X}|\boldsymbol{\theta})p(\boldsymbol{\theta})
\end{aligned}
\tag{3.9}
$$

In other words, we want

$$
\frac{\partial}{\partial \boldsymbol{\theta}}\left(p(\mathbf{X}|\boldsymbol{\theta})p(\boldsymbol{\theta})\right)\Big|_{\boldsymbol{\theta}=\boldsymbol{\theta}_{MAP}} = 0
\tag{3.10}
$$

Maximum likelihood and MAP estimates both produce a single best estimate for the parameters $\boldsymbol{\theta}$. In addition, they maximize the resulting function over the parameters by setting the gradients to zero. A better approach is to consider all plausible estimates of a parameter rather than relying on a single estimate. This will reduce the chances of finding biased estimates and thus avoids overfitting the data. This can be achieved by avoiding maximization altogether and estimate a *probability distribution* over the parameters given the data, $p(\boldsymbol{\theta}|\mathbf{X})$; using Bayes rule, we can write

$$
p(\boldsymbol{\theta}|\mathbf{X}) = \frac{p(\mathbf{X}|\boldsymbol{\theta})p(\boldsymbol{\theta})}{p(\mathbf{X})}
\tag{3.11}
$$

$$
p(\mathbf{X}) = \int p(\mathbf{X}|\boldsymbol{\theta})p(\boldsymbol{\theta})
\tag{3.12}
$$

where $p(\mathbf{X})$ is a normalizing constant to ensure that $p(\boldsymbol{\theta}|\mathbf{X})$ a valid posterior probability. The term $p(\mathbf{X}|\boldsymbol{\theta})$ can be computed using the data samples and the *i.i.d.* assumption:

$$
p(\mathbf{X}|\boldsymbol{\theta}) = \prod_{k=1}^{N} p(\mathbf{x}_k|\boldsymbol{\theta})
\tag{3.13}
$$

Eq. (3.11) involves an integral that can sometimes become intractable; in such cases, we need to use approximate inference. Having a posterior over parameters has a great inference power: for example, we can estimate the probability that a data point $\mathbf{x}$ is from the same group $\mathbf{X}$ by computing $p(\mathbf{x}\,|\,\mathbf{X})$. This can be done by integrating out the parameters, that is, making the inference by averaging over all settings of the parameters:

$$p(\mathbf{x} \mid \mathbf{X}) = \int p(\mathbf{x} \mid \boldsymbol{\theta}) p(\boldsymbol{\theta} \mid \mathbf{X}) d\boldsymbol{\theta} \tag{3.14}$$

3.2.2 Estimating parameters for individual densities

Case 1: Estimating the mean and variance of a normal distribution. The probability density function of a d-dimensional Gaussian distribution, $p(\mathbf{x})$, can be written as

$$p(\mathbf{x}; \boldsymbol{\mu}) = \mathcal{N}(\boldsymbol{\mu}, \boldsymbol{\Sigma}) \tag{3.15}$$

where parameters μ and Σ are the mean vector and covariance matrix of the density. Assuming *i.i.d.* samples (i.e., samples are independently drawn from an identical distribution), individual densities for each data sample $\mathbf{x_k}$ can be obtained using

$$p(\mathbf{x}_\mathrm{k}, \boldsymbol{\mu}) = \frac{1}{\sqrt[d]{2\pi}|\boldsymbol{\Sigma}|^{1/2}} \exp\left(-\frac{1}{2}(\mathbf{x}_\mathrm{k} - \boldsymbol{\mu})^\mathrm{T} \boldsymbol{\Sigma}^{-1} (\mathbf{x}_\mathrm{k} - \boldsymbol{\mu})\right) \tag{3.16}$$

The likelihood is a function of the parameters μ and can be expressed as the product of the corresponding individual densities of each sample $\mathbf{x_k}$ under the distribution:

$$\begin{aligned} \mathcal{L}(\boldsymbol{\mu}) &= \ln \prod_{k=1}^{N} p(\mathbf{x}_\mathrm{k}; \boldsymbol{\mu}) \\ &= \text{const.} - \frac{1}{2} \sum_{k=1}^{N} (\mathbf{x}_\mathrm{k} - \boldsymbol{\mu})^\mathrm{T} \Sigma^{-1} (\mathbf{x}_\mathrm{k} - \boldsymbol{\mu}) \end{aligned} \tag{3.17}$$

Differentiating with respect to μ and setting the expression to zero, we get the maximum likelihood solution as

$$\begin{aligned} \frac{\partial \mathcal{L}(\boldsymbol{\mu})}{\partial(\boldsymbol{\mu})} &= \sum_{k=1}^{N} (\mathbf{x}_\mathrm{k} - \boldsymbol{\mu}) = 0 \\ \Rightarrow \boldsymbol{\mu}_{ML} &= \frac{1}{N} \sum_{k=1}^{N} \mathbf{x}_\mathrm{k} \end{aligned} \tag{3.18}$$

Let us now compare the MAP and ML estimates for the mean of a Gaussian density $p(\mathbf{x}) = \mathrm{N}(\boldsymbol{\mu},\boldsymbol{\Sigma})$ from N *i.i.d.* samples $\mathbf{X} = \{\mathbf{x_1}, \mathbf{x_2}, \ldots, \mathbf{x_N}\}$. Assuming a Gaussian prior over the parameters, we can write

$$p(\boldsymbol{\mu}) = \frac{1}{\sqrt[d]{2\pi}\sigma_\mu} \exp\left(-\frac{\|\boldsymbol{\mu} - \boldsymbol{\mu}_0\|^2}{2\sigma_\mu^2}\right) \tag{3.19}$$

Using the *i.i.d.* assumption, we can write the derivative of the log likelihood times the prior with respect to the mean as

$$\frac{\partial}{\partial \boldsymbol{\mu}} \log\left(\prod_{k=1}^{N} p(\mathbf{x_k}|\boldsymbol{\mu})p(\boldsymbol{\mu})\right) = 0$$
$$\Rightarrow \sum_{K=1}^{N} \frac{1}{\sigma^2}(\mathbf{x_k} - \boldsymbol{\mu}) - \frac{1}{\sigma_\mu^2}(\hat{\boldsymbol{\mu}} - \boldsymbol{\mu}_0) = 0 \quad (3.20)$$

from which

$$\hat{\mu}_{MAP} = \frac{\boldsymbol{\mu}_0 + \frac{\sigma_\mu^2}{\sigma^2}\sum_{k=1}^{N} \mathbf{x_k}}{1 + \frac{\sigma_\mu^2}{\sigma^2}N} \quad (3.21)$$

Note that the MAP and the maximum likelihood estimates become equal as $N \rightarrow \infty$ or $\frac{\sigma_\mu^2}{\sigma^2} \gg 1$;

$$\hat{\boldsymbol{\mu}}_{MAP} = \frac{1}{N}\sum_{k=1}^{N} \mathbf{x}_k \quad (3.22)$$

We should also note that MAP estimation and maximum likelihood estimation produces approximately the same estimates of the parameters if the prior $p(\theta)$ is uniform, broad enough, or as the number of samples grows to infinity:

$$\hat{\boldsymbol{\theta}}_{MAP} \approx \hat{\boldsymbol{\theta}}_{ML} \quad (3.23)$$

This can be seen in the equation in the preceding text by letting $\frac{\sigma_\mu^2}{\sigma^2} \rightarrow \infty$ or letting $N \rightarrow \infty$, which results in

$$\hat{\boldsymbol{\theta}}_{MAP} \cong \hat{\boldsymbol{\theta}}_{ML} = \frac{1}{N}\sum_{k=1}^{N} \mathbf{x_k} \quad (3.24)$$

Let us now see what results we obtain for a Gaussian density. Assuming a univariate Gaussian prior over the "mean of the Gaussian, $p(\mu)$," and a Gaussian likelihood for the samples x:

$$p(\mu) = \mathcal{N}(\mu_0, \sigma_0^2) \quad (3.25)$$

$$p(x|\mu) = \mathcal{N}(\mu, \sigma^2) \quad (3.26)$$

Then the posterior over the mean is again Gaussian with posterior mean, μ_N, and posterior variance, ${\sigma_N}^2$,that is,$p(\mu|X) = \mathcal{N}(\mu_N, {\sigma_N}^2)$ where

$$\mu_N = \frac{N\sigma_0^2\mu + \sigma^2\mu_0}{N\sigma_0^2 + \sigma^2}$$
$$\sigma_N^2 = \frac{\sigma^2\sigma_0^2}{N\sigma^2 + \sigma^2} \quad (3.27)$$
$$\mu = \frac{1}{N}\sum_{k=1}^{N} x_k$$

Note that the parameters of the posterior depend on the number of samples N and the parameters of the prior and the likelihood. In fact, as $N \to \infty$, the posterior mean concentrates more and more about the true mean.

Modeling data as if they belong to a single density may not always be appropriate. For example, data can belong to clusters in the feature space; each cluster is a density of a specific form that we would like to identify. Mixture models can be used to handle this situation. Mixture model basically formulate the probability density as a parametric function of J densities with a parameter vector $\Theta = \{\boldsymbol{\theta}_1, \boldsymbol{\theta}_2, \ldots, \boldsymbol{\theta}_J\}$ as follows:

$$p(\mathbf{x}) = \sum_{j=1}^{J} p(\mathbf{x}/j; \boldsymbol{\theta}_j) P_j \tag{3.28}$$

where

$$\begin{aligned} &\sum_{j=1}^{J} P_j = 1; \\ &\int_{\mathbf{x}} p(\mathbf{x}|j) d\mathbf{x} = 1 \end{aligned} \tag{3.29}$$

As before, given a set of data observations sampled from a dataset $\mathbf{X} = \{\mathbf{x}_1, \mathbf{x}_2, \ldots, \mathbf{x}_N\}$ which are *i. i. d.* sampled from $p(\mathbf{x})$, our goal is to estimate the parameter vector, Θ, and the cluster weight priors $P_1, P_2, \ldots, P_j$. We can pose the problem as a maximum likelihood estimator—similar to what we did for individual densities:

$$\underset{\Theta, P_1 P_2, \ldots, P_j}{\arg\max} \prod P(\mathbf{x}_k; \boldsymbol{\theta}, P_1, \ldots, P_j) \tag{3.30}$$

However, this is a nonlinear problem because of the missing label information and requires a more involved optimization using the expectation-maximization (EM) algorithm.

3.2.3 Nonparametric and Kernel density estimation

Parametric density estimation requires that we specify a functional form of the probability density function in terms of a set of parameters $\boldsymbol{\theta}$. Maximum likelihood, MAP, and Bayesian estimation can then learn the parameters from data. Once the class-conditional densities are estimated, we can then choose the class label that has the largest posterior probability.

Assuming a specific functional form of class-conditional densities can sometimes be restricting. A different approach is to assume a mixture of densities models and learns the model parameters from data; this however is a bit involved and suffers from the identifiability problem. In this section, we adopt a nonparametric approach where instead of making assumptions about the underlying distribution, we estimate the density directly from the data, that is, let the data speak for itself! This may involve considering data topology, connectivity, and distance metrics that we define in the data domain and use that to understand local structures in the data.

3.2.3.1 Kernel density estimation

Nonparametric methods for density estimation eliminate the need for a parametric model of the assumed density. Suppose that we have N independently drawn data observations $[\mathbf{x}_1, \mathbf{x}_2, \ldots, \mathbf{x}_N]$ from a distribution that we would like to estimate. The probability that k of these samples fall inside a specific region R is given by the binomial distribution:

$$P_R(k) = \binom{N}{k} P^k (1-P)^{N-k} \tag{3.31}$$

where P is the probability that vector $\mathbf{x}$ lies inside the region (i.e., a success) and $(1-P)$ be the probability that it will fall outside R. A good estimate of P is the mean fraction of observations that fall within R:

$$P = k/N \tag{3.32}$$

the density at $\mathbf{x}$ is then

$$p(\mathbf{x}) \cong \frac{k}{N \times V} \tag{3.33}$$

where V is the volume containing $\mathbf{x}$.

Histograms estimate the density by dividing the sample space into a number of regions (or bins) that have a fixed size V and count the fraction of samples that lie in each bin. Histograms are the simplest form of nonparametric density estimation. However, they suffer from several drawbacks, for example, the shape of the histogram can significantly vary depending on the starting position, the orientation of the bins, and the number of bins used. Also, it is difficult to determine whether a discontinuity in a histogram is genuine or just an artifact because of our choice of hyper-parameters. As such, interpretation of the produced densities can sometimes be hard. Another drawback is that histograms provide us with a discrete distribution based on a fixed number of bins, rather than a continuous distribution, so it is only a rough approximation. The most severe and limiting drawback of histograms is that they suffer from the curse of dimensionality. As the number of dimensions in the data grows, the number of bins needed to model the density grows exponentially. This means that most bins will be empty! As such, the number of necessary training data will also tend to increase exponentially.

Parzen window estimators improve the histogram method by adopting a more flexible view of the sample space. Here, we do not have a clear bin-structure anymore; instead, we rely on kernels to define some neighborhood structure. The density at an arbitrary location $\mathbf{x}$ can be approximated by placing kernel functions $K(\mathbf{x}, \mathbf{x}_i)$ at every data point and compute an estimate using

$$p(\mathbf{x}) = \frac{1}{h^d N} \sum_{i=1} NK\left(\frac{\mathbf{x}_i - \mathbf{x}}{h}\right) \tag{3.34}$$

where h is a bandwidth or scale parameter which determines the range of influence (or sense of locality) of the kernel. The estimated pdf is affected by choice of the kernel function and on the bandwidth parameter. Valid kernels require that

$$K(\mathbf{x}) \geq 0, \int_{\mathbf{x}} K(\mathbf{x}) d\mathbf{x} = 1, \text{ and } K(\mathbf{x}) = K(-\mathbf{x}) \tag{3.35}$$

Examples of common kernels include the Parzen window kernel and Gaussian kernel. Parzen window kernel defines a hypercube of unit length centered at $\mathbf{x} = \mathbf{0}$:

$$K(\mathbf{x}_i) = \begin{cases} 1 & |\mathbf{x}_i| < \frac{1}{2} \\ 0 & \text{otherwise} \end{cases} \tag{3.36}$$

For example, the estimated density using Parzen window estimator will have discontinuities similar to those present in histograms; it weights all the points equally in the dataset that lies inside the window regardless of their distance to the point $\mathbf{x}$.

The estimated density $p(\mathbf{x})$ inherits the smoothness properties of the kernel functions used. Replacing the Parzen window with a smooth kernel provides us with continuous and smooth density estimates. The Gaussian window kernel defines a Gaussian bump centered at $\mathbf{x} = \mathbf{0}$:

$$K(\mathbf{x}_i) = \frac{1}{2\pi^{d/2}} \exp\left(-\frac{1}{2}\mathbf{x}_i^T \mathbf{x}_i\right) \tag{3.37}$$

Fig. 3.2 shows approximations to the density function for a dataset of 50 data points using a Gaussian kernel and different values for bandwidth h. Notice that h is a hyperparameter (smoothing parameter) whose value is chosen depending on the dataset. From the figure, we see that using a smooth kernel provides us with a smooth estimate of the underlying density. The estimate is a sum of Gaussian bumps placed at the data points.

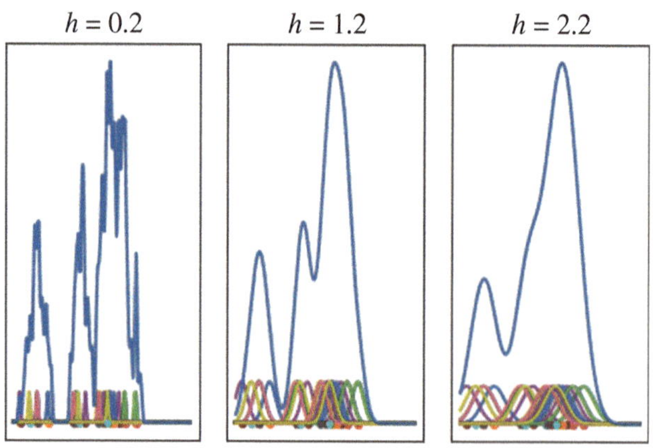

FIG. 3.2

The hyperparameter h acts as a smoothing parameter. A too small or too large value for h may fail to capture the underling density; as such, it is good to try different values.

3.2.3.2 Nearest neighbor density estimation

Kernel density estimation uses a fixed volume and estimates the density at location $\mathbf{x}$ by computing the contribution of all dataset observations that lie inside the window/kernel. The effect size at location $\mathbf{x}$, therefore, varies depending on the number of samples under the kernel function. In this section, we consider an alternative approach, where we let the volume vary so that it exactly contains k observations. This method is called k-nearest neighbor (kNN) density estimation. It can be shown that both kernel density estimation and kNN density estimation converge to the true probability density as $N \to \infty$, provided that V shrinks with N and k grows with N. In the kNN method, we grow the volume of a d-dimensional ball surrounding the estimation point $\mathbf{x}$ until it encloses k data points. The estimated density at our point is

$$p(\mathbf{x}) = \frac{k}{N} \frac{1}{V_d R_k^d(\mathbf{x})} \tag{3.38}$$

where $R_k(\mathbf{x})$ denotes the radius of such a ball that contains k points centered at $\mathbf{x}$ and V_d is the volume of the ball:

$$V_d = \frac{\pi^d/2}{(d/2)!} \tag{3.39}$$

Suppose we have five 1-D data points $\mathbf{X} = \{1, 2, 3.5, 4, 5\}$, and we want to estimate the density at $x = 2.5$ using $k = 2$. We first find the width of the region that contains the closest two data points to x based on the distances from $x = 2.5$ to each point in the dataset, that is, $d = \{1.5, 0.5, 1, 1.5, 2.5\}$. The width of the region is, therefore, $R_{k=2} = 1$. The density estimate is then

$$p(x = 2.5) = \frac{2}{5} \frac{1}{2.1} = 0.2 \tag{3.40}$$

The value of our estimate is prone to local noise and depends on the choice for k. Again, as with selecting a value for the smoothness hyperparameter h in kernel density estimation, the same applies for choosing k in kNN density estimation. Also, similar to Parzen and histogram methods, the density estimates produced by the kNN method can suffer from discontinuities since $R_k(\mathbf{x})$ is nonsmooth and nondifferentiable function.

3.3 Classification analysis

The goal in classification is to solve the problem of predicting categorical response variables that correspond to specific data observations. Data observations are represented by data matrix, $\mathbf{X}$ and a separate vector, and $\mathbf{y}$ used to store the class labels. Each row in $\mathbf{X}$ corresponds to a single observation (class instance) having a set of D features (measurements). Fig. 3.3 shows an example of a classification problem. In this case the scatter plot shows 2-D data instances from two classes, the red x's (class 1) and blue +'s (class 2). We can see that there is a linear decision boundary that can separate class 1 instances from class 2 instances. Classification algorithms utilize labeled data to learn a decision boundary that can separate the classes. Various real-world problems have more complex or nonlinear decision boundaries, much higher dimensional feature spaces, and perhaps hundreds or thousands of different classes, not just two!

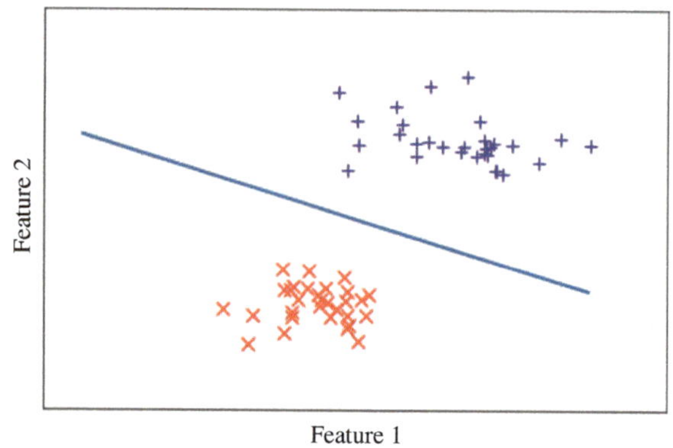

FIG. 3.3

Supervised learning: a two-class classification problem where supervised learning is used to find a line that can separate the classes.

3.3.1 Bayes classifier

Bayes decision theory formulates the classification problem using a flexible probabilistic framework that allows us to integrate various independent sources of information. Bayes decision theory produces optimal decision boundaries that produce the minimum total number of misclassifications. Assume you were asked to predict whether an X-ray image will be diagnosed as having cancer, $\omega = 1$ or otherwise normal, $\omega = 0$. Unless you are a trained radiologist, you will not have any information on how to make an accurate diagnosis. Hence, your best choice is to flip a coin and choose class ω_1 if you got heads or class ω_0 if you got tails. You are essentially assigning a chance probability ($P = 0.5$) for the presence of cancer. Now suppose that I told you that the X-ray image was picked randomly from a collection where 95% of the images are normal. Guided with this new information, your best choice is to label the image as belongs to ω_0 (i.e., normal) since 95% of the images in the collection are normal. The decision rule now favors the majority class as the most likely prediction. The probability of making an error is only 5% in this case.

When no information was available, the best choice was to choose the class label at random, assigning a chance probability to the predicted class. If we know the priori class information, then choosing the majority class is the optimal choice. The previous rules so far are independent of the evidence provided by our measurement (i.e., the X-ray image represented by the feature vector, $\mathbf{x}$). They only consider information provided by the empirical prior on class distribution, $p(\omega_i)$. Obviously, we need a rule that decides the class label based on the observed feature vector $\mathbf{x}$. If we have a good observation model for data instances in each class, $p(\mathbf{x} \mid \omega_i;\boldsymbol{\theta})$ (this also referred to as the class-conditional density or conditional likelihood of observations given the class label), then we can make predictions that now depend on the observation we want to predict. Our decision rule becomes to select the class that has the largest probability under the observation model:

$$\mathbf{x} \mapsto \omega_i \text{ if } p(\mathbf{x}|\,\omega_i) > p(\mathbf{x}|\,\omega_j) \tag{3.41}$$

This rule, however, is optimal only if the class priors are equal. If one class is more frequent than the other, then our decision must also consider this information. In this case, given a test observation **x**, we select the class that has the largest joint distribution, that is,

$$\begin{aligned} &\mathbf{x} \mapsto \omega_i \text{ if } p(\mathbf{x}, \omega_i) > p(\mathbf{x}, \omega_j) \text{ or} \\ &p(\mathbf{x}|\,\omega_i)p(\omega_i) > p(\mathbf{x}|\,\omega_j)p(\omega_j) \\ &\Rightarrow \frac{p(\mathbf{x}|\,\omega_i)}{p(\mathbf{x}|\,\omega_j)} > \frac{p(\omega_j)}{p(\omega_i)} \end{aligned} \tag{3.42}$$

It should be noted that this also corresponds to selecting the class that has the largest posterior probability. This is called Bayes decision rule or the maximum a posteriori (MAP) decision rule. We can calculate the posterior probability using Bayes rule as

$$P(\omega_i|\,\mathbf{x}) = \frac{p(\mathbf{x}|\,\omega_i;\boldsymbol{\theta})P(\omega_i)}{p(\mathbf{x})} \tag{3.43}$$

where,

$$p(\mathbf{x}) = \sum_{i=1}^{M=2} p(\mathbf{x}|\,\omega_i)P(\omega_i) \tag{3.44}$$

Here, $p(\mathbf{x})$ is the evidence or marginal likelihood—it is just a normalizing constant to ensure that $p(\omega|\mathbf{x})$ is a valid probability distribution. The posterior probability gives us how confident we are in our choice, that is, class label. For example, if $p(\omega_1|\mathbf{x}) = 0.9$, then this tells us that the model is willing to give a 90% score to this prediction. This is appealing since we can use this to reject the prediction if the confidence is below a specific threshold, for example, 80% as shown in Fig. 3.4.

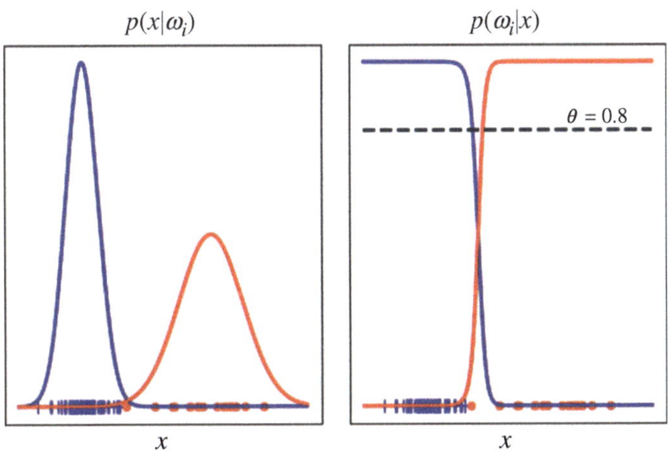

FIG. 3.4

Bayes rule can be used to convert the class-conditional densities into a posterior probability. A threshold can be used to indicate a reject region that determines whether to accept or reject a test case for classification.

Bayes decision rule splits the feature space $\mathbf{x}$ into regions $R_i(\mathbf{x}), i = 1\ldots C$, each specific to one class. Decision errors occur when we choose the wrong class, for example, if we choose class ω_i whereas the true class was ω_j. We can express the probability of error, $P_{\text{error}|x}$, as the integrand at every $\mathbf{x}$ drawn from $p(\mathbf{x})$. Fig. 3.5 shows two-class classification problem where we have assumed equal class priors and 1-D class-conditional likelihoods. We can see that the decision boundary can be fully specified by a scalar threshold x_0. The probability of error can be computed from the total shaded area using

$$\begin{aligned} P_{error} &= \int_{-\infty}^{\infty} P_{error|x}\, p(x)dx \\ &= \int_{-\infty}^{x0} p(x|\,\omega_2)dx + \int_{x0}^{\infty} p(x|\,\omega_1)dx \end{aligned} \tag{3.45}$$

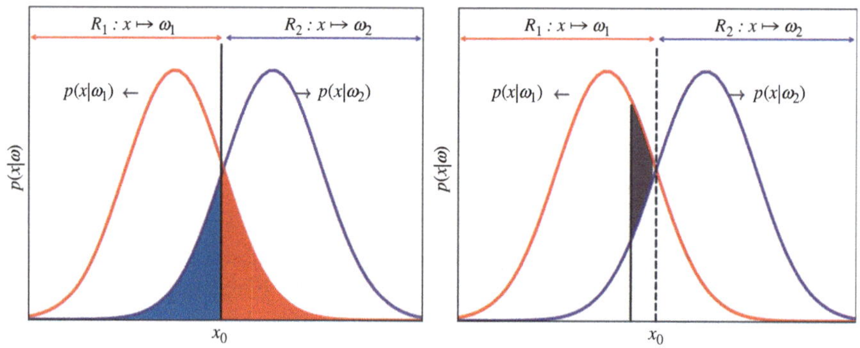

FIG. 3.5

Bayes decision rule selects a threshold x_0 that produces the lowest probability of error. Note that moving the threshold to the left will increase the probability of error by the extra *gray*-shaded area.

Bayes decision rule provides us with optimal decision regions that produce the lowest probability of error. This can be readily verified by inspecting Fig. 3.5 where it is easy to see that moving the threshold to the left will increase the probability of error by the extra gray-shaded area.

In real-life applications, some decisions are more critical and costly than others: for example, classifying an X-ray image incorrectly as normal (false negative) may cause loss of life, while classifying a normal image as positive (false positive) would incur unnecessary further testing and increased costs. Because the consequences of a false negative can be very severe, we rather want to minimize a weighted loss function instead of minimizing the total number of mistakes. Bayes decision theory allows us to incorporate custom misclassification *costs* associated with wrong decisions. A penalty term can penalize wrong predictions differently for each class. Let λ_{ij} indicating the penalty for misclassifying a pattern from class ω_i as class ω_j. The *loss* with respect to misclassifying ω_i as ω_j is obtained by weighting the probability of error by λ_{ij}. The loss for misclassifying class ω_i can be described by

$$\text{loss}(\omega_i|\,\mathbf{x}) = \sum_j \lambda_{ij}\, p\left(\omega_j|\,\mathbf{x}\right) \tag{3.46}$$

Here the optimal decision rule should minimize the Bayes loss; for example, for $M = 2$, we have

$$\mathbf{x} \mapsto \omega_i \text{ if } \frac{p(\mathbf{x}|\,\omega_i)}{p\left(\mathbf{x}|\,\omega_j\right)} > \frac{p\left(\omega_j\right)\lambda_{ij}}{p(\omega_i)\,\lambda_{ji}} \tag{3.47}$$

3.3.1.1 MVN discriminant functions

Bayes decision theory allowed us to make optimal decisions and MAP observations to classes via

$$\mathbf{x} \mapsto \omega_i \text{ if } P(\omega_i|\,\mathbf{x}) > P\left(\omega_j|\,\mathbf{x}\right) \tag{3.48}$$

This gives rise to a Bayes discriminant function (since it is expressed in terms of posterior class probabilities) $g(\mathbf{x})$:

$$g_{ij}(\mathbf{x}) = P(\omega_i|\,\mathbf{x}) - P\left(\omega_j|\,\mathbf{x}\right) \tag{3.49}$$

where we choose $\mathbf{x} \mapsto \omega_i$ if g is positive (+) and $\mathbf{x} \mapsto \omega_j$ if g is negative (−). The decision boundary can be obtained by setting $g_{ij}(\mathbf{x}) = 0$. The complexity of the induced decision surfaces depends on the observational model (i.e., class-conditional likelihood). In this section, we consider a multivariate normal class-conditional likelihood and examine the resulting decision surfaces.

The multivariate normal for d-dimensional observations $\mathbf{x} \in R^d$ can be written as

$$p(\mathbf{x}|\,\omega_i) = \frac{1}{(2\pi)^{\frac{d}{2}}\left|\sum_i\right|^{\frac{1}{2}}} \exp\left(-\frac{1}{2}(\mathbf{x}-\boldsymbol{\mu}_i)^{\mathrm{T}} \sum_i^{-1} (\mathbf{x}-\boldsymbol{\mu}_i)\right) \tag{3.50}$$

where μ_i and Σ_i are the mean vector and the covariance matrix for class ω_i.

$$\boldsymbol{\mu}_i = E[\mathbf{x}|\,\omega_i];\in R^d \tag{3.51}$$

$$\Sigma_i = E\left[(\mathbf{x}-\boldsymbol{\mu}_i)(\mathbf{x}-\boldsymbol{\mu}_i)^{\mathrm{T}}\right];\in R^{d\times d} \tag{3.52}$$

Applying a monotonic function $f(.) = \text{In}(.)$ to the Bayes discriminant function still gives the same discriminant since it does not affect the functional form of the decision region, that is,

$$\begin{aligned} g_{ij}(\mathbf{x}) &= \text{In}P(\omega_i|\,\mathbf{x}) - \text{In}P(\omega_j|\,\mathbf{x}) \\ &= \text{In}\frac{P(\omega_i|\,\mathbf{x})}{P(\omega_j|\,\mathbf{x})} \end{aligned} \tag{3.53}$$

This allows us to simplify the math; we can write our MVN density as

$$\begin{aligned} g_i(\mathbf{x}) &= \text{In}(p(\mathbf{x}|\,\omega_i)P(\omega_i)) = \text{In}\,p(\mathbf{x}|\,\omega_i) + \text{In}\,P(\omega_i) \\ &= -\frac{1}{2}(\mathbf{x}-\boldsymbol{\mu}_i)^{\mathrm{T}}\sum\nolimits_i^{-1}(\mathbf{x}-\boldsymbol{\mu}_i) + \text{In}\,P(\omega_i) + C_i \end{aligned} \tag{3.54}$$

where

$$C_i = -\frac{d}{2}\text{In}(2\pi) - \frac{1}{2}\text{In}\left|\sum\nolimits_i\right| \tag{3.55}$$

Our discriminant then becomes

$$\begin{aligned} g_{ij}(\mathbf{x}) &= \text{In}\,P(\omega_i|\,\mathbf{x}) - \text{In}\,P(\omega_j|\,\mathbf{x}) \\ &\sim (\mathbf{x}-\boldsymbol{\mu}_i)^{\mathrm{T}}\sum\nolimits_i^{-1}(\mathbf{x}-\boldsymbol{\mu}_i) + (\mathbf{x}-\boldsymbol{\mu}_j)^{\mathrm{T}}\sum\nolimits_j^{-1}(\mathbf{x}-\boldsymbol{\mu}_j) + C_{ij} \end{aligned} \tag{3.56}$$

where

$$C_{ij} = \text{In}\frac{P(\omega_i)}{P(\omega_j)} - \frac{1}{2}\text{In}\left|\sum\nolimits_i\right| + \frac{1}{2}\text{In}\left|\sum\nolimits_j\right| \tag{3.57}$$

Case I Shared diagonal covariance. The induced decision regions depend on the structure of the covariance matrix for each class. For example, if the class-conditional densities for both classes were equal and diagonal, that is,

$$\begin{aligned} \sum &= \sigma^2 I \\ &= \begin{bmatrix} \sigma^2 & 0 \\ 0 & \sigma^2 \end{bmatrix} \end{aligned} \tag{3.58}$$

then (3.56) becomes

$$g_{ij}(\mathbf{x}) = (\mathbf{x}-\boldsymbol{\mu}_i)^{\mathrm{T}}(\mathbf{x}-\boldsymbol{\mu}_i) + (\mathbf{x}-\boldsymbol{\mu}_j)^{\mathrm{T}}(\mathbf{x}-\boldsymbol{\mu}_j) \tag{3.59}$$

The quadratic terms are not involved in comparisons since they will cancel out:

$$g_{ij}(\mathbf{x}) = \mathbf{w}^{\mathrm{T}}\mathbf{x} - \mathbf{x}_0 \tag{3.60}$$

where

$$\begin{aligned} \mathrm{w} &= \boldsymbol{\mu}_i - \boldsymbol{\mu}_j \\ \mathbf{x}_0 &= \frac{1}{2}(\boldsymbol{\mu}_i + \boldsymbol{\mu}_j) - \sigma^2\text{In}\frac{P(\omega_i)}{P(\omega_j)}\frac{\boldsymbol{\mu}_i - \boldsymbol{\mu}_j}{\|\boldsymbol{\mu}_i - \boldsymbol{\mu}_j\|^2} \end{aligned} \tag{3.61}$$

The decision surface is now a hyperplane that is perpendicular to the lines connecting the class means as shown in Fig. 3.6.

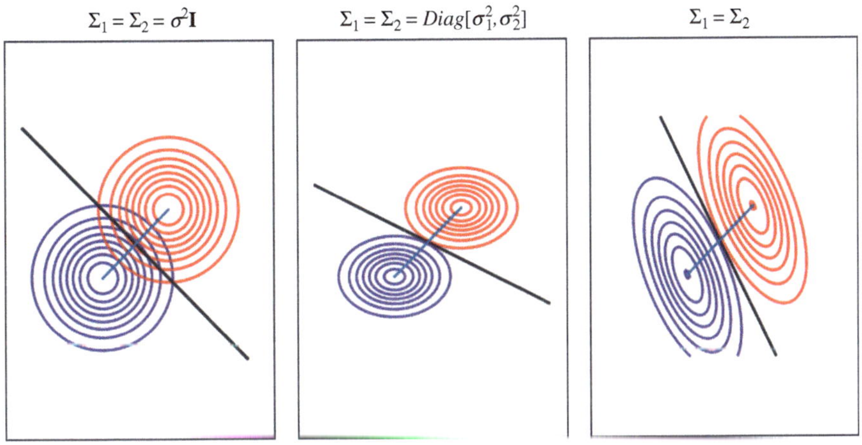

FIG. 3.6

When the classes share the same covariance structure, the resulting discriminant will produce a linear decision surface that is perpendicular to the lines connecting the class means.

The resulting classifier is a minimum distance classifier that decides the class label according to the closest Euclidean distance between the observation and class means. If we further assume that the classes are equiprobable, that is, $P(\omega_i) = P(\omega_j)$, then

$$\begin{aligned} &g_i(\mathbf{x}) = (\mathbf{x} - \boldsymbol{\mu}_i)^{T}\Sigma^{-1}(\mathbf{x} - \boldsymbol{\mu}_i) \\ &\mathbf{x} \mapsto \omega_i \text{ if } \|\mathbf{x} - \boldsymbol{\mu}_i\| \text{ is smaller} \end{aligned} \tag{3.62}$$

Case II Shared nondiagonal covariance. If the individual covariances were shared but not diagonal, that is, $\Sigma_i = \Sigma_j = \Sigma$, then the discriminant function becomes

$$\begin{aligned} g_{ij}(\mathbf{x}) &= (\mathbf{x} - \boldsymbol{\mu}_i)^{\mathrm{T}}\Sigma^{-1}(\mathbf{x} - \boldsymbol{\mu}_i) + (\mathbf{x} - \boldsymbol{\mu}_j)^{\mathrm{T}}\Sigma^{-1}(\mathbf{x} - \boldsymbol{\mu}_j) \\ &= \mathbf{w}^{\mathrm{T}}\mathbf{x} + \omega_0 \end{aligned} \tag{3.63}$$

where

$$\begin{aligned} &\mathrm{w}_i = \sum\nolimits^{-1}(\boldsymbol{\mu}_i - \boldsymbol{\mu}_j) \\ &\omega_0 = \mathrm{In}\frac{P(\omega_i)}{P(\omega_j)} - \frac{1}{2}\left(\boldsymbol{\mu}_j^{\mathrm{T}}\Sigma^{-1}\boldsymbol{\mu}_j\right) - \frac{1}{2}\left(\boldsymbol{\mu}_i^{\mathrm{T}}\Sigma^{-1}\boldsymbol{\mu}_i\right) \end{aligned} \tag{3.64}$$

Again, we have a linear decision boundary, but this time the hyperplane **w** is not perpendicular lines connecting class means; instead, it is perpendicular to $\Sigma^{-1}(\mu_i - \mu_j)$. This is also a minimum distance classifier. However, the distance measure is now based on the Mahalanobis distance metric:

$$\begin{aligned} &g_i(\mathbf{x}) = (\mathbf{x} - \boldsymbol{\mu}_i)^{\mathrm{T}}\Sigma^{-1}(\mathbf{x} - \boldsymbol{\mu}_i) \\ &\mathbf{x} \mapsto \omega_i \text{ if } (\mathbf{x} - \boldsymbol{\mu}_i)^{\mathrm{T}}\Sigma^{-1}(\mathbf{x} - \boldsymbol{\mu}_i) \text{ is smaller} \end{aligned} \tag{3.65}$$

Case III Distinct nondiagonal covariance. If the individual covariances were distinct and not diagonal, that is, $\Sigma_i \neq \Sigma_j$, then the discriminant function can be written as

$$g_{ij}(\mathbf{x}) = (\mathbf{x}-\boldsymbol{\mu}_i)^{\mathrm{T}}\Sigma_j^{-1}(\mathbf{x}-\boldsymbol{\mu}_i) + (\mathbf{x}-\boldsymbol{\mu}_j)^{\mathrm{T}}\Sigma_j^{-1}(\mathbf{x}-\boldsymbol{\mu}_j) \tag{3.66}$$

This time we have quadratic decision boundaries as shown in Fig. 3.7.

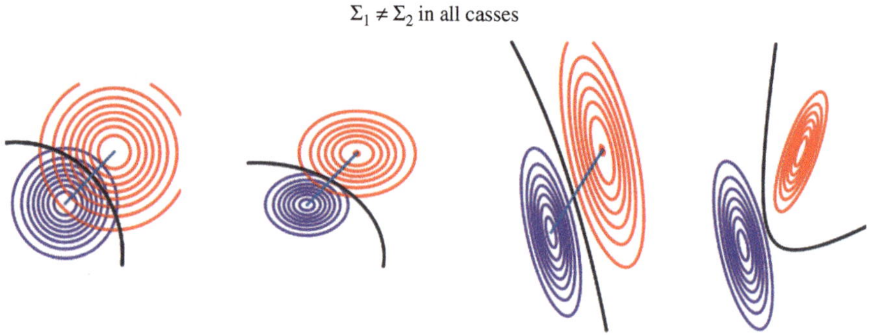

FIG. 3.7

The discriminant function is quadratic $\in R^d$ due to unequal covariance structures of the class-conditional densities.

3.3.1.2 Naive Bayes classifier

The Bayes classifier in the previous section assumed Gaussian class-conditional densities. We saw that if the covariances of the classes were shared and diagonal and if the classes were equiprobable, then the Bayes classifier is linear and corresponds to the minimum Euclidean distance classifier. If the covariances were equal but not diagonal, the Bayes classifier is still linear, and we have the minimum Mahalanobis distance classifier. In general the decision surfaces for nonequal class covariance are quadratic.

Let $\mathbf{x} \in R^d$; our goal is to estimate $p(\mathbf{x}|\omega_i)$; $i = 1, 2, \ldots, M$. Assuming MVN class conditionals allows us to capture dependencies between any two features of the d-dimensional feature vector. However, if the data are high dimensional, then the number of parameters required to express the MVN becomes very large as we need to learn d parameters for each of the class means and $d + \frac{d(d+1)}{2}$ parameters for each class covariance. Therefore, if the number of training examples in a dataset is small with respect to the total number of parameters, then the MVN Bayes classifier could easily overfit the data. This renders that Bayes MVNs unable to generalize in high dimensions.

The idea behind naive Bayes classifier is to *naively* assume that the class-conditional likelihoods can factorize into a product of univariate d-dimensional distributions. In other words, given the class label, the individual features will be independent. The naive Bayes assumption allows us to compute the class conditional densities in terms of a product of univariate densities $P(x(d)|\omega_i)$:

$$p(\mathbf{x}|\,\omega_i) = \prod_{j=1}^{d} P(x_j|\,\omega_i) \tag{3.67}$$

The discriminant function for naive Bayes classifier, therefore, involves

$$P(\omega_i)\prod_{k=1}^{d} P(x_k|\,\omega_i) \tag{3.68}$$

This is a much easier problem than estimating the full multivariate density $P(\mathbf{x}|\omega_i)$ and reduces the total number of parameters to just $M \times d$, where M is the number of classes. As such the naive Bayes assumption reduces model flexibility since it restricts the class conditional densities to be axis aligned, which is not really true, but nevertheless less works very well in most settings (e.g., see Fig. 3.8).

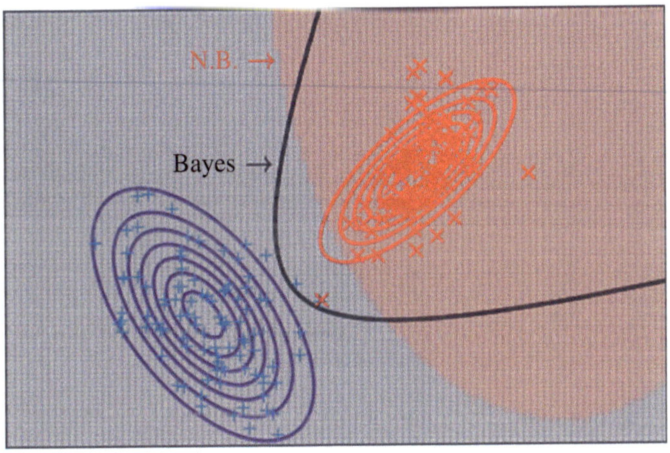

FIG. 3.8

Although the naive Bayes assumption is very simplistic, however, it does a pretty good job in approximating the class-conditional densities.

3.3.1.3 Nonparametric Bayes classifier

Bayes classifier requires that we specify a functional form of the class densities. Maximum likelihood principle can then be used to estimate the parameters of the class conditionals and then use Bayes rule to compute the posterior class probabilities. We then select the class with the largest posterior probability. Alternatively, we can use a nonparametric density estimation method, such as the kernel or nearest neighbor density estimation. For example, to design a Bayes classifier based on Parzen window density estimation, we choose a kernel function along with the kernel width, h. We then estimate the class-conditional densities for each class using

$$p(\mathbf{x}|\,\omega_i) = \frac{1}{h^d N_i}\sum_{\mathbf{x}_i \in \omega_1} K\left(\frac{\mathbf{x}_i - \mathbf{x}}{h}\right) \tag{3.69}$$

Assuming zero-one loss, we classify a test case using the maximum a posteriori rule:

$$
\begin{aligned}
\mathbf{x} \mapsto \omega 1: \text{ if } \frac{p(\mathbf{x}|\,\omega_1)}{p(\mathbf{x}|\,\omega_2)} &> \frac{p(\omega_2)}{P(\omega_1)} = \gamma \\
&> \frac{N_2 \Sigma_{x_i \in \omega_1} K\left(\frac{\mathbf{x}_i - \mathbf{x}}{h}\right)}{N_1 \Sigma_{x_i \in \omega_2} K\left(\frac{\mathbf{x}_i - \mathbf{x}}{h}\right)}
\end{aligned}
\tag{3.70}
$$

Alternatively, we can use the kNN density estimator to estimate the class-conditional densities and then compute the posterior class probability. It turns out that the resulting classifier leads to a straightforward formulation and interesting properties. This classifier is called k-nearest neighbor classifier, kNN, and is shown in Fig. 3.9 for two settings of the hyperparameter $k = 1$ and $k = 100$, respectively.

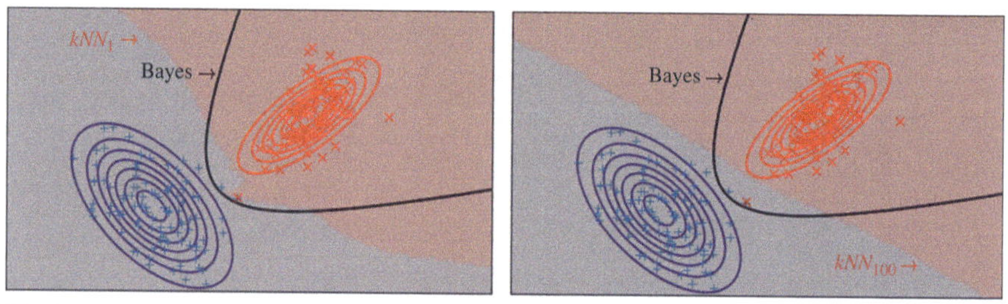

FIG. 3.9

Bayes decision boundary *(black line)* is optimal in the sense that it minimizes the probability of error. The kNN algorithm (*red*- and *blue*-shaded regions) however only relies on local geometry and seems to do a good job in separating the classes.

The kNN algorithm relies on local geometry of the data to estimate the class density in a given region of the feature space. Given N_i examples from class ω_i, we estimate the class-conditional density for an observation $\mathbf{x}$ by computing the volume surrounding $\mathbf{x}$ that contains k_i observations from ω_i:

$$
p(\mathbf{x}|\,\omega_i) = \frac{k_i}{N_i} \frac{1}{V_d R_k^d(\mathbf{x})}
\tag{3.71}
$$

where $R_k(\mathbf{x})$ is the distance between the estimation point $\mathbf{x}$ and its kth closest neighbor. The marginal density $p(\mathbf{x})$ is computed by fixing $R_k(\mathbf{x})$ and counting the total number of examples, k_t from all classes that fall in the volume surrounding $\mathbf{x}$. Now, we can use Bayes rule to estimate the posterior class probability as

$$
\begin{aligned}
p(\omega_i|\,\mathbf{x}) &= \frac{p(\mathbf{x}|\,\omega_i) p(\omega_i)}{p(\mathbf{x})} \\
&= \frac{k_i}{k_t}
\end{aligned}
\tag{3.72}
$$

The kNN algorithm can easily handle multiple classes since it relies on the local geometry of the training data as shown in Fig. 3.10. Notice how the decision boundaries are affected by the choice of k. In general the smaller the value of k the more flexible the decision boundaries become as shown in Fig. 3.11.

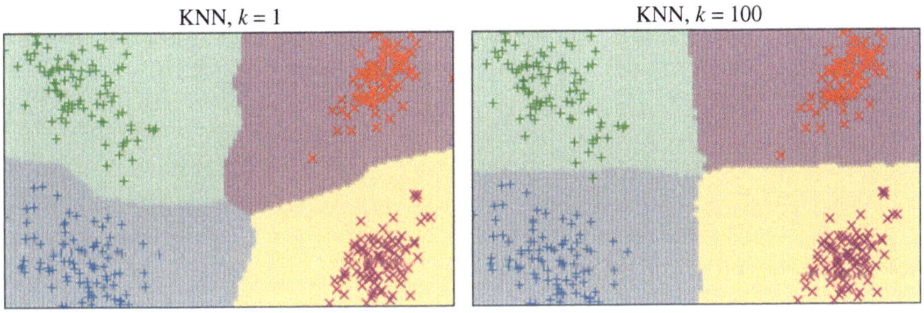

FIG. 3.10

The kNN algorithm can easily handle multiple classes since it relies on the local geometry of the training data.

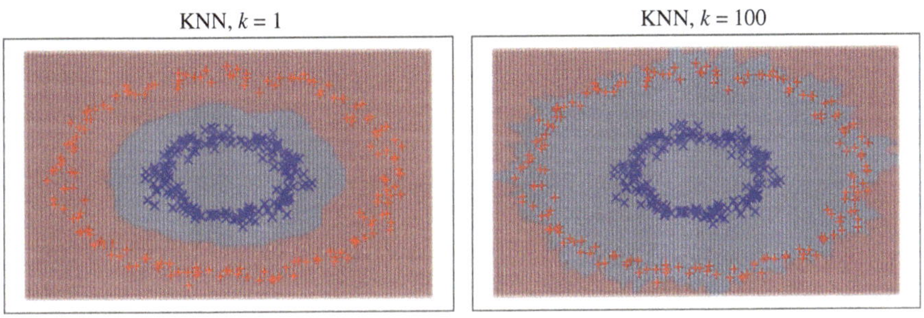

FIG. 3.11

As we increase k for the kNN model, the decision boundaries fail to capture the structure in the data. As such, it is recommended that several values for k are to be tested.

The kNN classifier suffers from a number of ailments; kNN classifier is known to be sensitive to noisy features especially in high dimensions. As such, it is recommended to perform feature selection to remove the noninformative features; also, it is recommended to scale the features to have zero mean and unit variance before running the KNN algorithm as this improves the accuracy of the results; finally, it should be noted that if the feature space is high dimensional, then the Euclidian distance metric becomes inappropriate; therefore it is recommended to adopt an alternative distance metric that considers the geometry of the manifold that the actual data lie on.

3.3.2 Discriminant functions

A *linear discriminant* is a function of the form $g(\mathbf{x}) = \mathbf{w}^{\mathrm{T}}\mathbf{x} \in R$. The decision boundaries are linear in the feature space $\mathbf{x}$:

$$g(\mathbf{x}) = \mathbf{w}^T\mathbf{x} = \omega_1 x_1 + \omega_2 x_2 + \ldots + \omega_d x_d + \omega_0 1 \tag{3.73}$$

Here, $\mathbf{w} \in R^d$ defines a d-dimensional hyperplane that lives in the feature space spanned by $\mathbf{x} = \{x_1, x_2, \ldots, x_d\} \in R^d$. This model is linear in both the parameters and the inputs (i.e., features). A *kernel discriminant* produces nonlinear decision boundaries by transforming the inputs into new spaces $\mathbf{x} \mapsto \varphi(\mathbf{x})$:

$$g(\mathbf{x}) = \mathbf{w}^T\varphi(\mathbf{x}) \tag{3.74}$$

Essentially, this creates new synthetic features from the original features $\mathbf{x}$ using the nonlinear function $\varphi(.)$. The decision boundary is no longer linear in the original feature space, however still linear in the new feature space, $\varphi(\mathbf{x})$. The decision boundary can be obtained by setting $g(\mathbf{x}) = 0$, that is,

$$g(\mathbf{x}) = \mathbf{w}^T\mathbf{x} = 0 \tag{3.75}$$

and for kernel discriminant functions,

$$g(\mathbf{x}) = \mathbf{w}^T\varphi(\mathbf{x}) = 0 \tag{3.76}$$

Discriminant functions can be further extended by introducing nonlinear activation functions $f(g(\mathbf{x}))$. If the discriminant is linear, that is, $g(\mathbf{x}) = \mathbf{w}^T\mathbf{x}$, then applying a nonlinear activation produces outputs y that are nonlinear both in $\mathbf{x}$ and $\mathbf{w}$; however, the decision surfaces are still linear in the original features, $\mathbf{x}$. These modes are called *generalized linear discriminants* since they can produce continuous and discrete responses. For example, to produce discrete outputs, we can apply a hard-thresholding function using

$$y = f(g(\mathbf{x})) = \text{sign}\left(\mathbf{w}^T\mathbf{x}\right) \tag{3.77}$$

or

$$y = f(g(\mathbf{x})) = \text{unitstep}\left(\mathbf{w}^T\mathbf{x}\right) \tag{3.78}$$

The first operation reduces the responses to either 0 or 1, while the second function reduces the y responses to either ± 1. In other words, using sign(.) activation separates the feature space into two distinct regions: the region to the right of the hyperplane, $g(\mathbf{x}) = \mathbf{w}^T\mathbf{x} \geq 0$; that is, $\mathbf{x}$ is in class ω_1, and the region to the left of the hyperplane $g(\mathbf{x}) = \mathbf{w}^T\mathbf{x} < 0$; that is, $\mathbf{x}$ is in class ω_2. If $g(\mathbf{x}) = 0$, we cannot tell what is the label of the observation as it lies on the decision boundary. We can also use activation functions that produce bounded continuous responses. For example,

$$y = f(g(\mathbf{x})) = \tanh\left(\mathbf{w}^T\mathbf{x}\right) \tag{3.79}$$

and

$$y = f(g(\mathbf{x})) = \sigma\left(\mathbf{w}^T\mathbf{x}\right) \tag{3.80}$$

where the sigmoid function is defined as

$$\sigma(x) = \frac{1}{1 + \exp(-x)} \tag{3.81}$$

The first operation defines a soft-thresholding rule where responses are now squashed in the interval [−1,+1], while the second operation uses the sigmoid function to squash the output in the interval [0,1]. For example, in logistic regression, we use the sigmoid function to interpret the responses y as the posterior class probabilities, for example, $y = 0.9$ means that the input has 90% chance of belonging to class ω_1 and 10% chance of belonging to class ω_2. Generalized linear discriminants of the form $y = f(\mathbf{w}^T\mathbf{x})$ produce nonlinear responses y but still produce linear decision boundaries even if $f(.)$ is nonlinear. The decision boundary can be obtained by two ways: for example, if we use the logistic sigmoid, the decision boundary can either be obtained by setting $\mathbf{w}^T\mathbf{x} = 0$ or $\sigma(\mathbf{w}^T\mathbf{x}) = 0.5$.

Generalized kernel discriminants use both nonlinear activations and nonlinear transformations of the inputs $\mathbf{x}$, that is,

$$y = f(g(\mathbf{x})) = \sigma\left(\mathbf{w}^T\varphi(\mathbf{x})\right) \tag{3.82}$$

This is used in kernel logistic regression. Here the outputs are nonlinear; the decision boundaries are nonlinear in $\mathbf{x}$ but still linear in $\varphi(\mathbf{x})$. Given a known parameter vector $\mathbf{w}$, the decision boundary can be obtained by setting

$$\mathbf{w}^T\varphi(\mathbf{x}) = 0 \tag{3.83}$$

or

$$\sigma\left(\mathbf{w}^T\varphi(\mathbf{x})\right) = 0.5 \tag{3.84}$$

We can again extend our discriminants further, this time we will call them *multilayer discriminants*, for example,

$$y = f\left(\mathbf{w}_1^T g_1\left(\mathbf{w}_2^T g_2(g(\mathbf{x};\, \mathbf{w}))\right)\right) \tag{3.85}$$

The difference here is that the model is of high flexibility and complexity. It is nonlinear in the parameters and the inputs. The decision boundaries are also nonlinear even when $g(\mathbf{x};\mathbf{w})$ is linear.

As a final extension, we consider the case of K-class problems. We can try to learn K separate discriminant functions using *one-versus-rest* or *one-versus-one* methodology. However, this will result in ambiguous regions. Instead, it is better to define a single discriminant comprising K linear functions, for example,

$$g_k(\mathbf{x}) = \sigma\left(\mathbf{w}_k^T\mathbf{x}\right) \tag{3.86}$$

and then assigning class ω_k if $g_k(\mathbf{x}) > g_j(\mathbf{x}) \forall j \neq k$, that is, we are now using the magnitude of $g(\mathbf{x})$ not just the sign. This solves the problem of ambiguous regions and results in convex singly connected decision regions. Alternatively, we can use *multidimensional discriminant functions* such as the *softmax*, where the output is a vector of K-real numbers that sum to 1.

3.3.3 Linear discriminants

Learning a discriminant function is about finding the weights $\mathbf{w}$ that best separates the classes. Depending on what "best" means we get different flavors for classification models, for example, "best" could mean finding the weights that minimize the total number of misclassified examples, maximize class separability, minimize the sum of squared errors between the predicted and true responses, or producing a decision boundary that has maximum margin. This is translated as an objective function (also called cost or loss function) that quantifies how good/bad a set of parameters are compared with others. The objective function can then be used to train our model and find the optimal parameters. Once a model is fitted, we can use it to make predictions on new test data.

3.3.3.1 Perceptron discriminant

The perceptron rule aims to find the weights of a separating hyperplane that minimizes the number of misclassified examples. However, as we will see, the algorithm only converges if the classes are linearly separable. For a linear discriminant, we expect $\mathbf{w}^T\mathbf{x} > 0$ for observations that belong to class ω_1 and $\mathbf{w}^T\mathbf{x} < 0$ for all observations that belong to class ω_2. As such an error is made if an observation that belongs to class ω_1 is incorrectly predicted, making $\mathbf{w}^T\mathbf{x} < 0$, or if an observation that belongs to class ω_2 is incorrectly predicted, making $\mathbf{w}^T\mathbf{x} > 0$. Let δ_x be an indicator variable where $\delta_x = -1$ if $\mathbf{x}$ is *misclassified* and originally belong to class ω_1, and $\delta_x = +1$ if $\mathbf{x}$ is *misclassified* but originally belong to class ω_2. This makes the product $\delta_x\mathbf{w}^T\mathbf{x} > 0$ for all misclassified instances $\mathbf{x} \in \mathbf{Z}$.

The perceptron learning rule, therefore, uses the following loss function:

$$J(\mathbf{w}) = \sum_{\mathbf{x} \in Z} \delta_x \mathbf{w}^T\mathbf{x} \tag{3.87}$$

where Z is the subset of instances wrongly classified for a given choice of $\mathbf{w}$. Note that the cost function, $J(\mathbf{w})$, is a piecewise linear function since it is a sum of linear terms, also $J(\mathbf{w}) \geq 0$ (it is zero when $Z = \Phi$, i.e., the empty set).

Minimizing the loss can be achieved using gradient descent: differentiating $J(\mathbf{w})$ with respect to the parameters, we get

$$\begin{aligned} \frac{\partial J(\mathbf{w})}{\partial w} &= \frac{\partial}{\partial w}\left(\sum_{\mathbf{x} \in Z} \delta_x \mathbf{w}^T\mathbf{x}\right) \\ &= \sum_{\mathbf{x} \in Z} \delta_x \mathbf{x} \end{aligned} \tag{3.88}$$

To find the optimal $\mathbf{w}$, we update the current estimate of the parameters by moving in the direction opposite to the gradient at $\mathbf{w} = \mathbf{w}_n$:

$$\begin{aligned} \mathbf{w}_{n+1} &= \mathbf{w}_n - \eta \left.\frac{\partial J(\mathbf{w})}{\partial w}\right|_{\mathbf{w}=\mathbf{w}_n} \\ &= \mathbf{w}_n - \eta \sum_{\mathbf{x} \in z} \delta_x \mathbf{x} \end{aligned} \tag{3.89}$$

where η is the learning rate. Note that updating $\mathbf{w}$ with respect to a misclassified input will lower the error for that particular input; however, the error for other inputs may increase. This means that the total error will not decrease monotonically at every iteration. Also the perceptron is usually slow, and even when it converges to a solution, it yields a nonunique solution because the objective function is not convex.

The perceptron learning rule is very simple and converges after a finite number of update steps have passed provided that the classes are linearly separable. However, if the classes are nonseparable, the perceptron rule iterates indefinitely and fails to converge to a solution. Fig. 3.12 shows an example of a linear perceptron where the classes are not linearly separable. One way to stop the algorithm for iterating indefinitely is to store a record of the classification accuracy in previous steps and report the best performance after some iterations have passed.

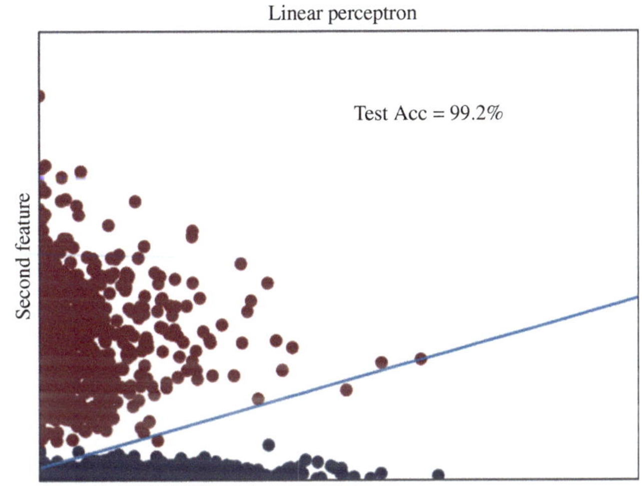

FIG. 3.12

Linear perceptron: Here the classes are not linearly separable; as such the perceptron fails to converge. One way to stop the algorithm for iterating indefinitely is to store a record of the classification accuracy in previous steps and report the best performance after some iterations have passed.

3.3.3.2 Least squares methods

The least squares classifier constructs a cost function using the mean squared errors between the true responses, y and the predictions $\hat{y}$, that is,

$$\hat{\mathbf{w}} = \underset{\mathbf{w}}{\arg\min}\, E\left[\left(\mathrm{y} - \mathbf{w}^{\mathrm{T}}\mathbf{x}\right)^2\right] \tag{3.90}$$

Unlike the loss function of a perceptron, this is a convex function and has a unique and simple closed-form solution. The optimal solution can be obtained by taking the gradients of (3.90) and solving for $\mathbf{w}$:

$$\begin{aligned} \frac{\partial J(\mathbf{w})}{\partial w} &= \frac{\partial}{\partial w} E\left[\left(\mathrm{y} - \mathbf{w}^{\mathrm{T}}\mathbf{x}\right)^2\right] = 0 \\ & 2E[\mathbf{x}(\mathrm{y} - \mathbf{x}^{\mathrm{T}}\mathbf{w})] = 0 \\ & E[\mathbf{x}\mathbf{x}^{\mathrm{T}}]\mathrm{w} = E[\mathbf{x}\mathrm{y}] \\ & \Rightarrow \hat{\mathbf{w}} = R_x^{-1} E[\mathbf{x}\mathrm{y}] \end{aligned} \tag{3.91}$$

where $\mathbf{R}_x$ is the autocorrelation matrix and $E[\mathbf{x}\hat{\mathbf{x}}]$ and $E[\mathbf{x}\mathrm{y}]$ are the cross-correlation vectors. It should be noted that while least squares is guaranteed to achieve a global minimum, however, this is not necessarily the best solution. It is only best in terms of achieving the lowest sum of squared errors, but the solution does not guarantee small probability of error. It is, in fact, possible that least squares fails to find the separating hyperplane even when the classes are separable. For example, the presence of outliers in the data causes the decision boundary to swing toward the outliers. This is because least squares approximates the conditional expectation of the targets given the inputs, $E[\mathbf{y}|\mathbf{x}]$, as such too positive predictions will cause the expectation to be greatly affected by outliers. Linear activations are not suitable for binary data as the classifier produces numbers that can be too positive or too negative (linear activations cause the outputs to become outside the [0, 1] interval), and hence the square errors can become very large even for correct predictions. As such, we conclude that least squares classifier with linear activations is not a good choice for a classification model.

3.3.3.3 Fisher's linear discriminant

Linear discriminant functions can be solved in the context of dimensionality reduction. The problem of a two-class classification becomes finding the projection $\mathbf{w}$ that maximizes the separation between the projected classes. Let us assume that our data are $2d$ and we want to find a $1d$ projection direction (embedded in the original $2d$ space) such that the separation between the projected classes is maximum. Geometrically the separation between classes is a measure that depends on the projected means and the projected scatter of the two classes; the further the classes are from each other, the larger the distance between their centroids, and the larger the separation. Similarly the smaller the scatter within each class, the further apart they become (and, therefore, the minimum the overlap between classes). We can use the ratio of class separation to total class scatter as a measure (objective) for class separation. This is called the Fisher criterion:

$$J(\mathbf{w}) = \frac{(\mathrm{m}_1 - \mathrm{m}_2)^2}{s_1^2 + s_2^2} \tag{3.92}$$

where

$$\begin{aligned} m_i \in R &= \mathrm{w}^{\mathrm{T}} \frac{1}{N_i} \sum_{n \in Ci} \mathbf{x}_n \\ s_k^2 \in R &= \sum_{n \in Ci} (\mathrm{y}_n - m_i)^2, \ldots\ i = 1,2 \end{aligned} \tag{3.93}$$

where $y_n \in R = \mathbf{w}^{\mathrm{T}}\mathbf{x}_n$ is the 1d projection of original data $\mathbf{x}$ and s_k^2 is the kth within-class variance (we use variance since data is now 1d). Equivalently, we can rewrite the criterion in terms of the within-class scatter, $\mathbf{S}_W$, and between-class scatter, $\mathbf{S}_B$:

$$J(\boldsymbol{w}) = \frac{\mathbf{w}^{\mathrm{T}} \mathrm{S}_{\mathrm{B}} \mathbf{w}}{\mathbf{w}^{\mathrm{T}} \mathrm{S}_W \mathbf{w}} \tag{3.94}$$

where

$$S_B = (m_2 - m_1)(m_2 - m_1)^T$$
$$S_W = \sum_{\in C_1} (x_n - m_1)(x_n - m_1)^T + \sum_{\in C_2} (x_n - m_2)(x_n - m_2)^T \tag{3.95}$$
$$m_i \in R^d = \frac{1}{N} \sum_{n \in C_i} x_n$$

It can be shown that maximizing Eq. (3.94) with respect to **w** results in the following solution:

$$\omega \propto \mathbf{S}_w^{-1}(m_2 - m_1) \tag{3.96}$$

This is called the Fisher's linear discriminant. It can be shown that if the class distributions are MVNs with shared covariance, then the within-class scatter is nothing but a scaled MVN covariance matrix, Σ. If the classes were further isotropic, then the Fisher linear discriminant will result in the following solution:

$$\omega \propto (m_2 - m_1) \tag{3.97}$$

This is the same as the minimum distance classifier.

3.3.4 Generalized discriminants

3.3.4.1 Logistic regression

Logistic regression is a common theme for classification and belongs to the generalized linear model category. Generalized linear discriminants, for example, $g(\mathbf{x}) = f(\mathbf{w}^T\mathbf{x})$, and generalized kernel discriminants, for example, $g(\mathbf{x}) - f(\mathbf{w}^T\varphi(\mathbf{x}))$, apply activation functions f(.) to obtain nonlinear responses, y. Generalized linear discriminants will therefore have linear decision boundaries.

The goal of logistic regression is to design a linear classifier, that is, a linear decision boundary while producing predictions, y, between 0 and 1 that represent the posterior class probabilities. Logistic regression models the log-odds ratio of two classes using a linear model while making sure that the sum of all class probabilities adds to 1, that is,

$$\text{In}\left(\frac{P(\omega_1|\mathbf{x})}{P(\omega_2|\mathbf{x})}\right) = \mathbf{w}^T\mathbf{x} \tag{3.98}$$

$$P(\omega_1|\mathbf{x}) + P(\omega_2|\mathbf{x}) = 1 \tag{3.99}$$

It can be shown that this is equivalent to applying a sigmoidal nonlinearity to the linear model that effectively squashes the response variable so that it is between 0 and 1. Specifically, Eq. (3.98) can be written in terms of posterior class probabilities using

$$P(\omega_2|\mathbf{x}) = \frac{1}{1 + \exp(\mathbf{w}^T\mathbf{x})} \tag{3.100}$$

where the parameters $\mathbf{w}$ can be estimated by maximizing the likelihood. The posterior class probabilities are finally computed using

$$P(\omega_1|\,\mathbf{x}) = 1 - P(\omega_2|\,\mathbf{x}) \\ = \frac{\exp(\mathbf{w}^{\mathrm{T}}\mathbf{x})}{1+\exp(\mathbf{w}^{\mathrm{T}}\mathbf{x})} \tag{3.101}$$

Logistic regression

Binary and categorical cross entropy. Binary cross entropy or negative log loss is commonly used for training and evaluating probabilistic binary classifiers such as naive Bayes and logistic regression. It is defined as

$$\text{Log loss} = -\frac{1}{N}\sum_i y_i \log p_i + (1-y_i)\log(1-p_i) \tag{3.102}$$

The cross entropy measures the extent to which the predicted probabilities match the true labels. In other words, it takes into account the uncertainty in the predictions to measure the goodness of the model. Suppose we have an instance with a class label as $y = 1$ is predicted by the model as $p = 1$, then the log loss for this case depends only on the first term since the second term of zero. The first term becomes $-\log p$, and since $p = 1.0$, then the incurred loss is zero.

If $p = 0$, then the loss will be very high. For $M > 2$ classes the categorical cross entropy is simply defined as

$$\text{Log loss} = -\frac{1}{N}\sum_i\sum_j y_{ij}\log(p_{ij}) \tag{3.103}$$

where y_{ij} is a one-shot encoding of the labels where $y_{ij} = 1$ at the jth position if the class of the ith instance is ω_j and zero elsewhere.

3.3.4.2 Kernel discriminants

Linear discriminants allow us to find a linear decision boundary that separates the data in the original feature space. However, real-world data are often nonlinearly separable. The idea behind kernel discriminants is to create synthesized nonlinear features by using nonlinear mapping functions $\varphi(\mathbf{x})$. The probability of finding a linear decision boundary in the new feature space is higher as we increase the number of synthetic features. The new feature space may consist of the raw features and/or nonlinear mappings of the original features and combinations of the original features: $\mathbf{x} \in R^l \mapsto \mathbf{z} = \phi(\mathbf{x}) \in R^k;\ k \gg l$. The price for such flexibility is increased model complexity and potentially overfitting the data. This results in poor generalization, especially as the number of model parameters becomes greater than the number of observations. For example, a 2D feature space can be transformed to a 3D space using the following mapping:

$$\mathbf{x} = [x_1, x_2]^{\mathrm{T}} \in R^2 \mapsto \mathbf{z} = \begin{bmatrix} x_1^2 \\ \sqrt{2}x_1x_2 \\ x_2^2 \end{bmatrix} \in R^3 \tag{3.104}$$

We then proceed normally with writing our model as a linear model in the new feature space:

$$\begin{aligned} y &= w_0 + w_1z_1 + w_2z_2 + w_3z_3 \\ &= w_0 + w_1x_1^2 + w_2\sqrt{2}x_1x_2 + w_3x_3^3 \end{aligned} \tag{3.105}$$

The transformation defined by Eq. (3.104) can be used to obtain kernel logistic regression model:

$$\begin{aligned} \log\left(\frac{P(y=1|\,\mathbf{z},\mathbf{w})}{P(y=0|\,\mathbf{z},\mathbf{w})}\right) &= w_0 + w_1z_1 + w_2z_2 + w_3z_3 \\ &= w_0 + w_1x_1^2 + w_2\sqrt{2}x_1x_2 + w_3x_2^2 \end{aligned} \tag{3.106}$$

This turns out to produce a linear decision boundary in the transformed feature space, $\mathbf{z}$, but a nonlinear decision boundary in the original feature space, $\mathbf{x}$, with scaled responses, y.

3.3.5 Constrained discriminant functions

For separable classes, there can be infinitely many decision boundaries that can perfectly separate the classes. Fig. 3.13 shows two linearly separable classes and two decision boundaries (hyperplanes) that perfectly separate the classes. The blue decision

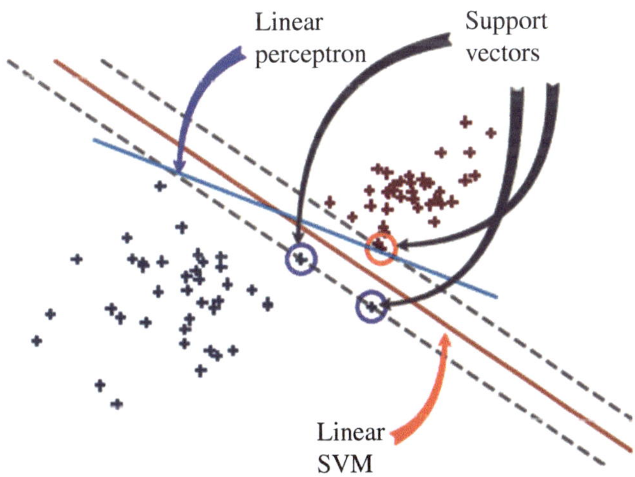

FIG. 3.13

The *blue* decision boundary is obtained using the perceptron algorithm, while the *red* decision boundary is produced by the SVM classifier. The *blue* and *red* circles are called support vectors, which uniquely define the parametric form of the decision boundary.

boundary, $\mathbf{w_1}$, was obtained by the perceptron algorithm discussed earlier (each run of the algorithm will find one of the infinitely many linear separators), while the red decision boundary, $\mathbf{w_2}$, was obtained by the support vector machine algorithm. But which decision boundary is better? It seems that the decision boundary defined by $\mathbf{w_1}$ produces less confident predictions for points that are near the decision boundary—there is almost 50% chance that the classifier predicts either way. Classifier $\mathbf{w_1}$ seems to be less confident in predicting class 1 examples (red +'s) compared with class 2 examples (blue +s) since the data points of class 1 are closer to the decision boundary than class 2 examples. However, classifier $\mathbf{w_2}$ seems to have the right balance: the decision boundary is equally and maximally distant from both class examples. Intuitively, this is the best classifier because it is less prone to overfitting (the maximal margin/distance constraint reduces the possible choices of such a line compared with the infinitely possible linear separators) and produces fewer misclassification errors, especially for points near the decision surface.

3.3.5.1 Support vector machines

Support vector machines still use linear models, but constrain the choice of the separating hyperplane, $\mathbf{w}$, as the one that is maximally far away from any data point on both sides of the decision surface. In addition the decision boundary is specified in terms of a small subset of the original data referred to as the support vectors. The decision boundary has fewer degrees of freedom and good generalization properties. A large margin (i.e., a fat separator between classes) reduces the choices of $\mathbf{w}$, hence reduces the chances of overfitting and also reduces memory capacity of the model.

For a decision boundary *that separates the classes*, the margin is defined as twice the *distance* from the nearest point from each class to the decision surface in the direction *perpendicular* to $\mathbf{w}$. Therefore the decision surface leaves the same distance from the nearest points from each class. This makes the classifier equally sensitive near the decision surface to test data that lie close to it from both sides. In binary SVMs, we use +1 or −1 instead of 0/1 for the class labels. Hence, we require that $\mathbf{w}^T\mathbf{x} \geq +1$ for all points in class 1 and $\mathbf{w}^T\mathbf{x} \leq -1$ for all points in class 2. For any point $\mathbf{x}$, that lies on a decision boundary, the distance in the direction *perpendicular* to $\mathbf{w}$ is

$$g(\mathbf{x}) = \frac{\mathbf{w}^T\mathbf{x}}{\|\mathbf{w}\|} = 0 \tag{3.107}$$

Let $\mathbf{x}_1$ denote the nearest point from class 1 to the decision boundary. The distance from $\mathbf{x}_1$ to the hyperplane is now given by

$$d_{\mathbf{x}_1} = \frac{\mathbf{w}^T\mathbf{x}}{\|\mathbf{w}\|} \tag{3.108}$$

The discriminant function for this point $\mathbf{w}^T\mathbf{x}_1 \geq +1$ since the point belongs to class 1. Note also that if we scale $\mathbf{w}$ by a positive constant, the output of the discriminant function will remain ≥ 1, that is, it is not affected by scaling $\mathbf{w}$ by a constant. This allows us to simplify the objective by scaling $\mathbf{w}$ so that the nearest points from each class will make the discriminant function either ± 1. The margin now becomes

$$2\frac{1}{\|\mathbf{w}\|} \quad (3.109)$$

SVMs aim to find a separating hyperplane that maximizes the margin. The optimization problem can be expressed using

$$\begin{aligned} &\arg\min_{\mathbf{w}} \frac{1}{2}\|\mathbf{w}\|^2 \\ &\text{st.} y_n\left(\mathbf{w}^{\mathrm{T}}\mathbf{x}_n\right) \geq 1, \forall n \end{aligned} \quad (3.110)$$

Here, we are minimizing kwk that is equivalent to maximizing the margin 2/**w**. This is a constrained quadratic optimization problem that does not have a closed-form analytical solution. To solve it, we need to create a new unconstrained objective function through a set of Lagrange multipliers and use numerical methods to minimize the function. The new objective function will have the same optimum as the original problem and is given by

$$\begin{aligned} &\arg\min_{\mathbf{w},\alpha} \frac{1}{2}\mathbf{w}^{\mathrm{T}}\mathbf{w} - \sum_{i=1}^{N} \alpha_i \left[y_i\left(\mathbf{w}^{\mathrm{T}}\mathbf{x}_i\right) - 1\right] \\ &\text{st.}: \alpha_i \geq 0, \forall n \end{aligned} \quad (3.111)$$

It can be shown that the optimal solution satisfies the following two identities:

$$\mathbf{w} = \sum_{i=1}^{N} \alpha_i y_i \mathbf{x}_i \quad (3.112)$$

$$\alpha \geq 0, \sum_{i=1}^{N} \alpha_i y_i = 0 \quad (3.113)$$

The closest vectors $\mathbf{x}_s$ from each class to the classifier's decision boundary having $\alpha_s \neq 0$ are known as support vectors. They uniquely define the decision boundary $\mathbf{w}$. In fact, if we remove all data except the support vectors from both classes and retrain the model, we will get the same decision boundary.

For nonseparable classes, there is no hyperplane such that $\mathbf{w}^{\mathrm{T}}\mathbf{x} \geq 1$. We need to relax the constraint to allow points to lie within the margin even if they get misclassified. This can be done by using slack variables $\zeta_n \geq 0$ such that

$$y_n\left(\mathbf{w}^{\mathrm{T}}\mathbf{x}_n\right) \geq 1 - \zeta_n, \forall n \quad (3.114)$$

If $0 \geq \zeta_n \leq 1$, then a point $\mathbf{x}_n$ is correctly classified; however, if $\zeta_n > 1$, this means that the point lies on the wrong side of the boundary. The optimization problem now aims at maximizing the margin and at the same time minimizing the number of misclassified examples (i.e., those with $\zeta_i > 1$):

$$\begin{aligned} &\arg\min_{\mathbf{w}} \frac{1}{2}\|\mathbf{w}\|^2 + C\sum_{i=1}^{N}\zeta_i \\ &\text{st.}: \zeta_i \geq 0 \text{ and} \\ &y_n(\mathbf{w}^{\mathrm{T}}\mathbf{x}_n) \geq 1-\zeta_i \forall_i \end{aligned} \tag{3.115}$$

The only difference with the separable class case is the existence of a constant C term that controls to what extent we allow points to sit within the margin or be misclassified. The optimization problem becomes

$$\begin{aligned} &\arg\max_{\mathbf{w}} \sum_i \alpha_i - \frac{1}{2}\sum_{i,j}\alpha_i\alpha_j y_i y_j \mathbf{x}_i^{\mathrm{T}}\mathbf{x}_j \\ &\text{st.}: \sum_{i=1}^{N}\alpha_i y_i = 0 \text{ and } 0 \leq \alpha_i \leq C, \forall i \end{aligned} \tag{3.116}$$

Training SVM classifiers is in general computationally demanding. However, the solutions tend to be sparse, generalize very well, and require low storage capacities to store the trained model. Fig. 3.14 shows the effect of different values of C in the case of nonseparable classes. Note that higher values of C result in smaller margins and fewer support vectors inside the margin. Finally, SVM extensions to multiclass problems exist; however, in practice, such problems are viewed as M-one against all two-class problems.

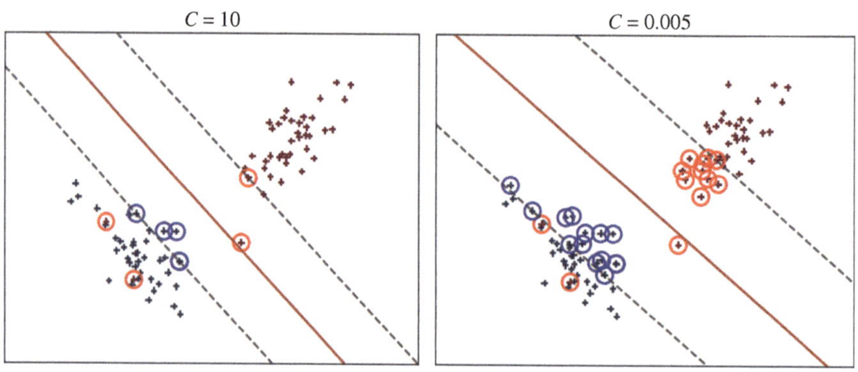

FIG. 3.14

Linear SVM with two choices for the capacity C. Higher values of C results in smaller margins and fewer support vectors inside the margin.

3.3.5.2 Kernel support vector machines

Kernel SVMs allow us to generalize SVM learning algorithm to deal with nonlinear decision boundaries. Similar to what we did for unconstrained discriminants, the raw data can be either explicitly or implicitly transformed into a new feature space

$\mathbf{x} \rightarrow \mathbf{z} \in R^k$ using a user-specified kernel. The SVM optimization problem in the new feature space becomes

$$\arg\max_{\alpha} \left(\sum_{i=1}^{N} \alpha_i - \frac{1}{2} \sum_{ij} \alpha_i \alpha_j y_i y_i \mathbf{z}_i^{\mathrm{T}} \mathbf{z}_j \right) \tag{3.117}$$

The final classifier, $\mathbf{w}$, can be expressed in terms of inner products in a high-dimensional space:

$$\begin{aligned} g(\mathrm{y}) &= \mathbf{w}^{\mathrm{T}} \mathbf{z} \\ &= \sum_{i-1}^{N_s} \alpha_i y_i \mathrm{z}_i \mathrm{z} \end{aligned} \tag{3.118}$$

Eq. (3.118) requires that we compute inner products between each transformed training sampled, $\mathbf{z}_i$, and the test sample, $\mathbf{z}$. This is a very complex computation as the feature space can be very high dimensional. To compute Eq. (3.118), we can rely on Mercer's theorem that allows us to implicitly perform inner products. Mercer's theorem stats that if $\mathbf{x} \mapsto \Phi(x) \in H$, then the inner product in H reduces to a kernel function computed on the data points:

$$\sum_r \Phi_r(\mathbf{x}) \Phi_r(\mathbf{x}') = K(\mathbf{x}, \mathbf{x}') \tag{3.119}$$

A valid kernel must satisfy

$$\int K(\mathbf{x}, \mathbf{x}') g(\mathbf{x}) g(\mathbf{x}') d\mathbf{x} d\mathbf{x}' \geq 0 \tag{3.120}$$

and for any $g(\mathbf{x}),\mathbf{x}$,

$$\int g^2(\mathbf{x}) d\mathbf{x} < +\infty \tag{3.121}$$

The opposite is also true. Any kernel, with the previous properties, corresponds to an inner product in some space. For example, $\mathbf{z}_i^{\mathrm{T}} \mathbf{z}_j = (\mathbf{x}_i^{\mathrm{T}} \mathbf{x}_j)^2$ corresponds to the mapping:

$$\mathbf{x} = [x_1, x_2]^{\mathrm{T}} \in R^2 \rightarrow \mathrm{z} = \begin{bmatrix} x_1^2 \\ \sqrt{2} x_1 x_2 \\ x_2^2 \end{bmatrix} \in R^3 \tag{3.122}$$

Examples of kernels include polynomials, radial basis functions, and hyperbolic tangent:

$$K(\mathbf{x}, \mathbf{x}') = \exp\left(-\frac{\|\mathbf{x} - \mathbf{x}'\|^2}{\sigma^2} \right) \tag{3.123}$$

$$K(\mathbf{x}, \mathbf{x}') = (\mathbf{x}^{\mathrm{T}} \mathbf{x}' + 1)^q, q > 0 \tag{3.124}$$

$$K(\mathbf{x}, \mathbf{x}') = \tan h(\beta \mathbf{x}^{\mathrm{T}} \mathbf{x}' + \gamma) \tag{3.125}$$

The kernel trick allows us to avoid computing inner products; as such, our kernel SVM formulation becomes

$$\arg\max_{\lambda} \left(\sum_i \lambda_i - \frac{1}{2} \sum_{i,j} \lambda_i \lambda_j y_i y_j K(\boldsymbol{x}_i, \boldsymbol{x}_j) \right)$$

subject to

$$\begin{aligned} & 0 \le \lambda_i \le C, i = 1, 2, \ldots, N \\ & \sum_i \lambda_i y_i = 0 \end{aligned} \tag{3.126}$$

The final solution also takes an implicit combination:

$$\mathbf{w} = \sum_{i=1}^{N} \lambda_i y_i \varphi(x_i) \tag{3.127}$$

$$\omega_1(\omega_2) \text{ if } g(\mathbf{x}) = \sum_{i=1}^{N} \lambda_i y_i K(\mathbf{x}_i, \mathbf{x}) + w_0 > (<) 0 \tag{3.128}$$

Fig. 3.15 shows the decision boundary of a kernel support vector machine. Note that the induced diction boundary is not linear (C acts as a regularizer that controls how much we tolerate classification errors).

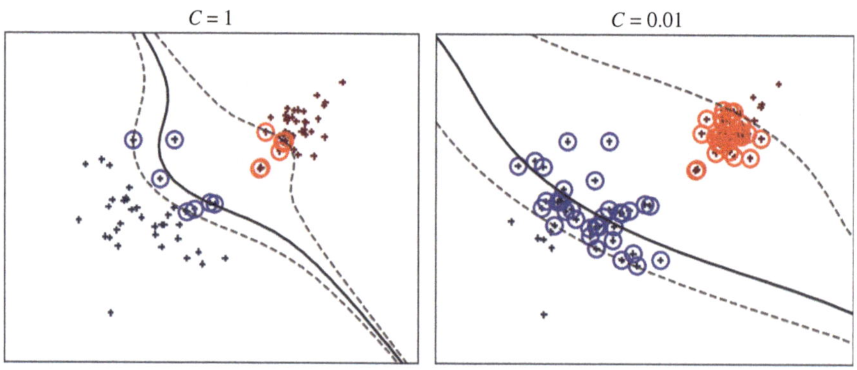

FIG. 3.15

Kernel support vector machines express the decision boundary in terms of support in the transformed space. Note that C acts as a regularizer and controls how much we tolerate classification errors.

3.4 Training and generalization performance

In this section, we discuss closely related concepts in machine learning that is generalization performance, underfitting, and overfitting. Suppose you have trained a model on a training dataset and now you want to test the model. There are many factors that affect the ability of the model to make accurate predictions such as the amount of training data used to train the model; the more the data, the better the predictions. Other factors include the quality of the data and the flexibility of the model. A highly flexible model is able to memorize all data points. Such a model can make 100% accuracy on the training data. However, it turns out that such a model overfits the data and is useless. This is because it cannot make accurate predictions on a new test data. This is a case of poor generalization. On the other hand, if the model is too simple, then it will fail to capture enough structure in the data. This is also a case of poor generalization due to underfitting. In fact, regardless of how many data are used to train the model, such a model will always produce bad performance on both the training data and the test data.

Generalization refers to the ability of the model to make accurate predictions on new never seen before data. To accurately estimate the true performance, we will need to test the model using infinite data resources (i.e., data generated from an assumed generating density $p(\mathbf{x})$). However, in practice, data resources are scarce, thus limiting our ability to model $p(\mathbf{x})$ accurately. Also, for obvious reasons, we cannot rely on training data used during model fitting to test the performance because it provides biased and overconfident predictions. As such, we need to use available data in a way that gives us approximately unbiased estimates of the true accuracy.

Overfitting means very low training error and high test error, while underfitting means both high training and high test errors. Therefore there must be a point between underfitting and overfitting. This point is what we are interested to find and use as the basis to select the best model. One technique to find such a point is by splitting the data into training and validation data. This can be done using various techniques such as hold out split, resampling and cross-validation. The holdout approach is also called train-test split method; here, given N training examples, we randomly split it into N_1 training points and N_2 test points, where $N = N_1 + N_2$. A common choice is to randomly take 80% of the data for training and 20% for testing. The model is then iteratively fitted on the training data where at each iteration, we compute the training error and validation error. It is expected that the training error goes down over time as the algorithm becomes better and better in learning and the test error is also shrinking on the test dataset. The reduction in test error will go on until reaching a point where it starts to rise up again. This is an indication that we trained the model for too long and overfitting the data. Therefore this is when we must stop training, that is, just before the test error rises again (see Fig. 3.16).

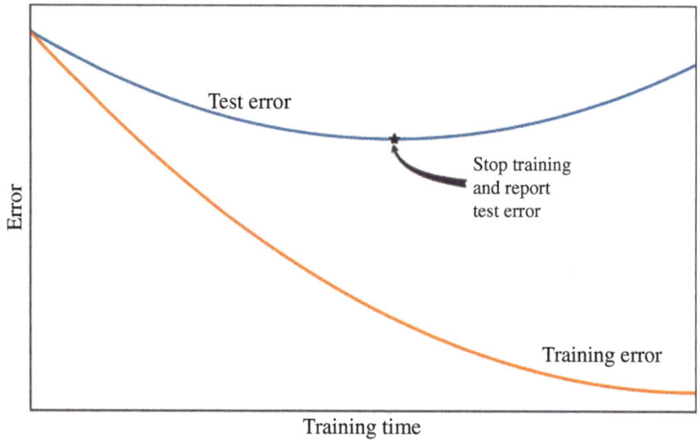

FIG. 3.16

Initially the training and testing error are both large since the model has still not learned anything from the data. If the model is very complex we will start to note that the training error shrinks to zero as we train the model over longer periods of time. However, the validation error shows a different trend, thus indicating that training need to stop. The testing error in this case might be high indicating that this model probably cannot learn much.

The holdout approach works well if the amount of data is large and both the training and testing data distributions come from the same generating distribution. However, if data are little, then problems might arise as splitting the data in this way leaves fewer data both for training and testing. It is likely that our estimates will be biased because of information lost from unused data. In addition, we could have a low test error just by chance, especially if the number of models we are comparing is very large. As such, we should not rely on the test set alone for evaluating the model (also in choosing the best model) as there is a risk that we might overfit the test data.

To obtain less biased estimates of the generalization performance, a three-way split of the data into training, validation, and test sets can be used. Here the test set is left to the last stage in model selection and never used at all for hyperparameter tuning. Again, data splitting based on three-way splits might not always be suitable; for example, performance evaluation could be unreliable as the accuracy for one test set can be very different on another test set.

One way to solve such a problem is to use K-fold cross-validation (CV). K-fold CV is a resampling technique that involves dividing the data into K disjoint folds; using $(K - 1)$ partitions for training and one for validation while ensuring that each fold is used as a validation only once. The higher the value of K, the smaller the bias (and the larger the variance) in the estimated model performance. The lower value of K, the method produces similar results to the train-split method. K-fold CV requires training and testing the model K-times ensuring that every observation from the original dataset appears in training and test sets.

K-fold CV can be summarized in Algorithm 3.1.

Algorithm 3.1 K-fold cross validation.

1. Select a value for K that is not too small or too large (as it might lead to overfitting due to high variance), typically 5- to 10-folds depending on the size of the data.
2. Randomly split the data into K folds while maintaining empirical data representation (i.e., producing stratified folds).
3. Fit the model using data from the $(K - 1)$ folds and validate it on the remaining Kth fold.
4. Repeat this process until every K-fold has been used as the test set.
5. Compute the score of the model by averaging the scores for the K experiments.

K-fold CV is especially useful if we have a limited supply of training data. However, if data are large, implementing K-fold CV becomes computationally intensive because we need to train the model K-times. An extreme case of K-fold CV is when we set $K = N$. Here, each time $N - 1$ samples are used for training the model leaving only one sample to test the model. This is good in the sense that we eventually use all data for testing and training but is computationally demanding, especially in high dimensions.

3.5 Evaluating performance

Evaluating the performance of machine learning algorithms allows us to compare different algorithms. The best model can then be selected based on its generalization performance. Various performance metrics could be used to evaluate classifiers on a given prediction task. Examples of commonly used metrics include the probability of error, expected Bayes risk, log loss, cross entropy, accuracy, confusion matrix, precision, recall, false positive rate, false negative rate, F1 score, Cohen's Kappa, Matthews correlation coefficient (MCC), and receiver operating characteristics–area under curve (ROC-AUC). In general, performance measures often evaluate a classifier from certain perspectives but might fail to account for the big picture.

The choice of a suitable metric is both application and data dependent. It is often guided by several factors including class imbalance, the number of available classes, and relative class importance. Choosing the right metric provides us with unbiased goodness estimates for selecting the optimal classifier. In the succeeding text, we discuss several commonly used performance measures.

Confusion matrices are commonly used for both binary and multiclass classification problems. They are good at showing whether there is a significant overlap in class properties that could render a model confused and making prediction errors.

Suppose that we have trained a classifier to predict the outcome of a binary classification problem as to whether a test image has cancer (positive) or normal otherwise (negative). The output of the classifier can be positive or negative, and the prediction made can be correct or wrong. We can summarize this information in a two-dimensional matrix: the actual classifications shown as columns, while the predicted classifications shown as rows.

Confusion matrices capture the performance of the model from several perspectives. It provides information on various metrics such as true positives (TP), true negatives (TN), false positives (FP), false negatives (FN), precision, recall, and classification accuracy. The TP cell indicates the number of cases where the predictions made were positive and correctly predicted, the TN cell indicates the number of cases where the predictions made were negative and also correctly predicted, the FP cell indicates the cases where the predictions made were incorrectly predicted as positive, and FN cell indicates the cases that were incorrectly predicted as negative. From the confusion matrix, we can compute the following performance metrics:

Accuracy: This is simply the proportion of correct predictions made by the model:

$$\text{Accuracy} = \frac{TP + TN}{TP + TN + FP + FN} \tag{3.129}$$

Accuracy is a good indicator only when the classes are nearly balanced in the dataset and have equal costs for misclassification. In general, accuracy is a biased estimate toward the majority class.

Precision: Precision measures the ratio of true positive predictions and all positive predictions:

$$\text{P} = \frac{TP}{TP + FP} \tag{3.130}$$

Recall: Recall or sensitivity measures the ratio of true positive predictions and actual positive cases ($TP + FN$):

$$\text{R} = \frac{TP}{TP + FN} \tag{3.131}$$

Note that if the false positives were 0, then precision will be 100%, while if false negatives were 0, then recall = 100

Specificity: Specificity is opposite of recall and measures the ratio of true negatives and all negative cases:

$$\text{Specificity} = \frac{TN}{TN + FP} \tag{3.132}$$

Weighted F metric: This score manages the trade-off between precision and recall and is defined using

$$F_\beta = \left(1 + \beta^2\right)\frac{PR}{\beta^2 P + R} \tag{3.133}$$

F1 Score: The F1 score combines precision (P) and recall (R) into a single metric using the harmonic mean:

$$\text{F1 Score} = 2\frac{PR}{P + R} \tag{3.134}$$

The F1 score can be used for both binary and multiclass classification problems. It is a normalized metric between 0 and 1, where a high F1 score indicates a good model having both high recall and precision. Thanks to the harmonic mean, the F1 score is useful for detecting cases where either P or R is small (e.g., $P = 3\%$, $R = 97\%$ or $P = 97\%$, $R = 3\%$). This is because the harmonic mean is biased more toward the smaller number, as such the F1 Score will always be small if either P or R is small, hence indicating a bad model.

Once a model is finalized, performance metrics can be used to summarize the model performance. One such metric is the receiver operating characteristics (ROC) curve. The ROC curve is simply the plot of the sensitivity versus 1 − specificity, as we vary a threshold:

$$\begin{aligned} \text{Sensitivity} &= TPR = \text{Recall} = TP/(TP+FP) \\ 1-\text{Specificity} &= FPR = FP/(TN+FP) \end{aligned} \tag{3.135}$$

Fig. 3.17 shows how ROC curves can be used to select the optimal classification threshold which gives the best trade-off between the FPR and TPR. The ROC curve can result in different thresholds for different classifiers; each optimal threshold gives the best FPR and TPR. This will make it harder to compare different models; as such, the area under the curve (AUC) can be used in this case. The AUC is commonly used for model selection and to compare the performance of different classifiers. This is because the AUC score is independent of classification thresholds and indicates how well the probabilities from the positive classes are separated from the negative classes.

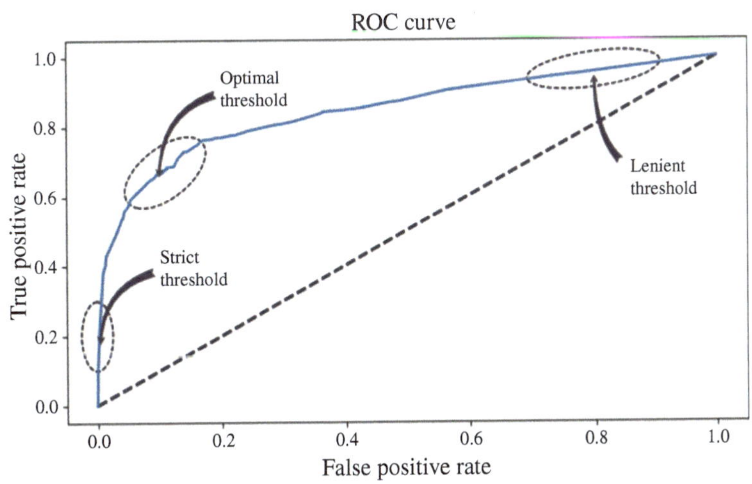

FIG. 3.17

The ROC curve is a plot of the false positive rate (i.e., 1 − specificity) versus the true positive rate (i.e., sensitivity). The bottom-left and top-right corners are bad choices for selecting a threshold.

3.6 Summary

This chapter presented a brief introduction to supervised and unsupervised learning. Although this chapter only skimmed the surface of an enormous subject, the content presented here is sufficient for the reader to develop a reasonable understanding of the main concepts. The first sections introduced unsupervised learning in the context of parametric and non-parametric density estimation. Next, supervised learning for classification are introduced, such as linear discriminants, generalized linear models, kernel models for classification, and support vector machines. The chapter concludes with addressing a few performance metrics for classification, such as sensitivity, specificity, the ROC curve and the area under the curve.

Further reading

H. Abdi, L.J. Williams, Principal component analysis, WIREs Comput. Stat. 2 (4) (2010) 433–459.

A. Ali, S.M.H. Shamsuddin, A.L. Ralescu, Classification with class imbalance problem: a review, in: SOCO 2015, 2015.

S. Angra, S. Ahuja, Machine learning and its applications: a review, in: '2017 International Conference on Big Data Analytics and Computational Intelligence (ICBDAC), 2017, pp. 57–60.

S. Balakrishnama, A. Ganapathiraju, 'Linear Discriminant Analysis—A Brief Tutorial', (1998), p. 9.

D. Barber, Bayesian Reasoning and Machine Learning, Cambridge University Press, Cambridge, 2011.

C.M. Bishop, Pattern Recognition and Machine Learning, Information Science and Statistics, Springer, New York, 2006.

M.W. Browne, Cross-validation methods, J. Math. Psychol. 44 (1) (2000) 108–132.

K. Chomboon, P. Chujai, P. Teerarassammee, K. Kerdprasop, N. Kerdprasop, An empirical study of distance metrics for k-nearest neighbor algorithm, in: The 3rd International Conference on Industrial Application Engineering 2015 (ICIAE2015), 2015.

O. Isafiade, O. Isafiade, A. Bagula, Data Mining Trends and Applications in Criminal Science and Investigations, first ed., IGI Global, Hershey, PA, 2016.

M.J. Islam, Q.M.J. Wu, M. Ahmadi, M.A. Sid-Ahmed, Investigating the performance of naive Bayes classifiers and K-nearest neighbor classifiers, in: 2007 International Conference on Convergence Information Technology (ICCIT 2007), 2007, pp. 1541–1546.

Jain, A. K. & Ramaswami, M. D. (1988), Classifier Design with Parzen Windows (Research supported by NSF grant ECS-8603541), *in* E. S. Gelsema & L. N. Kanal, eds, 'Machine Intelligence and Pattern Recognition', vol. 7 of *Pattern Recognition and Artificial Intelligence*, North-Holland, pp. 211–228.

V. Labatut, H. Cherifi, Accuracy Measures for the Comparison of Classifiers, 2012.

R. Longadge, S. Dongre, Class Imbalance Problem in Data Mining Review, 2013.

M.E. McCue, A.M. McCoy, The scope of big data in one medicine: unprecedented opportunities and challenges, Front. Vet. Sci. 4 (2017).

S. Mika, G. Ratsch, J. Weston, B. Scholkopf, K. Mullers, Fisher discriminant analysis with kernels, in: Neural Networks for Signal Processing IX: Proceedings of the 1999 IEEE Signal Processing Society Workshop (Cat. No.98TH8468), IEEE, Madison, WI, USA, 1999, pp. 41–48.

K.P. Murphy, Machine Learning: A Probabilistic Perspective, first ed., The MIT Press, Cambridge, MA, 2012.

A.Y. Ng, M.I. Jordan, On discriminative vs. generative classifiers: a comparison of logistic regression and naive Bayes, in: T.G. Dietterich, S. Becker, Z. Ghahramani (Eds.), Advances in Neural Information Processing Systems 14, MIT Press, 2002, pp. 841–848.

V.B.S. Prasath, H.A.A. Alfeilat, A.B.A. Hassanat, O. Lasassmeh, A.S. Tarawneh, M. B. Alhasanat, H.S.E. Salman, Distance and similarity measures effect on the performance of K-nearest neighbor classifier—a review, Big Data 7 (4) (2019) 221–248.

F.P. Ramsey, J.W. Pratt, H. Raiffa, R.O. Schlaifer, R. Schlaifer, Introduction to Statistical Decision Theory, MIT Press, 1995.

R.A. Redner, H.F. Walker, Mixture densities, maximum likelihood and the EM Algorithm, SIAM Rev. 26 (2) (1984) 195–239.

I. Rish, An empirical study of the naive bayes classifier, in: Proceedings of IJCAI01 Workshop on Empirical Methods in AI, International Joint Conference on Artificial Intelligence, American Association for Artificial Intelligence [1507], 2001, pp. 41–46. Online available at http:/www.cc.gatech.edu/~isbell/ classes/reading/papers/Rish.pdf.

P. Sharma, M. Kaur, Classification in Pattern Recognition: A Review, (2013).

A. Singh, N. Thakur, A. Sharma, A review of supervised machine learning algorithms, in: 2016 3rd International Conference on Computing for Sustainable Global Development (INDIACom), 2016, pp. 1310–1315.

M. Sokolova, N. Japkowicz, S. Szpakowicz, Beyond accuracy, F-score and ROC: a family of discriminant measures for performance evaluation, in: A. Sattar, B.-H. Kang (Eds.), AI 2006: Advances in Artificial Intelligence, Lecture Notes in Computer Science, Springer, Berlin, Heidelberg, 2006, pp. 1015–1021.

S. Theodoridis, Classifiers based on Bayes decision theory, in: Matlab Introduction to Pattern Recognition, Elsevier, 2010, pp. 1–27.

X. Wang, P. Tino, M.A. Fardal, S. Raychaudhury, A. Babul, Fast parzen window density estimator, in: 2009 International Joint Conference on Neural Networks, 2009, pp. 3267–3274.

J. Ye, R. Janardan, Q. Li, Two-dimensional linear discriminant analysis, in: L.K. Saul, Y. Weiss, L. Bottou (Eds.), Advances in Neural Information Processing Systems 17, MIT Press, 2005, pp. 1569–1576.

CHAPTER

Machine learning in biomedical signal processing with ECG applications

4

Dr. Bashar Rajoub

Faculty of Engineering Technology and Science, Higher Colleges of Technology, Dubai, United Arab Emirates

4.1 Introduction

The human body comprises a complex network of subsystems that perform vital physiological processes. For example, the circulatory system is composed of the heart, arteries, capillaries, and veins. The heart consists of four chambers: two ventricles for pumping blood and two atria for collecting blood. The repolarization and depolarization of the atrial and ventricular chambers cause the heart to contract and expand, pumping blood and delivering oxygen and nutrients throughout the body.

The heart's electrical activity controls heart operation and regulates the contractions and relaxations of the heart's muscles. Disturbances in the heart rate, popularly known as arrhythmias, can indicate abnormalities in heart function. According to the World Health Organization, cardiovascular diseases are the main reason for deaths worldwide, 2015. Electrocardiogram (ECG) analysis is an effective tool for diagnosing CVD. Electrocardiograms represent the electrical activity of the heart and provide useful information about potential underlying pathologies.

Manual analysis of ECG signals typically involve an expert cardiologist that examines a printout of the ECG signal, looking at individual ECG beat shapes, heart rate variability, and heart rhythm, and decides if the signal contains cardiac arrhythmias or normal otherwise. However, this process is time-consuming, requires expert training, and is prone to error due to human factors (e.g., subjective judgments and fatigue due to dealing with long-term ECG recordings).

This process is lengthy and resource intensive. Therefore the need for automatic ECG classification has grown significantly over the past few years; the main aim of which is to provide us with reliable detection of cardiac arrhythmias.

4.1.1 Automated ECG signal analysis

Computer processing and analysis of ECG signals rely on a variety of interdisciplinary research activities, from signal acquisition to digital signal processing and pattern recognition. Advances in digital signal processing and machine learning enabled the

Biomedical Signal Processing and Artificial Intelligence in Healthcare. https://doi.org/10.1016/B978-0-12-818946-7.00004-4

development of automatic computer-aided diagnosis (CAD) systems for biomedical ECG signal interpretation.

In medicine, CAD systems assist clinicians in detecting CVDs and heart abnormalities, predicting the onset of a heart condition, and reduce the overall time required to make a diagnosis. ECG analysis has been used for evaluating heart rate variability, detecting heart abnormalities, early detection of cardiovascular diseases, sleep apnea detection, fetal heart rate detection, home-care monitoring, telemedicine, monitoring of patients in intensive care units (ICUs), and arrhythmia recognition.

ECG analysis can be used for emotion recognition as it can reveal stress levels and cognitive load. Here, ECG features are used to establish a baseline that can discriminate between different cognitive workloads. Emotion recognition can be achieved by training a model to differentiate between ECG signals at different stress situations, such as truth telling versus lying during interviews, and driver alertness/drowsiness detection.

Biometric recognition is another application for ECG signal analysis. Biometric recognition requires universal features that work on people regardless of their skin color, gender and race, and robust against intrusion attacks. ECG signals can be used to provide us with unique physiological characteristics that are specific for a given individual. The assumption is that the heart's physiological and electrical characteristics of an individual (e.g., the electrical paths within the heart, QRS electrical axis, and heart's tissue thickness and size) result in unique temporal relationships and shape of ECG signals for a given individual. Finally, ECG in sports has been used to monitor heart rate and estimate calories consumed during activity and physical activity recognition.

Computer-aided diagnosis for monitoring cardiac health offers cardiologists diagnostic aid and improves medical decision-making. A considerable amount of research has been dedicated to address automated early-stage detection of cardiac arrhythmia.

This chapter is concerned with ECG analysis for the diagnosis of cardiovascular diseases. The main aim of this chapter is to help the biomedical engineer to build a machine learning model to perform automatic classification of ECG beats. I will start with an overview of machine learning for automated classification of ECG beats. A case study is then implemented to design a classifier for detecting ECG beats.

4.2 The electrocardiogram

Repolarization and depolarization patterns produce small electrical changes that can be detected and recorded by performing electrocardiography (ECG). Electrocardiography (ECG) provides us with a graphic representation of the heart's electrical activity. The electrocardiogram uses electrodes, that is, conductive pads, on the surface of the body to measure cardiac potentials of the heart. An electrocardiographic lead is a recording electrode or a pair of recording electrodes at a specified location. An ECG lead provides us with a "view" of the heart's electrical potential between the locations corresponding to the electrode(s) positions.

The standard 12-channel ECG serves as the basis of clinical ECG diagnoses. It records the overall magnitude and direction of the heart's electrical depolarization and repolarization potentials from 12 different angles or "leads." Ten electrodes are used: three limbs, one reference limb, and six chest electrodes.

Three limb electrodes placed on the right arm, left arm, and left leg form an equilateral triangle (with the heart at the center). This triangle is called the "Einthoven's triangle"—in honor of the Dutch doctor Willem Einthoven who described the relationship as three leads enclosing a central source of cardiac potential (i.e., the heart) placed at the center of the triangle in the early 1900s. The placement of the three limb electrodes is flexible since the limbs serve as electrical cables; as such, they can be attached to the end of the limb (i.e., wrists or ankles) or at the origin of the limb (i.e., shoulder or upper thigh). A fourth limb electrode placed on the right leg is used as the ground electrode for recording purposes. Six additional chest electrodes are placed on the surface of the chest over different regions to provide a different view of the electrical activity within the heart.

The three limb electrodes generate 6 views (i.e., 6 leads), while the 6 chest electrodes generate the remaining 12 view "leads." Specifically, limb electrodes generate views of the electrical activity along the frontal plane of the heart: the views comprise three bipolar standard leads I, II, and III and three unipolar augmented leads aVR, aVL, and aVF. Meanwhile, chest electrodes generate another six views of the electrical activity of the heart in a plane perpendicular to the frontal plane. The generated chest views are labeled V1–V6 (Fig. 4.1).

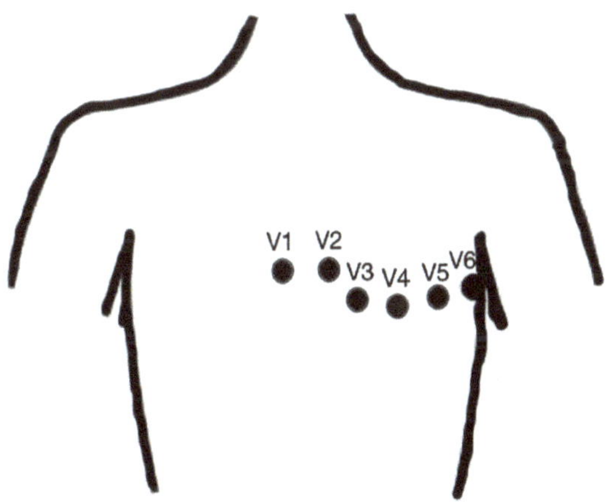

FIG. 4.1

ECG electrode placements for 12-lead ECG. Chest leads are indicated by the labels V1–6.

4.2.1 Standard bipolar limb leads

Limb leads provide us with a view of cardiac electrical potentials along the frontal plane of the heart. The left arm, right arm, and left leg are used to place limb leads I, II, and III. Lead I measures the potential difference between the two arms with the positive electrode placed on the left arm and the negative electrode on the right arm; lead II has the positive electrode on the left leg and the negative electrode on the right arm, and lead III has the positive electrode on the left leg, while the negative electrode on the left arm. Limb leads are bipolar since they detect the change in electric potential between two electrodes—one electrode on the skin surface acts as the positive pole, while the other acts as the negative pole.

A wave due to a depolarization heading *toward* a positive electrode creates a *positive* deflection in that lead. *Maximum positive* ECG deflection is observed when the wave of depolarization travels *toward* the positive electrode in a direction parallel to the axis between negative and positive electrodes in that lead (or view). Similarly a wave due to a depolarization heading *away from* a positive electrode creates a *negative* deflection in that lead. *Minimum negative* ECG deflection is observed when the wave of depolarization travels *away from* the positive electrode in a direction parallel to the axis between negative and positive electrodes in that lead (or view).

We can visualize standard limb leads as electrical vectors, using what is known as the axial reference system, where leads are superimposed over the heart. Here the positive electrode for lead I (RA-LA axis) forms the positive X-axis. The positive electrode for lead II (RA-LA axis) makes +60 degrees relative to lead I axis. In contrast the positive electrode for lead III (LA-LL axis) makes +120 degree relative to the lead I axis. This helps us identify the direction of travel of a depolarization wave: for example, a wave traveling at 0 degree produces the greatest positive deflection in lead I; while a wave of depolarization oriented +90 degree relative to the heart produces equally positive deflections in both lead II and III but zero deflection in lead I (this is because the wave is heading perpendicular to lead I axis). It is also interesting to show that the three bipolar limb leads maintain a mathematical relationship explained by the Einthoven's law, which states that II=I+III. As such, this law allows us to validate the ECG recording and helps us determine whether the limb electrodes are correctly placed.

4.2.2 Augmented unipolar limb leads

The same three leads that form the standard leads also form the three unipolar leads known as the augmented leads. Augmented limb leads are "unipolar" leads since a single electrode on the skin surface acts as the positive (+) pole, while the reference is a combination of the other limb electrodes, also known as Wilson's central terminal—a theoretical null point at the center of the Einthoven's triangle.

ECG signal from unipolar limb leads represents the potential difference between the center of the Einthoven's triangle (i.e., a virtual null point that is neutral and insensitive to cardiac potentials) and the electrode of each augmented lead. The flow of electricity is therefore measured from the heart to either the right arm (aVR), left arm (aVL), or left foot (aVF), where lowercase "a" denotes augmented, V denotes vector, R denotes right, L denotes left, and F denotes foot (see Fig. 4.2). The null point for each lead is obtained by adding the potential from the other two leads. For example, in lead aVR, the electric potential of the right arm is compared with a null point, which is obtained by adding together the potential of lead aVL and lead aVF.

Like standard bipolar leads, augmented unipolar limb leads also record a change in electric potential along the frontal plane of the heart. We can visualize augmented unipolar leads aVR, aVL, and aVF on the axial reference system used for leads I, II, and III as a vector oriented at −150, −30, and +90 degrees, respectively. The interpretation of ECG signals follows a similar approach to interpreting standard limb leads: a wave of depolarization traveling downward toward the aVF electrode will elicit a positive deflection, and this deflection is maximized if it is in the direction of the aVF lead, that is, +90 degrees. If a wave of depolarization is moving from left to right at +150 degrees, then aVL will show the greatest negative deflection.

4.2.3 Precordial (chest) leads

Standard and augmented limb leads record cardiac potentials along the frontal plane of the heart. Chest leads, on the other hand, provide a different view of the electrical activity along the cross-sectional plane of the heart. A total of six unipolar chest leads

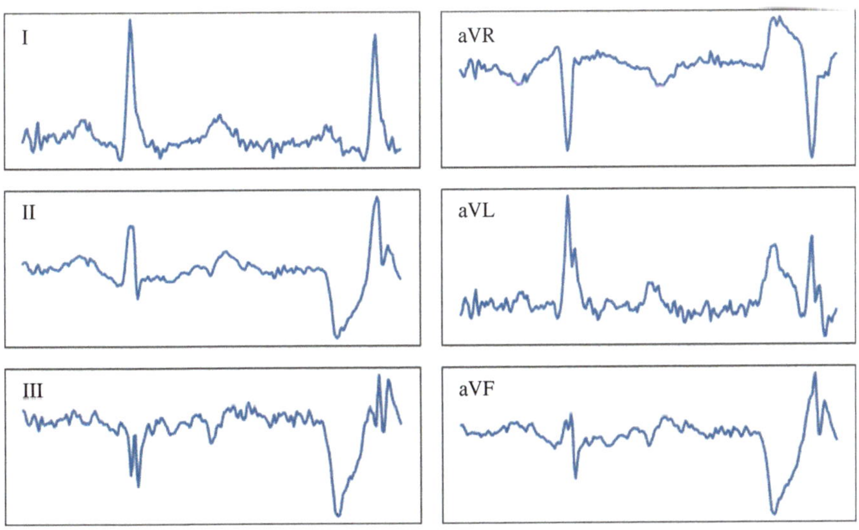

FIG. 4.2

Bipolar standard limb leads I, II, and II and the unipolar augmented limb leads aVR, aVL, and aVF.

are placed in standardized positions on the chest. The leads, labeled V1–V6, record the electrical variations that occur directly under the electrode.

Chest leads measure the absolute potential of a lead relative to a virtual reference. The reference, known as Wilson's central terminal, is formed by combining the left arm, right arm, and left leg electrodes. Cardiac defects, such as left ventricle abnormalities, especially of the anterior and posterior walls of the heart, can be detected by analyzing the wave shapes from chest leads. Interpretation of ECG waveform for chest leads is similar to interpreting waves from the limb leads; that is, a wave of depolarization traveling toward a particular electrode on the chest surface will elicit a positive deflection.

Chest leads VI and V2 are best for monitoring activity in the right half of the heart. Lead V1 registers potentials from the atria, part of the septum, and the right ventricle anterior wall. Because initial ventricular depolarization is from left to right across the septum, the QRS complex is formed by a small R wave (septum depolarization) followed by a deep S wave as the anterior and lateral walls of the left ventricle depolarize (ventricle activation). A normal ECG appears predominantly negative in lead V1. Lead V2 electrode rests over the right ventricle wall. Similar to V1 lead, a normal ECG in V2 has a predominately negative QRS complex with an R wave that is slightly bigger than in V1, followed by a deep S wave.

Chest leads V3 and V4 depict septal activity best. The electrode for lead V3 rests over the interventricular septum. It is a transitional lead between the electrocardiogram left and right potentials. The QRS complex in this lead is biphasic since the R and S waves are almost identical. The electrode for chest lead V4 rests over the left ventricle apex, where the walls are thicker. The QRS complex in V4 is positive and is characterized by a tall R wave followed by a small S wave (right ventricle depolarization).

Chest leads V5 and V6 are best for monitoring left ventricular activity as they are situated over the left ventricle myocardium. The QRS complex in leads V5 and V6 shows a large net positive QR. The R wave is preceded by a small Q wave (septum depolarization); however, it is not as tall as the R wave in lead V4 since the left ventricle myocardium has thinner walls than in V4. In addition, the waveforms from leads V5 and V6 are almost opposite in polarity from V1 since the electrodes are viewing the opposite sides of the heart (Fig. 4.3).

4.3 Clinical ECG features

ECG signals appear as a series of beats (i.e., cardiac cycle; see Fig. 4.4). Each cycle in the ECG signal consists of distinctive structures of upward and downward deflections, called P, Q, R, S, T, and U, which are joined in order along the isoelectric line of the signal. These structures have physiological and clinical significance; for example, the P wave represents the depolarization of the atria, the QRS complex represents the depolarization of the ventricles, and the T wave represents the repolarization of the ventricles.

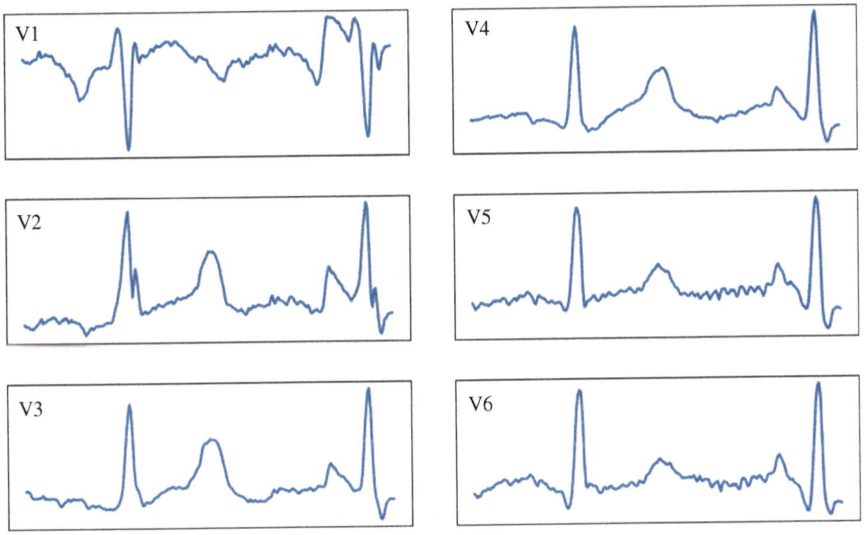

FIG. 4.3

Chest leads V1–V6 provide a different view of the electrical activity along the cross-sectional plane of the heart.

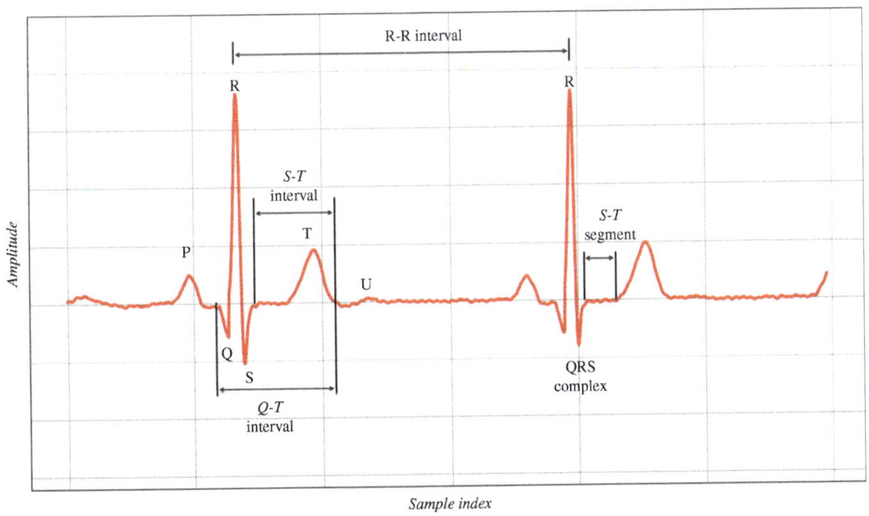

FIG. 4.4

Typical ECG signal. The signal consists of a number of segments. The QRS complex is one of the most important features.

A segment in an ECG is the region between two waves. For example, the PR segment starts at the beginning of the P wave and ends at the start of the Q wave. An interval in an ECG is a duration of time that includes one segment and one or more waves. For example, the PR interval contains the P wave plus the PR segment, while the QT interval includes the ST segment and the Q, R, S, and T waves.

Fig. 4.4 shows a typical ECG signal and the main waveforms, segments, and intervals. The P wave is the first wave of the cardiac cycle that is attributed to atrial contraction (i.e., depolarization). The PR segment begins at the beginning of the P wave and ends at the onset of the QRS complex. The PR segment corresponds to the depolarization of the AV node. It is a flat line indicating a pause in electrical activity to ensure the completion of the blood transfer from the atria to the ventricles. The PR interval denotes the conduction of the impulse from the upper part of the atrium through the AV node and ends just before it activates the ventricles to depolarize.

The QRS complex is a structure that contains a combination of the Q, R, and S waves. The Q wave is generated as a result of ventricular septal depolarization. A Q wave on the ECG appears as an initially negative deflection that precedes the R wave of the QRS complex. The R wave is produced as a result of early ventricular muscle depolarization. The R is seen on the ECG trace as a sharp upward deflection of around one millivolt in amplitude. The S wave is the first negative deflection of the QRS complex following the large R wave. The S wave represents depolarization in the Purkinje fibers (they spread out into the ventricles and enable fast and synchronized impulse conduction of the action potentials to the whole myocardium).

The QRS complex represents rapid left and right ventricular depolarization (contraction). The beginning of the QRS complex is the start of ventricular systole and goes until the end of the T wave. Ventricular diastole starts when the T wave ends. The main features to consider for QRS complex include the width of the complex and the voltage amplitude (height). The QRS interval covers the QRS complex from beginning to end. The QRS width is useful in determining the origin of the complex (e.g., sinus, atrial, junctional, or ventricular).

The interval between two R waves (R-R interval) is often used to measure the heart rate and heart rate variability. This interval is controlled by the autonomous nervous system, which adjusts heart output depending on the state of the subject (e.g., during a specific activity such as sleep, exercise, and when fighting infections).

The T wave corresponds to ventricular repolarization (relaxation). In general a normal T wave is asymmetric (i.e., with an ascending portion that is slower than the descending one), and it has a smaller amplitude than the QRS complex. The ST segment is located between the end of the QRS complex and the beginning of the T wave. It represents the heart's electrical activity immediately after all the ventricular myocardium is depolarized, that is, after both the left and right ventricles have pumped blood to the body. During this period, little or no electricity is flowing through the myocardium to allow ventricular muscle cells to relax and get ready for the next cardiac pulse.

The QT interval starts at the start of the QRS and ends at the end of the T wave. It denotes the electrical systole of the heart. It covers the entire ventricular activity beginning from ventricular depolarization through the plateau phase and finally to the ventricular repolarization. As such, it represents the time taken for ventricular depolarization and repolarization.

The ST segment reflects the plateau in the myocardial action potential. Observing acute elevation/depression of ST segment in at least two adjacent leads may indicate myocardial injury, complete coronary artery occlusion, myocardial infarction, or myocardial ischemia.

The U wave is hypothesized to be caused by the repolarization of Purkinje fibers—specialized muscle cells that can conduct electricity quite rapidly. It usually appears predominantly in precordial leads following the T wave as a low amplitude wave, but more often, it is entirely absent.

The TP segment begins at the end of the T wave and ends at the start of the next P wave. The TP segment represents the time when the heart muscle cells are electrically silent and hence appears as an isoelectric interval on the ECG trace. It is good to consider the TP segment as a reference to determine whether the ST segment is elevated or depressed since there is no pathology that is known to elevate or depress the TP segment. It is also good to closely examine the TP segment for the presence of U waves. If the heart rhythm is fast, for example, during exercise, the TP segment shortens and have T wave merge with the P wave of the next cycle.

4.4 Cardiac arrhythmia

During each heartbeat a pattern of depolarization and repolarization spreads across the cardiac muscle fibers. A healthy beat starts by initiating a depolarization wave from the sinoatrial node of the heart (i.e., the natural pacemaker of the heart because it adjusts the heart rate based on activity and body needs). The depolarization wave spreads throughout the atrium and passes through the atrioventricular node down into the bundle of His and into the Purkinje fibers, spreading down and to the left throughout the ventricles.

Cardiac arrhythmia is a heart condition that alters the regular rhythmic activity of heart, for example, resulting in faster, slower, or irregular heartbeats. Most arrhythmias are harmless, but sometimes they can be due to a serious illness. The types of cardiac arrhythmia depend on the originating site of the beats and the frequency of the generated signals. For example, abnormalities in the sinoatrial (SA) node of the heart or the presence of abnormal/additional pacing activity from other parts of the heart may result in ectopic beats.

4.4.1 Life-threatening arrhythmias

Cardiac arrhythmias can be divided into two groups: life-threatening arrhythmias (e.g., ventricular fibrillation and tachycardia, atrial fibrillation, myocardial ischemia, and myocardial infarction) and arrhythmias that are not harmful but may require preventative therapy.

Ventricular fibrillation is a rapid and irregular electrical activity that causes the ventricles to fail to contract in a synchronized manner, resulting in cessation of cardiac output. Atrial fibrillation (AF) is the most common type of irregular heartbeat. It is caused by a very rapid and random disturbance to the atrium, causing the atria to quiver and unable to effectively move blood into the ventricles. Ventricular tachycardia causes the heart to beat faster than normal and out of sync with the upper chambers. This reduces the amount of blood in the chambers as they will not have enough time to fill appropriately due to the fast and out of sync beats. Myocardial ischemia is caused by the reduced blood supply to a part of the heart muscles due to a block in the coronary arteries. In contrast, myocardial infarction is caused by a complete cutoff of blood supply to myocardial tissue. The tissue dies and becomes incapable of contraction.

4.4.2 The AAMI standard

The Association for the Advancement of Medical Instrumentation (AAMI) standard (ANSI/AAMI EC57:1998/(R)2003) groups cardiac arrhythmia into five superclasses: normal (N), supraventricular ectopic beat (S), ventricular ectopic beat (V), fusion beat (F), and unknown beats (Q). The five superclasses contain 15 different classes of heartbeats. It is outside the scope of this book to discuss all arrhythmias in each category. As such, only a brief description of a subset of the arrhythmias is presented in Table 4.1.

Normal (N) category: A normal rhythm category (N) generates heartbeats from the sinoatrial (SA) node located in the right atrium. This category includes various types of heartbeats such as left/right bundle branch block (LBBB and RBBB) and escape and atrial nodal beats (AE and NE). A bundle branch consists of Purkinje fibers that spread out through the ventricles enabling fast impulse conduction to the ventricles. Bundle branch block occurs when the left/right bundle branch is unable to transmit the impulse fast enough. Therefore the QRS duration is prolonged.

Supraventricular ectopic beats (S): This category corresponds both to atrial and supraventricular premature beats, and its variants include atrial premature beat, aberrated premature beat (APB), nodal premature beat, and supraventricular premature beat. Atrial premature (AP—A) beat (i.e., atrial ectopic or premature atrial contraction) is an extra heartbeat originating from an abnormal site in the atria just before a normal heartbeat occurs. They are harmless and are often perceived as a skipped beat or a jolt in the chest. However, frequent APBs could be an early symptom of heart failure and may precede atrial fibrillation.

Ventricular ectopic beats (V): This category includes premature ventricular contraction and ventricular escape beats. Premature ventricular contraction (PVC—V) is an extra heartbeat originating in the ventricles, which result in chaotic contraction of the ventricles. This arrhythmia may be caused by physical or emotional stress and excessive caffeine in the bloodstream. Ventricular escape beats result from self-generated electrical discharge that usually occurs after a long pause in ventricular

Table 4.1 ECG class description using AAMI standard.

AAMI superclass		**MIT-BIH heartbeat types**			
Normal beat (N)	**Normal beat (N)**	**Left bundle branch block beat (L)**	**Right bundle branch block beat (R)**	**Atrial escape beat (e)**	**Nodal (junctional) escape beat (j)**
Supraventricular ectopic beat (S)	Atrial premature beat (A)	Aberrated atrial premature beat (a)	Nodal (junctional) premature beat (J)	Supraventricular premature beat (S)	
Ventricular ectopic beat (V)	Premature ventricular contraction (V)	Ventricular escape beat (E)			
Fusion beat (F)	Fusion of ventricular and normal beat (F)				
Unknown beat (Q)	Paced beat (/)	Fusion of paced and normal beat (f)	Unclassified beat (Q)		

rhythm (around 2–3 s) to prevent cardiac arrest (e.g., due to the failure of an electrical impulse to reach the ventricles).

Fusion beats (F): Fusion beats can occur when either the atria or the ventricles are activated by different sources at the same time, for example, from the heart's SA node and atrial ectopic beat or from an external pacemaker.

Unclassified beats (Q): Unclassified heartbeats are outlier beats that should be removed from training data. Examples of unclassified heartbeats include artifacts, poor electrode connections, or heartbeats originated by pacemakers.

Several databases of ECG recordings are available for the research community for studying and evaluating automatic ECG analysis methods. PhysioBank is one of the widely used data sources that hosts well-characterized, documented, and labeled ECG signals from healthy subjects and patients with pathological conditions (e.g., heart failure, myocardial infarction, and sleep apnea). One of the most commonly used databases is the MIT-BIH database. The database is available to the scientific community via the PhysioNet website. The MIT-BIH database contains several ECG datasets: arrhythmia dataset, normal sinus rhythm dataset, atrial fibrillation dataset, supraventricular arrhythmia dataset, the long-term ST dataset, and the QT dataset (refer to PhysioNet website for a full list of ECG datasets).

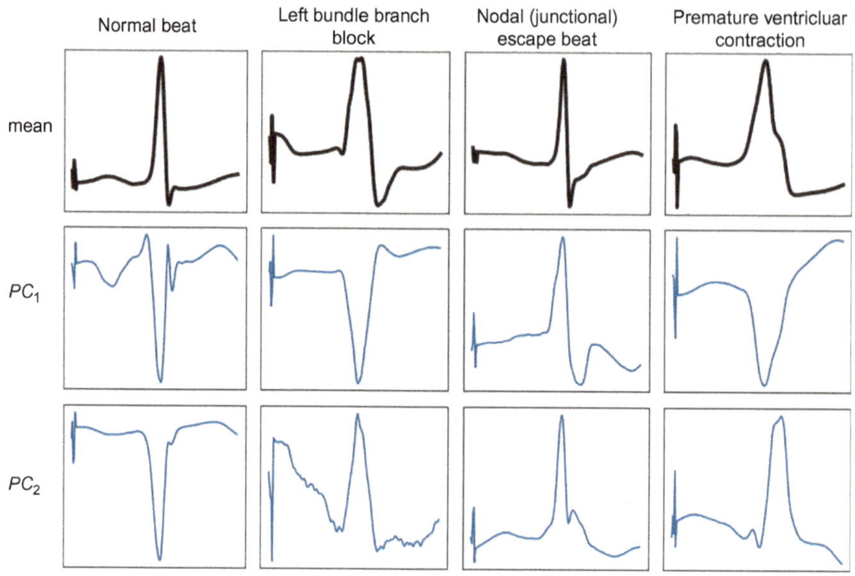

FIG. 4.5

The mean shape of heartbeats from four AAMI class types along with the largest two eigenvectors obtained by applying principal component analysis.

Fig. 4.5 shows four AAMI classes (represented in terms of mean components and the first and second eigenvectors following PCA analysis).

4.5 ECG heartbeat classifier

ECG analysis is an important resource for cardiovascular pathology diagnosis. Heart rhythm disorders in ECG waveforms are evidence of underlying cardiovascular problems. Manual analysis of ECG signals is difficult and time-consuming and requires professionals who are well trained to detect and categorize different waveform morphologies in the signal.

Several machine learning algorithms can be used for heartbeat classification, such as support vector machine (SVM), Bayesian classification, neural networks, LDA, k-nearest neighbor (kNN), and decision trees. In this section the SVM classification model is used to classify ECG beats. SVMs find a decision boundary that maximizes the margin between the different classes. SVMs have excellent generalization properties because it provides sparse solutions expressed in terms of a small number of support vectors (i.e., training samples that are closest to the decision boundary).

4.5.1 ECG signal descriptor

A typical heartbeat consists of a distinctive number of structures such as the P wave, QRS complex, and T wave. Each structure has its own morphology, amplitude, duration, and frequency content. ECG signal descriptors combine several features in a hope to capture various aspects of the signal. This provides us with appropriate representation of the signals and allows us to train more accurate and reliable classifiers. In this section a feature descriptor is built by combining several features to characterize ECG signals. The descriptor will then be used to train a classifier for the detection of cardiac arrhythmias.

An ECG signal is a time-series signal that reflects the time evolution of the heart's electrical activity. The quality of ECG signals may be degraded due to high- and low-frequency distortions. For example, dc offsets, low-frequency interference from power lines, high-frequency interference due to contraction of the muscles, baseline wandering due to respiratory movements, and noise due to poor electrode contact.

Noise can result in a false diagnosis of arrhythmia. Therefore the main goal of signal preprocessing is to remove noise and reject artifacts from ECG recordings. To remove the dc offset, the ECG record is subtracted from its mean, which makes the global signal baseline at level zero. Power line interference can be suppressed by using a band-stop filter centered at 50 Hz (or 60 Hz depending on the country) and its harmonics. Noise from patient's muscle contractions can be reduced by using a low-pass k-point moving average filter (e.g., $k=11$).

The QRS complex is a distinctive feature for segmenting cardiac cycles in ECG signals. The accuracy of QRS detection algorithms is affected by various factors such as the natural variability in QRS complex morphology and duration and noise sources such as motion artifact and baseline wandering. QRS segmentation methods mainly consist of two stages: a signal preprocessing and threshold-based QRS detector. One of the widely used algorithms for beat segmentation is proposed by Pan and Tompkins [1]. The background noise is first removed; then the ECG signal is squared to amplify the QRS complex. Finally, several adaptive thresholds are applied to detect the peaks of the filtered signal.

In this section the ECG signal is passed through a preprocessing stage to remove unwanted noise and remove the ECG baseline. Baseline wandering, as shown in Fig. 4.6, is an artifact that is due to chest movements. It appears as a low-frequency component in the corrupted ECG signal and can be removed by using low-frequency suppression to attenuate low frequencies. One common method for removing baseline wandering is by cascading two moving median filters using two different window sizes (e.g., applying a moving median filter using a window size of 57 followed by another moving median filter of size 151). The positions of the R waves provided from the annotated MIT-BIH records are used to obtain QRS positions in the ECG signal. ECG beats are then segmented by extracting samples around the R wave position using a widow of fixed size w.

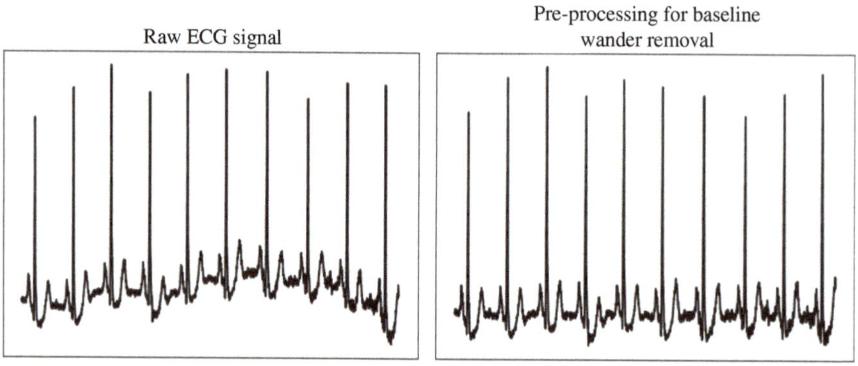

FIG. 4.6

Baseline wander removal using signal preprocessing. The preprocessed signal is generated by applying a two-stage median filter with window lengths of 57 and 151 samples, respectively.

4.5.2 Intra- and interpatient paradigms

Creating training and testing datasets is an important concept in data science, which is used to improve generalization and minimize overfitting. One way to generate test data is to split our data into two subsets: training data and testing data. The model is then fitted using the training data and tested on the unseen test data.

There are several ways one can use to split the data. In the context of ECG heartbeat classification, two data splitting paradigms are commonly used: intra- and interpatient paradigms.

The intrapatient paradigm generates training and testing subsets from the dataset based on the beat type. One of the main limitations of this scheme is that it results in an overoptimistic estimate of the actual classifier performance. This is because heartbeats from the same patient can appear in both training and test datasets. A more robust split uses the interpatient paradigm; here the patients used to train the classifier are different from the patients used to evaluate it. This ensures that beats from the same patient are not present in the training and test sets. It also takes into account the interindividual variation and therefore provides nonbiased estimates of the classification performance.

In this section the performance of a heartbeat classifier will be evaluated using the interpatient test paradigm (see [2]). The following datasets are created from the MIT-BIH database: DS1 = [101, 106, 108, 109, 112, 114, 115, 116, 118, 119, 122, 124, 201, 203, 205, 207, 208, 209, 215, 220, 223, 230] and DS2 = [100, 103, 105, 111, 113, 117, 121, 123, 200, 202, 210, 212, 213, 214, 219, 221, 222, 228, 231, 232, 233, 234]. Records [102, 104, 107, and 217] are paced recordings and are excluded from the training and test datasets; furthermore, only MLII lead is extracted for training and testing the models. Finally, class labels are extracted based on the AAMI beat classification standard (however, class-5, i.e., Q-class or "unclassified category," is not used).

4.5.3 Feature generation

Accurate heartbeat classification is considered the first step toward detecting cardiac arrhythmia. The procedure for heartbeat classification is composed of the following steps: preprocessing, beat segmentation, feature engineering, feature processing, classification, and evaluation. Heartbeat classification generally relies on extracting features from heartbeat segments. Several attributes of the extracted ECG beats can be used as features for a classification model. These features can be grouped into categories depending on the methods used: for example, statistical, temporal, frequency, wavelet, and morphological features. Feature selection and dimensionality reduction are usually performed before training a particular machine learning model. This reduces computational costs and improves generalization.

Statistical features are useful for extracting summary statistics from ECG signal amplitude variations in the time domain. Standard features include the mean; median; maximum; minimum; and higher-order statistical moments such as variance, kurtosis, and skewness.

Temporal features involve interval-based measurements of an ECG waveform, for example, computing the previous and next RR intervals (RRI); the average, minimum, and maximum duration of the previous/next 10 RR intervals; and the width of the QRS complex.

Morphological feature extraction uses information of signal profile to model local geometry. For example, local binary patterns (LBP) have been used to extract morphological features. For example, for each segment, we apply an eight-sample neighborhood operator that compares the center sample with the samples in the neighborhood; a binary stream of 1's and 0's is generated to indicate whether a sample is greater than center sample, otherwise output a zero. The binary numbers are converted to a decimal, and a histogram is computed using k-bins. The features are then the k-bin LBP histogram for that beat or even some summary statistics of the produced histogram such as the mode, mean, median, skewness, and kurtosis.

4.5.4 Ranking individual feature subsets

Performance of any machine learning algorithm depends highly on the proper selection of features. In this section an SVM classifier was independently trained using the full training set (DS1) and tested over the evaluation set (DS2) for each feature subset category to measure the goodness of the individual features.

The following statistical metrics are often used to measure a classifier performance: sensitivity (Se), positive predictive value (PPV), and specificity (Sp):

$$Se = TP/(TP + FN) \tag{4.1}$$

$$PPV = TP/(TP + FP) \tag{4.2}$$

$$Sp = TN/(TN + FP) \tag{4.3}$$

where TP is the number of correct positive predictions, TN is the number of correct negative predictions, FN is the number of incorrect predictions for positive cases, and FP is the number of incorrect predictions for negative cases.

Sensitivity measures how many of the actually positive cases are predicted as positive. Specificity is the proportion of negatively predicted cases to the total number of actual negative cases. Finally the precision (or positive predictivity) is the proportion of the positive results that are true positives (i.e., measures the relevancy of the positively predicted cases).

Similarly, arithmetic accuracy (Acc) can also be defined as the ratio of correct predictions (both positive and negative cases) to the number of total classified cases:

$$Acc = (TP + TN)/(TP + TN + \mathrm{FP} + \mathrm{FN}) \tag{4.4}$$

However, if the dataset is hugely imbalanced, the arithmetic accuracy will be biased toward the majority class. An alternative measure that can account for class imbalance in the dataset is the geometric mean accuracy, $gmAcc$:

$$gmAcc = \sqrt{Se \times Sp} \tag{4.5}$$

This metric is high only when both the sensitivity and specificity are also high.

In this section, individual feature subsets are used to train and test an SVM classifier for predicting heartbeat AAMI class. The following features are tested:

- Segmented ECG beat: here the preprocessed ECG beat is used itself as a $k \times 1$ feature vector, where k denotes the number of samples in the ECG beat.
- Subsampled ECG beat: using raw beats as features could result in high-dimensional features and affect the generalization performance of the classifier. To reduce the dimensionality, one can downsample the segmented beat to $m < k$ samples and use these as features.
- RR features: the RR features are extracted from the RRI intervals and are as follows: width of previous RR interval, $preRR$; width of next RR interval, $postRR$; average width of previous/next k RR intervals, $preRR_{avgk}$ and $postRR_{avgk}$; and the average width of k RRI intervals surrounding the current beat, $centerRRavg$ and $RR90sec\ avg$.
- Hermite coefficients: since low-order Hermite functions have similar morphology to the shape of the QRS complex, one can approximate ECG beats by fitting an nth order Hermite polynomial expansion to QRS complex. The resulting coefficients are used as features for the QRS complex.
- Higher-order statistics: the ECG beat is first segmented into k segments. Higher-order statistics (HOS) are then computed using the third- and fourth-order cumulants (i.e., skewness and kurtosis). This results in a $2 \times k$-dimensional feature for each beat.
- Local binary patterns: local binary patterns are widespread in the context of image descriptors. Since ECG is one-dimensional data, a 1D LBP is calculated for each data point in the segmented beat: here a neighborhood size is fixed around the current sample, x_0, and a binary code is produced for each sample in

the neighborhood x_i where i indicates $x_i > x_0$. The binary pattern is converted to decimal form, and a histogram over the patterns is built using m bins.
- Wavelet features: the discrete wavelet transform is used here to extract features from segmented ECG beats. Wavelet features are expected to have both spatial and temporal information from the QRS complex. The wavelet transform is applied to each beat signal using the Daubechies 3 family and a specific decomposition level. The approximation band coefficients are then used as wavelet features for the beat.

In this experiment the relevance of individual feature subsets from the segmented ECG beats is evaluated. A window of size 40 and 80 samples (before and after the R-peak) is used. The following features and associated parameters are tested:

- subsampled ECG waveform ($n_{samples}=20, 40, 60$),
- higher-order statistics (segment width$=5, 10, 20, 40$),
- Hermite features (order$=2, 3, 4$),
- local binary patterns (neighborhood size$=8$, $n_{bins}=30, 60, 100$),
- wavelet features ($family=db3$, $levels=1, 2, 3, 4, 5$),
- RR-interval features (num local beats$=10, 20, 40$),
- segmented ECG beat (ECG beat wave).

A multiclass SVM model is trained using one-versus-one classification scheme. This generates a decision function of shape ($n_{samples}$ and $n_{classes}$). Class weights are also calculated to reduce the effects of class imbalance. Each class is assigned a weight equal to the ratio between all training data (i.e., rest class) and the number of cases in each class. This will adjust the regularization parameter C of class i to $class_{weight}[i] \times C$. Table 4.2 shows a summary of the hyperparameters used for the model.

Table 4.3 shows the performance results for each feature subset using heartbeat segments of 80 samples wide. The sensitivity and positive predictive value for each AAMI class is computed. The average values are then pulled and reported, as shown in the table. The most important single feature with the highest average sensitivity of 65.22% is the wavelet feature obtained using "db3" wavelet family with two decomposition levels. On the other hand the most important single feature that achieves the best average predictive value of 40.68% is the subsampled ECG beat using only eight samples.

Table 4.2 Hyperparameters for the SVM classifier.

Hyperparameter	Description
Kernel	Radial basis function of degree 3
C	Regularization parameter, $C=0.05$
Gamma	Kernel coefficient, set to 1/*nfeatures*

Table 4.3 Performance of each feature subset. ECG beat=2×40=80 samples.

Feature	Parameters	avgSe	avgPPV
Subsample ECG	Resample 8	**64.62**	**40.68**
Subsample ECG	Resample 20	61.23	38.52
Subsample ECG	Resample 40	63.08	38.77
Subsample ECG	Resample 60	63.13	38.84
HOS features seglength	40	41.04	37.02
HOS features seglength	20	**47.83**	32.76
HOS features	Seglength 60	46.45	**38.24**
HOS features	Seglength 10	41.65	30.53
Hermite features	ords [2,3,4]	**47.68**	**33.95**
lbp	nbins 30 ne 8	46.92	34.76
lbp	nbins 60 ne 8	**48.08**	35.6
lbp	nbins 100 ne 8	47.86	**36.3**
Wavelet features	Family db3 level 3	60.49	39.35
Wavelet features	Family db3 level 4	61.76	42.02
Wavelet features	Family db3 level 5	54.29	**42.6**
Wavelet features	Family db3 level 2	**65.22**	38.87
Wavelet features	Family db3 level 1	64.23	38.8
RR features	*n* local beats 10	**64.48**	40.01
RR features	*n* local beats 20	62.09	40.29
RR features	*n* local beats 40	60.63	**40.64**
ECG beat wave		**63.21**	**38.87**

Notes: *The bold numbers indicate the parameters that produced the highest performance for each feature. For example, for the feature "lbp" the bins = 60, ne = 8 produced the best avgSe of 48.08%.*

The SVM model is now trained using the top two individual features. The resulting training data have a shape of 52,509 beats and 31 features for each beat. The test indicates that the average geometric mean accuracy for all AAMI classes is 75.38% and with an average sensitivity and average *PPV* of 66.75% and 39.08%, respectively.

Table 4.4 shows the performance results for each feature subset using heartbeat segments of 160 samples wide. The most important single feature with the highest average sensitivity of 64.13% is the wavelet feature obtained using "db3" wavelet family with four decomposition levels. On the other hand the most important single feature that achieves the best average predictive value is Hermite features (*PPV*=43.99%) of orders (2, 3, and 4).

The SVM model is now trained using the top two individual features. The resulting training data have a shape of 52,509 beats and 23 features for each beat. The test indicates that the average geometric mean accuracy for all AAMI classes is 73.89% and with an average sensitivity and average *PPV* of 67.27% and 36.93%, respectively.

Table 4.4 Performance of each feature subset. ECG beat=80×2=160 samples.

Feature	Parameters	avgSe	avgPPV
Subsample ECG	Resample 60	**58.4**	**39.29**
Subsample ECG	Resample 40	58.32	39.16
Subsample ECG	Resample 20	54.3	36.98
HOS features	Seglength 5	44.25	31.7
HOS features	Seglength 10	39.39	30.5
HOS features	Seglength 20	53.6	36.1
HOS features	Seglength 40	**56.23**	**39.88**
Hermite features	ords [2,3,4]	**52.31**	**43.99**
lbp	nbins 100 ne 8	38.8	30.43
lbp	nbins 30 ne 8	39.18	30.89
lbp	nbins 60 ne 8	**39.61**	**30.91**
Wavelet features	Family db3 level 1	59.31	**39.37**
Wavelet features	Family db3 level 2	58.98	39.18
Wavelet features	Family db3 level 3	61.3	38.24
Wavelet features	Family db3 level 4	**64.13**	37.6
Wavelet features	Family db3 level 5	62.37	35.06
RR features	*n* local beats 10	**63.18**	39.74
RR features	*n* local beats 20	60.2	40.28
RR features	*n* local beats 40	57.1	**40.32**
ECG beat wave		**58.81**	**39.31**

Notes: *The bold numbers indicate the parameters that produced the highest performance for each feature. For example, for the feature "lbp" the bins = 60, ne = 8 produced the best avgSe of 48.08%.*

4.5.5 Training and testing the final model

The mean and standard deviation of the features from dataset (DS1) are calculated. The training data are then standardized by subtracting the mean and dividing by the standard deviation obtained from the previous step. The test data are also standardized in the same way but using the same mean and standard deviation used for the training data.

Following the AAMI standard, a heartbeat classifier is trained by fusing a number of relevant feature subsets. Table 4.5 shows the average sensitivity and PPV values for different feature combinations. The best result was achieved using the following features:

- Beat segment length (160 samples),
- RR features (using up to 40 beats for local interval averaging—additionally beats spanning up to 90 seconds are used for the global average),
- Subsampled ECG beat (8 samples),
- Higher-order statistics (extracting statistical patterns using a segment length of 60 samples),

Table 4.5 Performance for five classifiers trained with different feature combinations.

winSize	avgSe	avgPPV	Features used
80	65.48	50.27	RR features (*n* local beats 40) Subsample ECG (resample 8) HOS features (seg length 60) lbp (nbins 30 ne 8) Wavelet features (family db3 level 2)
40	58.29	49.65	RR features (*n* local beats 40) Subsample ECG (resample 8) HOS features (seg length 60) lbp (nbins 30 ne 8) Wavelet features (family db3 level 2)
80	61.31	49.53	RR features (*n* local beats 10) Subsample ECG (resample 60) HOS features (seg length 40) lbp (nbins 60 ne 8) Wavelet features (family db3 level 1)
80	58.05	49.24	RR features (*n* local beats 10) Subsample ECG (resample 20) Hermite features (ords [2,3,4]) HOS features (seglength 20) lbp (nbins 30 ne 8) Wavelet features (family db3 level 3)
80	60.37	48.22	RR features (*n* local beats 10) Subsample ECG (resample 60) Hermite features (ords [2,3,4]) HOS features (seglength 40) lbp (nbins 60 ne 8) Wavelet features (family db3 level 1)

- Local binary patterns (using 30 bins for the histogram),
- Wavelet features (based on db3 wavelet family and two levels of decomposition).

4.6 Conclusions

Automated arrhythmia detection is a challenging problem due to the wide variability in ECG morphological and temporal features within the population. Several factors such as age, gender, the time of recordings, and previous physical activity affect the appearance of features in an ECG recording. Besides, confounding factors exist where different beat morphologies may be observed for the same disease or similar morphologies showing for different diseases. Other aspects include the need to process massive amounts of data. For example, sometimes, it is necessary to obtain extended ECG recordings spanning several hours to monitor the state of patients' health. Such scenarios bring the need for real-time monitoring and increased storage requirements.

References

[1] J. Pan, W. Tompkins, A real-time QRS detection algorithm, IEEE Trans. Biomed. Eng. 3 (1985) 230–236.

[2] P. Chazal, M. O'Dwyer, R. Reilly, Automatic classification of heartbeats using ECG morphology and heartbeat interval features, IEEE Trans. Biomed. Eng. 51 (7) (2004) 1196–1206.

Further reading

cablesandsensors (n.d.) 12-Lead ECG Placement Guide With Illustrations, https://www.cablesandsensors.com/pages/12-lead-ecg-placement-guidewith-illustrations.

E. Aramendi, U. Irusta, E. Pastor, A. Bodegas, F. Benito, ECG spectral and morphological parameters reviewed and updated to detect adult and paediatric life-threatening arrhythmia, Physiol. Meas. 31 (6) (2010) 749.

M. Arif, Robust electrocardiogram (ECG) beat classification using discrete wavelet transform, Physiol. Meas. 29 (5) (2008) 555.

C.J. Breen, G.P. Kelly, W.G. Kernohan, ECG interpretation skill acquisition: a review of learning, teaching and assessment. J. Electrocardiol. (2019) https://doi.org/10.1016/j.jelectrocard.2019.03.010.

J.T. Catalano, Guide to ECG Analysis, Lippincott Williams & Wilkins, 2002.

I. Christov, G. Gomez-Herrero, V. Krasteva, I. Jekova, A. Gotchev, K. Egiazarian, Comparative study of morphological and time-frequency ECG descriptors for heartbeat classification, Med. Eng. Phys. 28 (9) (2006) 876–887.

Electrocardiography (2020), Wikipedia. Page Version ID: 941133769

J. Francis, ECG monitoring leads and special leads, Ind. Pacing Electrophysiol. J. 16 (3) (2016) 92–95.

G. Garcia, G. Moreira, D. Menotti, E. Luz, Inter-patient ECG heartbeat classification with temporal VCG optimized by *PSO*, Sci. Rep. 7 (1) (2017) 10543.

G.D. Gargiulo, P. Bifulco, M. Cesarelli, A.L. McEwan, H. Moeinzadeh, A. O'Loughlin, I.M. Shugman, J.C. Tapson, A. Thiagalingam, On the einthoven triangle: a critical analysis of the single rotating dipole hypothesis, Sensors 18 (7) (2018) 2353.

A. Goshvarpour, A. Abbasi, A. Goshvarpour, An accurate emotion recognition system using ECG and GSR signals and matching pursuit method, Biomed. J. 40 (6) (2017) 355–368.

Heart (2019), Wikipedia. Page Version ID: 933179881

M.R. Homaeinezhad, S.A. Atyabi, E. Tavakkoli, H.N. Toosi, Ghaffari, A. & Ebrahimpour, R., ECG arrhythmia recognition via a neuro-SVM–KNN hybrid classifier with virtual QRS image-based geometrical features, Expert Syst. Appl. 39 (2) (2012) 2047–2058.

M.R. Homaeinezhad, A. Ghaffari, H. Najjaran Toosi, R. Rahmani, M. Tahmasebi, M.M. Daevaeiha, Ambulatory Holter ECG individual events delineation via segmentation of a wavelet-based information-optimized 1-D feature, Sci. Iran. 18 (1) (2011) 86–104.

B. Hopenfeld, H. Ashikaga, Origin of the electrocardiographic U wave: effects of M cells and dynamic gap junction coupling, Ann. Biomed. Eng. 38 (3) (2010) 1060–1070.

A.F. Hussein, A.K. AlZubaidi, A. Al-Bayaty, Q.A. Habash, An IoT real-time biometric authentication system based on ECG fiducial extracted features using discrete cosine transform, arXiv (2017) arXiv:1708.08189 [cs].

R.E. Ideker, W. Kong, S. Pogwizd, Purkinje fibers and arrhythmias, Pacing Clin. Electrophysiol. 32 (3) (2009) 283–285.

LearntheHeart.Com (n.d.) Introduction to ECG—Online 12-Lead ECG Interpretation Course, https://www.healio.com/cardiology/learn-the-heart/ecgreview/ecg-interpretation-tutorial/introduction-to-the-ecg.

H.J. Kim, J.S. Lim, Study on a biometric authentication model based on ECG using a fuzzy neural network, IOP Conf. Ser. Mater. Sci. Eng. 317 (2018) 012030.

P. Kligfield, L.S. Gettes, J.J. Bailey, R. Childers, B.J. Deal, E.W. Hancock, G. van Herpen, J.A. Kors, P. Macfarlane, D.M. Mirvis, O. Pahlm, P. Rautaharju, G.S. Wagner, Recommendations for the standardization and interpretation of the electrocardiogram: part I: the electrocardiogram and its technology: a scientific statement from the American Heart Association Electrocardiography and Arrhythmias Committee, Council on Clinical Cardiology; the American College of Cardiology Foundation; and the Heart Rhythm Society Endorsed by the International Society for Computerized Electrocardiology, Circulation 115 (10) (2007) 1306–1324.

S. Led, J. Fernandez, L. Serrano, Design of a wearable device for ECG continuous monitoring using wireless technology, in: The 26th Annual International Conference of the IEEE Engineering in Medicine and Biology Society, vol. 2, 2004, pp. 3318–3321.

A. Lyon, A. Minchole, J.P. Martınez, P. Laguna, B. Rodriguez, Computational techniques for ECG analysis and interpretation in light of their contribution to medical advances, J. R. Soc. Interface 15 (138) (2018).

S. Meek, ABC of clinical electrocardiography: introduction. II—basic terminology, BMJ 324 (7335) (2002) 470–473.

S. Meek, F. Morris, Introduction. I—leads, rate, rhythm, and cardiac axis, British Med. J. 324 (7334) (2002) 415–418.

physionet, (n.d.) MIT-BIH Arrhythmia Database v1.0.0, https://physionet.org/content/mitdb/1.0.0/.

H. Moeinzadeh, J. Assad, P. Bifulco, M. Cesarelli, A. O'Loughlin, I.M. Shugman, G.D. Gargiulo, Einthoven Unipolar Leads: Towards a better understanding of Wilson Central Terminal, in: 2019 International Conference on Electrical Engineering Research Practice (ICEERP), 2019, pp. 1–4.

Electrocardiography WikiLectures MEFANET: Czech and SlovakMedical Faculties Network (n.d.), https://www.wikilectures.eu/w/Electrocardiography.

M. Rahhal, Y. Bazi, H. AlHichri, N. Alajlan, F. Melgani, R. Yager, Deep learning approach for active classification of electrocardiogram signals, Inf. Sci. 345 (2016) 340–354.

A.H. Ribeiro, M.H. Ribeiro, G. Paixao, D. Oliveira, P.R. Gomes, J.A. Canazart, M. Pifano, W. Meira Jr., T.B. Schon, A.L. Ribeiro, Automatic diagnosis of short-duration 12-lead ECG using a deep convolutional network, arXiv (2019) arXiv:1811.12194 [cs, eess, stat].

G. Sannino, G. De Pietro, A deep learning approach for ECG-based heartbeat classification for arrhythmia detection, Futur. Gener. Comput. Syst. 86 (2018) 446–455.

Willem Einthoven (2020), Wikipedia. Page Version ID: 937823922

C. Ye, B. Kumar, M. Coimbra, Heartbeat classification using morphological and dynamic features of ECG signals, IEEE Trans. Biomed. Eng. 59 (10) (2012) 2930–2941.

J. Zheng, J. Zhang, S. Danioko, H. Yao, H. Guo, C. Rakovski, A 12-lead electrocardiogram database for arrhythmia research covering more than 10,000 patients, Sci. Data 7 (1) (2020) 1–8.

CHAPTER

Deep EEG: Deep learning in biomedical signal processing with EEG applications

5

Dr. J. Teye Brown and Dr. Walid Zgallai

Faculty of Engineering Technology and Science, Higher Colleges of Technology, Dubai, United Arab Emirates

5.1 EEG data basics

This chapter is not intended to be a comprehensive coverage of electroencephalogram (EEG) signals and its applications as this has been already covered in other literature. A brief introduction to EEG signal has been covered in Chapter 1, Section 1.2. The intention here, however, is to show detailed and practical applications for the reader to get an insight on how to process EEG signals using deep learning algorithms.

As introduced in Chapter 1 the electroencephalogram (EEG) signal records electrical activity noninvasively from the scalp via electrodes. EEG signals have maximum amplitude of 100 mV and a frequency range of 0–100 Hz. These signals are classified as delta, theta, alpha, beta, and gamma waves. Delta waves have the lowest frequency range, that is, 0–4 Hz. The frequency range of theta and alpha waves are 4–8 Hz and 9–13 Hz, respectively. Finally, beta waves have a frequency range of 14–30 Hz, while gamma waves have a frequency range of 30–100 Hz [1].

To use EEG signals to control robots, a brain-computer interface device (BCI) is used. A BCI is a system that uses human brain signals to control or communicate with an external device. A BCI system has four main functions: signal acquisition, signal processing, output control, and operating protocol [2]. In this chapter a new methodology is used to employ a deep learning neural network, to process the EEG signals captured from an Emotiv Pro headset, to control the movement of a wheelchair in four directions, left, right, forward, and stop.

5.2 Fundamentals of deep convolutional neural networks (DCNNs)

5.2.1 Why deep learning

Recently, there has been a conspicuous resurgence in the use of deep learning in scientific research and the media in general. Deep neural networks (DNNs) are the neural networks that have a large number of layers. There is no specific number of layers

Biomedical Signal Processing and Artificial Intelligence in Healthcare. https://doi.org/10.1016/B978-0-12-818946-7.00005-6

used to classify a deep neural network, but general consensus appears to be that they are neural networks with more than three hidden layers. Due to the larger network size, DNNs require a lot of computational power. Additionally, their performance generally improves with larger datasets.

The combination of larger neural networks and larger datasets (labeled datasets) substantially increases the performance of deep learning algorithms over other algorithms. Labeled datasets, including training sets with input values x and output values y, are used in deep learning. Thus the larger the training set, along with larger neural networks, the better the performance of the algorithm. When the data size of the training data is relatively small, there is no distinct/defined advantage of one algorithm over the other.

5.2.2 Basics of deep convolutional neural networks

An artificial neural network (ANN) is a subset of machine learning algorithms modeled after the human brain. An in-depth review of ANNs can be found in [3, 4]. Convolutional neural networks (CNNs) are a unique type of ANN whereby at least one network layer operates on input data via convolutions rather than general matrix multiplication [5]. CNNs consist of learnable weights w and biases b.

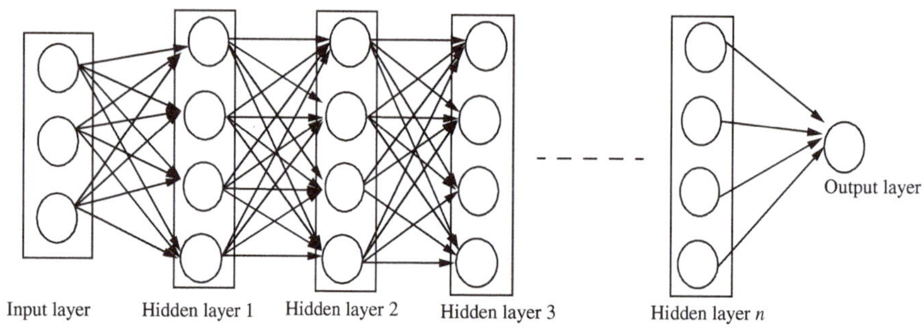

FIG. 5.1

Deep artificial neural network.

Fig. 5.1 is a representation of an artificial neural network. The circular nodes represent neurons, while the arrows represent the interconnectedness between the neurons. The initial layer is known as the input layer. The final layer is known as the output layer, while the layers between the two are called the hidden layers. Data such as stock prices, election data, audio files, image, and video data are passed into the input layer of the neural network. Each layer extracts features from the data allowing the network to "learn" a generalized pattern of higher level features associated with the data. The output layer classifies the data based on the features "learned" in the hidden layers.

5.2.3 The perceptron

The simplest case of an ANN is the perceptron shown in Fig. 5.2.

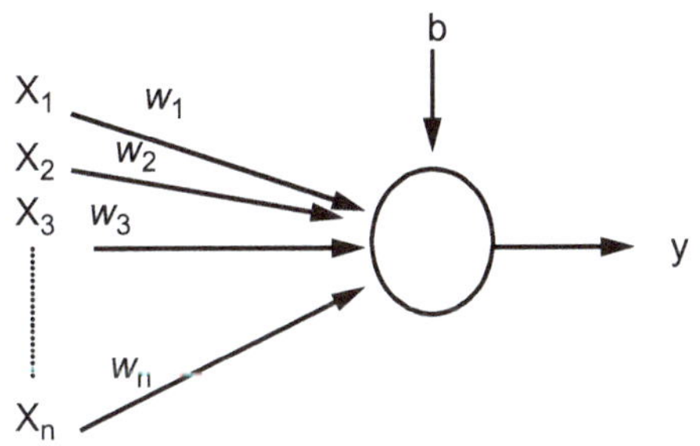

FIG. 5.2

Perceptron.

It is obvious from Fig. 5.2 that a perceptron is a neural network that has no hidden layers. X_1, X_2, etc. are the input data. The variables w_1, w_2, etc. are the weights associated with each input. The variable b is the bias. The numerical value of each of these weights is a measure of the relative importance of each input. The aim of the perceptron is to "learn" these weights.

The output y is determined in two main steps:

$$z = \sum_{i=1}^{n} w_i x + b \tag{5.1}$$

$$y = g(z) \tag{5.2}$$

The expression $g(z)$ represents the implementation of activation functions on the linear combination, z. These activation functions introduce nonlinearity into the network. The most common activation functions are tanh (x), sigmoid(x), relu(x), and softmax(x), which are defined in Eqs. (5.3)–(5.6), respectively:

$$Tanh : f(x) = \frac{e^x - e^{-x}}{e^x + e^{-x}} \tag{5.3}$$

$$\text{Sigmoid} : \sigma(x) = \frac{1}{1 + e^{-x}} \tag{5.4}$$

$$\text{Relu} : f(x) = \max(0, x) \tag{5.5}$$

$$\text{Softmax(x)} : f(x) = \frac{e^{x_i}}{\sum_{i=1}^{n} e^{x_i}} \tag{5.6}$$

Example 5.1 A perceptron receives as input $x_1 = 1, x_2 = 2, x_3 = 0.5$, with associated weights and bias $w_1 = 0.5$, $w_2 = 1$, $w_3 = 0.2$, $b = 0.1$.The activation function at the output layer is the sigmoid function. What is the output of this perceptron?

Solution

The sigmoid function is $\sigma(x) = \frac{1}{1+e^{-x}}$

So

$$z = \sum_{i=1}^{3} w_i x_i + b = [w_1\ w_2\ w_3]\begin{vmatrix} x_1 \\ x_2 \\ x_3 \end{vmatrix} + b = 0.5(1) + 1(2) + 0.2(0.5) + 0.1 = 2.7$$

$$y = \sigma(2.7) = \frac{1}{1+e^{-2.7}} = 0.937 > 0.5 = 1$$

At the output layer,

$$y = 0, \text{ if } \sigma(z) < 0.5 \text{ and } y = 1, \text{ if } \sigma(z) \geq 0.5. \quad (5.7)$$

5.2.4 CNN architecture

As aforementioned, CNNs are a special class of neural networks whereby at least one of the network layers is a convolutional layer. Additionally, CNNs are generally used for grid-like data such as images, videos, and time series. The architecture of CNNs therefore assumes the input data are two dimensional, for example, an image (or a series of images), and are therefore optimized to deal with such data. Regular neural networks do not scale well to full images since the number of learnable parameters will be too large for their fully connected layers. For a more in-depth discussion of this, refer to [6].

CNNs may possess the following layers: input layer, convolutional layer, activation layer, pooling layer, and fully connected output layer. The input layer may contain three-dimensional data in three-channel (RGB) format. The convolutional layer uses a two-dimensional filter that convolves across the width and height of the input layer producing a two-dimensional result of the response of the filter at every spatial position. The activation layer adds a nonlinearity to the input data and leaves the dimensionality unchanged. The most commonly used activation functions are described in Eqs. (5.3)–(5.6).

The sigmoid function is used in the outer layer in the case of binary classification (logistic regression), for example, forward and stop commands. The Softmax activation function is used in the case of multiclass classification such as left, right, forward, and stop.

The pooling layers perform a downsampling of the input, resulting in lower dimensionality. The main type of pooling used in max pooling where the maximum value in a localized grid is chosen to replace the entire grid. In the average pooling scheme, the average value in a localized grid is chosen to replace the entire grid. Examples 5.2 and 5.3 illustrate those two operations.

Example 5.2 Consider the 4 × 4 array of values representing a section of a 2-D image data shown in Fig. 5.3. Compute the output of a max pooling layer applied to this array.

2	23	12	30
102	0	122	2
0	7	22	0
5	4	11	0

FIG. 5.3

Sample 2-D data.

Solution

To use a 2 × 2 max pooling filter, slide across the two-dimensional array representation of the data starting at the top left. The max pooling then chooses the largest value, that is, 102. The entire grid is replaced with 102 as shown in Fig. 5.4.

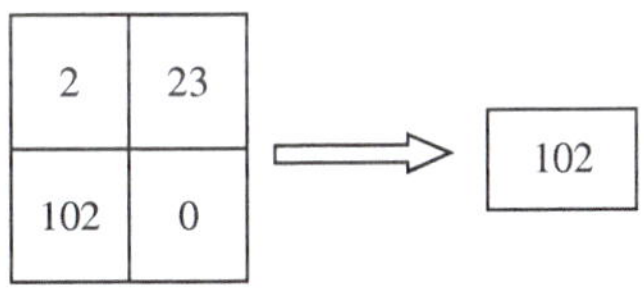

FIG. 5.4

Max pool operation.

The max pooling then slides two spaces to the right and repeats the operation as shown in Fig. 5.5.

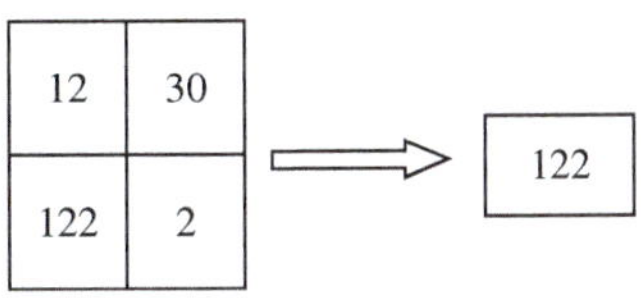

FIG. 5.5

Sample max pooling operation.

This process is repeated iteratively along the columns and rows. The final output is shown in Fig. 5.6.

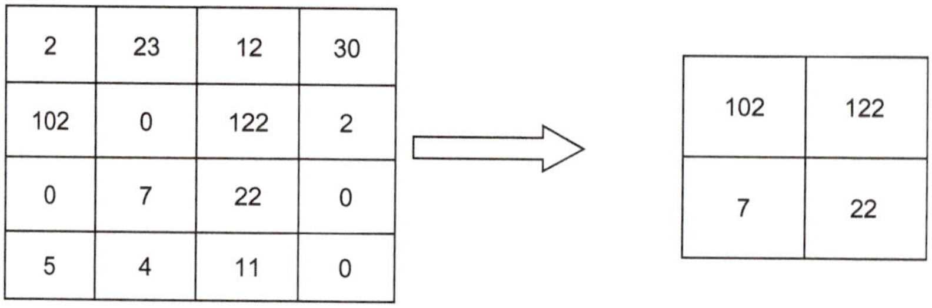

FIG. 5.6

Result of max pooling operation on 2-D data.

Example 5.3 Given the input shown in Fig. 5.7, provide the output of a 2×2 average pooling layer.

0	20	5	48	6	92
40	0	0	7	22	40
100	120	102	124	68	10
2	2	4	62	22	20
0	12	34	30	6	140
0	0	40	20	10	20

FIG. 5.7

2-D input data.

Solution

Beginning with the top left, we get the first result in Fig. 5.8 since the average of the four numbers, 0, 20, 40, and 0, is $(0 + 20 + 40 + 0) / 4 = 60 / 4 = 15$.

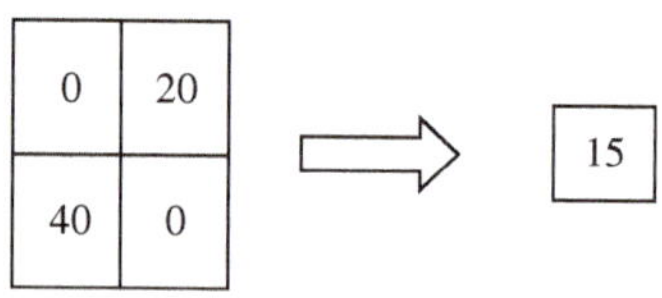

FIG. 5.8

Average pooling operation.

Sliding to the right the next output is shown in Fig. 5.9, $(5 + 48 + 0 + 7) / 4 = 60 / 4 = 15$.

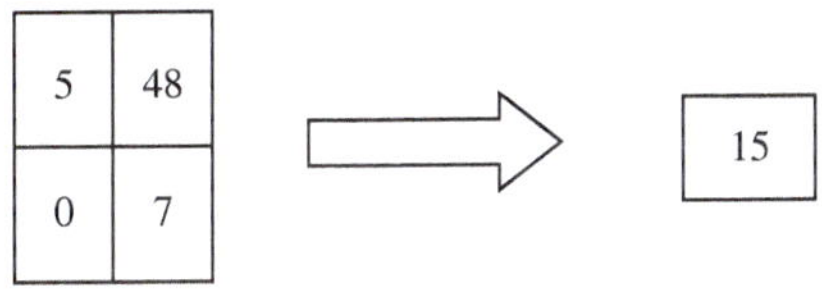

FIG. 5.9

Average pooling operation.

The final result is shown in Fig. 5.10.

15	15	40
56	73	30
3	31	44

FIG. 5.10

Result of average pooling on 2-D data.

5.2.5 Convolutions and the convolutional layer

We have discussed what the layers of a CNN are made up of, but here, we want to delve into the function that makes a neural network, a convolutional neural network. This function is known in the field of mathematics as a convolution.

A convolution is a type of linear operation that operates on two functions f, g, where both functions have real-valued arguments. The result is a new function, h, whose data show the extent to which one function affects the shape of the other. A convolution of $f$and g is expressed as $f * g$, while the result, h, is also called a convolution. More specifically,

$$h(t) = (f(t)^*g(t)) = \int_{-\infty}^{\infty} f(\tau)g(t-\tau)d\tau \tag{5.8}$$

As can be seen in Eq. (5.8), $g(t)$ is reflected and then shifted. The dummy variable τ theoretically spans all real numbers. This means that we slide over τ from $-\infty$ to ∞ and perform and compute an integral or multiplication wherever the two functions intersect.

Further exploration of the details of mathematical convolutions is beyond the scope of this book and can be found in [5]. We therefore redirect our discussion to its application in deep convolutional neural networks and, more specifically, to the convolutional layer. Firstly the range of the dummy variable is limited to the size of our two-dimensional array representation of the data. Secondly the function f may be considered to be the actual input data, X,that is, our two-dimensional array. The function g is called a filter or kernel. These two terms are interchangeable although kernel is used more in the field of image processing, while filter is more used in the field of deep learning.

Example 5.4 Consider an input X as shown in Fig. 5.11 and the corresponding filter f. Compute the output of the convolution.

2	0	1	2	9	7	4	1
3	5	6	3	3	1	0	2
2	0	1	2	9	0	4	8
2	0	1	2	0	7	10	8
5	6	12	2	9	3	4	9
2	0	1	6	9	1	4	7
3	3	1	2	4	6	14	6
5	4	9	3	2	5	4	9

X

*

−1	0	1
−1	0	1
−1	0	1

f

FIG. 5.11

Input data and 3 × 3 kernel.

Solution

Begin by sliding the filter over the top left 3 × 3 grid of X as shown in Fig. 5.12. Then perform an element-wise product.

2	0	1	2	9	7	4	1
3	5	6	3	3	1	0	2
2	0	1	2	9	0	4	8
2	0	1	2	0	7	10	8
5	6	12	2	9	3	4	9
2	0	1	6	9	1	4	7
3	3	1	2	4	6	14	6
5	4	9	3	2	5	4	9

X

*

−1	0	1
−1	0	1
−1	0	1

f

FIG. 5.12

First convolution operation.

The result is $2(-1) + 0(0) + 1(1) + 3(-1) + 5(0) + 6(1) + 2(-1) + 0(0) + 1(1) = 1$. We then slide one step to the right as shown in Fig. 5.13.

2	0	1	2	9	7	4	1
3	5	6	3	3	1	0	2
2	0	1	2	9	0	4	8
2	0	1	2	0	7	10	8
5	6	12	2	9	3	4	9
2	0	1	6	9	1	4	7
3	3	1	2	4	6	14	6
5	4	9	3	2	5	4	9

X

$*$

−1	0	1
−1	0	1
−1	0	1

f

FIG. 5.13

Second convolution operation.

The result is

$$0(-1)+1(0)+2(1)+5(-1)+6(0)+3(1)+0(-1)+1(0)+2(1)=2$$

Next

$$1(-1)+2(0)+9(1)+6(-1)+3(0)+3(1)+1(-1)+2(0)+9(1)=9$$

Eventually, we will have a row of six values. We then slide the filter downwards and repeat.

The result is clearly a 6×6 grid as shown in Fig. 5.14.

1	2	9	6	−18	4
1	2	4	1	2	10
5	0	4	4	0	15
5	0	4	1	0	13
4	1	8	0	0	12
1	4	4	1	7	10

FIG. 5.14

Output of convolutional operation.

Generally speaking, if the data size is $n \times n$, with a filter of size $f \times f$, then the size of the output of a convolution is

$$output\ size = (n - f + 1) \times (\mathrm{n} - \mathrm{f} + 1). \tag{5.9}$$

5.2.6 Padding

One important function typically used in convolutional neural networks is padding, also known as zero padding. Generally speaking, padding refers to the artificial inclusion of additional peripheral layers of pixels, uniformly around the 2-D data. This additional layer(s) is/are made up of zero-valued pixels. There is a very important reason for this in a convolutional neural network. Padding serves to maintain dimensionality in the data. Consider the grid representing an 8×8 array shown in Fig. 5.15.

FIG. 5.15

Sample 8 × 8, 2-D input data.

If one layer of padding is added, the data will now have a size of 10×10 as shown in Fig. 5.16.

This is important in convolutional neural networks. Section 5.2.5 shows that the convolutional layer results in a reduction of the dimensions of the image. Consider a situation where there are three or more convolutional layers. After each convolutional layer, the array size is reduced. For a large convolutional neural network, the size of the input data may be reduced to a point where it is too small. There is another effect caused by the reduction of the input data's dimensions in the convolutional layers. That is the loss of information on the edges of the data. Essentially the convolutional layers result in a potential disposal of information in the input data. By adding a padding layer, the layer just beneath the padding may be examined, involved in a convolution (see 6.2.5), at least one more time. This means more feature extraction and improved pattern recognition. This generally means improved accuracy by the CNN.

FIG. 5.16

Addition of one padding layer.

Example 5.5 Consider the situation of an 5 × 5 input array to a convolutional layer with a filter of size $f = 3$. How much padding (p) should be added to maintain the original image dimensions?

Solution

$$output\ \ size = (n - f + 1) \times (n - f + 1) = (5 - 3 + 1) \times (5 - 3 + 1) = 3 \times 3$$

There is a reduction of the image dimensions by 2, that is, 3 × 3. To offset this loss, it is necessary to add two more cells to the grid. However, it is important to consider the fact that the padding is included on each side of image symmetrically. Therefore add one layer of padding, that is, $p = 1$.

Generally speaking,

$$output\ \ size = (n - f + 2p + 1)\, x\, (n - f + 2p + 1) \tag{5.10}$$

In the development of a CNN, there are two main options for padding. Firstly, there may be no padding or zero padding. In this case the output dimension is given by Eq. (5.9). This is sometimes referred to as "valid convolutions." Furthermore the input data, after padding and convolutions, may result in an output of the same dimensions as the input. This is attained using the Eq. (5.10) and is referred to as "same convolutions." To ensure "same convolutions," we can use the following:

$$output\ \ size = (n - f + 2p + 1)x\,(n - f + 2p + 1) = n\,x\,n$$

So,

$$p = \frac{f - 1}{2} \tag{5.11}$$

5.2.7 Strided convolutions

Section 5.2.5 discussed the convolution operation as it pertains to convolutional neural networks. Additionally, padding as a key operation in the process was discussed. However, in Example 5.5, the filter was slid horizontally and sometimes vertically by one square. This is referred to as a stride of 1, that is, $s = 1$. Hence, stride is the amount by which the filter is slid after a convolutional operation, to compute another convolution.

Example 5.6 Using the data provided for X in Fig. 5.17 and the corresponding filter, f, determine the dimensions and output of a convolutional layer using a stride of 2, with no padding.

4	0	9	8	7	7	2
8	1	1	3	5	5	6
5	0	2	2	3	1	9
9	1	0	4	2	7	9
0	1	1	9	4	8	6
2	8	5	3	2	9	4
9	7	6	6	3	3	7

X

$*$

1	1	1
0	0	0
–1	–1	–1

f

FIG. 5.17

Input data and 3 × 3 filter.

Solution:

As show in Fig. 5.18, begin with the top left corner.

The result is $4(1) + 0(1) + 9(1) + 8(0) + 1(0) + 1(0) + 5(-1) + 0(-1) + 2(-1) = 6$.

Next, take a stride of 2 as shown in Fig. 5.19.

The result is $9(1) + 8(1) + 7(1) + 1(0) + 3(0) + 5(0) + 2(-1) + 2(-1) + 3(-1) = 17$.

Fig. 5.20 shows the next step.

The result is

$$7(1)+7(1)+2(1)+5(0)+5(0)+6(0)+3(-1)+1(-1)+9(-1)=3.$$

Eventually the output has dimensions of 3 × 3. This can be determined using

$$output\ size = \frac{n+2p-f}{s}+1 \tag{5.12}$$

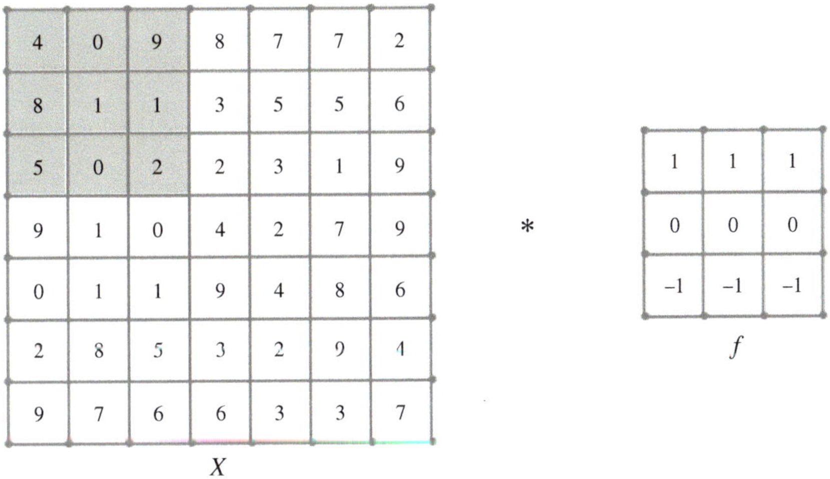

FIG. 5.18

Convolution operation first step.

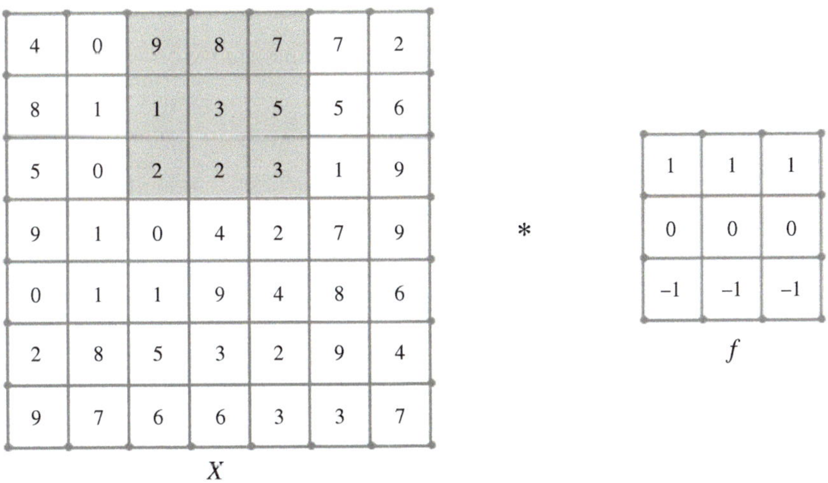

FIG. 5.19

Convolution operation with stride 2.

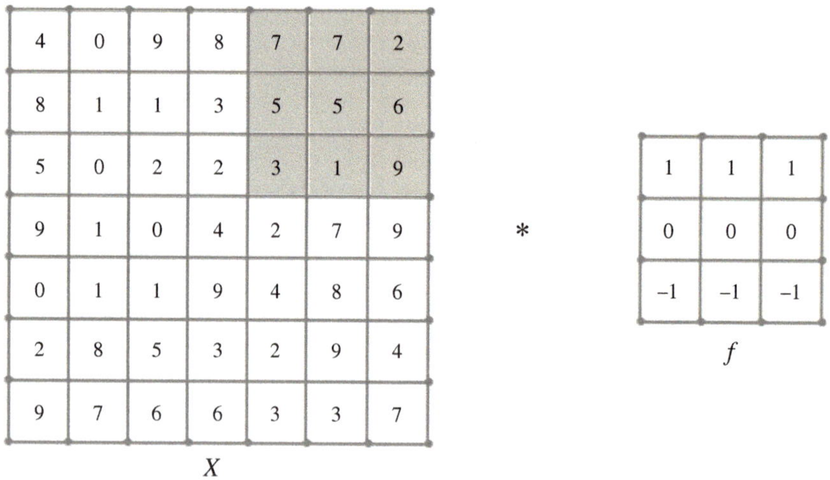

FIG. 5.20

Next convolution operation with stride 2.

Example 5.7 Repeat Example 5.6 using "same convolution" operation as described in Section 5.2.6.

Solution

$$output = \frac{n + 2p - f}{s} + 1 = n$$

$$p = \frac{s(n-1) + f - n}{2} \tag{5.13}$$

$$p = \frac{2(6) + 3 - 7}{2} = 4$$

This means we need to add 4 layers of zero padding, before beginning the convolutions. The resulting output will have a dimension of 7 × 7, since $\frac{7+2(4)-3}{2} + 1 = 7$. We therefore begin with the setup in Fig. 5.21.

We can then repeat the steps used in Example 5.6 to obtain the results. The reader is encouraged to complete this on his/her own.

5.2.8 Loss and optimization: Updated weights and biases

In Sections 5.2.1–5.2.2, it was discussed that the weights and biases (w, b) are parameters that are "learned" during the training process. To do so the network compares its decisions at the output layer with the labeled input data. This results in an estimation of an error. Let $\hat{y}$ represent the output decision by the network, and let y represent the true/correct label. The error estimate is referred to as the model error and is determined using a loss/cost function. There are several cost functions:

Mean absolute error (MAE):

$$loss = L(y, \hat{y}) = \frac{\sum_{i=1}^{n} |y_i - \hat{y}_i|}{n} \tag{5.14}$$

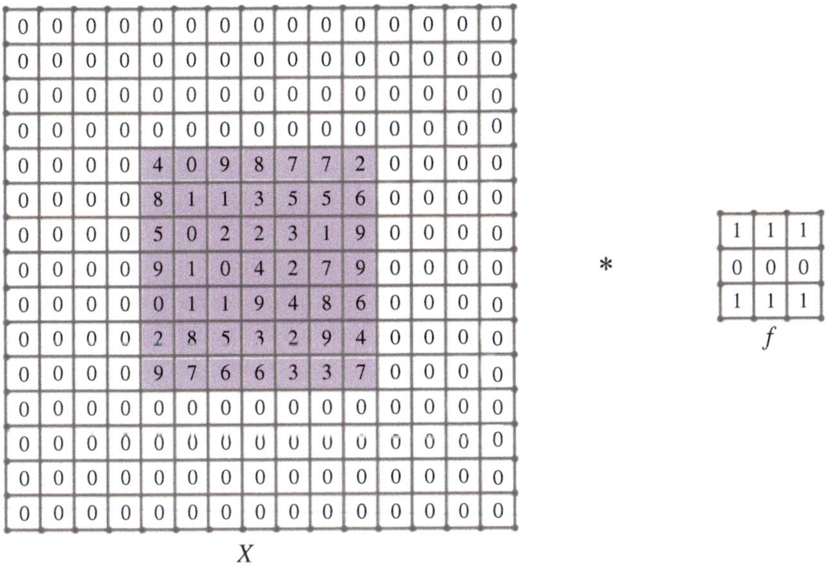

FIG. 5.21

Input padded 2-D data and 3 × 3 kernel.

Mean square error (MSE):

$$loss = L(y, \hat{y}) = \frac{\sum_{i=1}^{n} (y_i \quad \hat{y}_i)^2}{n} \tag{5.15}$$

Binary cross entropy loss:

$$loss = L(y, \hat{y}) = \frac{1}{n} \sum_{i=1}^{n} -y_i \log(\hat{y}_i) - (1 - y_i) \log(1 - \hat{y}_i) \tag{5.16}$$

Binary cross entropy loss is used for binary classification networks.

There are other loss functions used in deep learning, but the aforementioned are among the most commonly used. The general aim of the network is to minimize the total loss. In the case of binary cross entropy, the aim is to maximize the cost function since this minimizes the loss.

5.2.9 Optimization algorithms

When the loss is determined, the next step is to update the weights and bias. This is the actual "learning" process, where the network fine-tunes the weights, thus minimizing the loss. This is done through the use of several optimization algorithms.

5.2.9.1 Minibatch gradient descent and stochastic gradient descent (SGD)

The input to a neural network can be a very large dataset such as 10 million or even 1 billion. Typically, vectorization is used to accelerate training [7]. However, for very large datasets, vectorization may not suffice in terms of speed. For example, if m = 15,000,000, where m represents the size of the dataset or the number of training examples. In such a case, it is better to split the data into "minibatches" of, for example, 5000, then compute forward and backward propagations on each dataset iteratively (in a loop).

If the minibatch size is 1, then the process is called stochastic gradient descent.

The cost function for minibatch gradient descent has a general downward slope as for a regular batch gradient descent; however, there is noise in the function plot. Typically, minibatch sizes that are powers of 2, that is, 2^n is used. Therefore good minibatch sizes are 64, 128, 256, 512, and 1024.

5.2.9.2 Gradient descent with momentum

Initially,

$$v_{dw} = 0, \; v_{db} = 0$$

$$v_{dw} = \beta v_{dw} + (1-\beta)dw \tag{5.17}$$

$$v_{db} = \beta v_{db} + (1-\beta)db \tag{5.18}$$

Then update the weights and biases,

$$w = w - \alpha v_{dw} \tag{5.19}$$

$$b = b - \alpha v_{db} \tag{5.20}$$

The variables α, β are called hyperparameters since they are parameters whose values are set before training begins, as opposed to regular parameters (such as w, b) whose values are learned during the training. The most commonly used value of β is 0.9.

5.2.9.3 Root mean square prop (RMSprop)

$$v_{dw} = \beta_2 v_{dw} + (1-\beta_2)dw^2 \tag{5.21}$$

$$v_{db} = \beta_2 v_{db} + (1-\beta_2)db^2 \tag{5.22}$$

The squares dw^2, db^2 are element-wise computations.

Then, we update the weights and biases using

$$w = w - \frac{\alpha dw}{\sqrt{v_{dw} + \varepsilon}} \tag{5.23}$$

$$b = b - \frac{\alpha db}{\sqrt{v_{db} + \varepsilon}} \tag{5.24}$$

The parameter *db* is relatively large compared with *dw*, so *vdb* is relatively large compared with *vdw*. As a result, *w* will be updated quickly, while b will be updated slowly; see Eqs. (5.23)–(5.24). Hence, gradient descent is accelerated more in the *w* direction than in the *b* direction. The variable ε is a small number included to prevent division by zero. Typically, $\varepsilon = 10^{-8}$.

5.2.9.4 Adam optimization (adaptive moment estimation)

This algorithm combines gradient descent with momentum and RMS prop. As usual, we initialize the key variables as zeros:

$$V_{dw} = 0,\ V_{db} = 0;\quad S_{dw} = 0,\quad S_{db} = 0$$

Then, we update them using the familiar formulae:

$$Vdw = \beta_1 Vdw + (1 - \beta_1)dw \tag{5.25}$$

$$Vdb = \beta_1 Vdb + (1 - \beta_1)db \tag{5.26}$$

Typically,

$$\beta_1 = 0.9;\ \beta_2 = 0.999;\ \varepsilon = 10^{-8}$$

$$Sdw = \beta_2 Sdw + (1 - \beta_2)dw^2 \tag{5.27}$$

$$Sdb = \beta_2 Sdb + (1 - \beta_2)db^2 \tag{5.28}$$

Bias correction is then used to improve the accuracy of the algorithm [8]:

$$V_{dw}^{corrected} = \frac{V_{dw}}{1 - \beta_1{}^t} \quad V_{db}^{corrected} = \frac{V_{db}}{1 - \beta_1{}^t} \tag{5.29}$$

$$S_{dw}^{corrected} = \frac{S_{dw}}{1 - \beta_2{}^t} \quad S_{db}^{corrected} = \frac{S_{db}}{1 - \beta_2{}^t} \tag{5.30}$$

Finally, we update the weights and biases

$$w := w - \frac{\alpha V_{dw}^{corrected}}{\sqrt{S_{dw}^{corrected}} + \varepsilon} \qquad b := b - \frac{\alpha V_{db}^{corrected}}{\sqrt{S_{db}^{corrected}} + \varepsilon} \tag{5.31}$$

Regardless of which optimization technique is used, learning rate decay may be employed to accelerate training. Let one epoch equals one training pass through the data, then

$$\alpha = \frac{1}{1 + kt}\alpha_0 \tag{5.32}$$

where $\alpha_0 =$ *initial learning rate*, $k =$ *decay rate*, $t =$ *epoch number*.

For a more detailed overview on these optimization algorithms, the reader is encouraged to refer to [8, 9].

5.3 TensorFlow and keras for deep convolutional neural networks

5.3.1 Deep learning frameworks

The main goal of this chapter is to present the practical aspects of developing deep neural network software systems. The application of deep learning to electroencephalogram (EEG) data is of particular interest. Inevitably the chapter delves into the theoretical aspects of neural networks and, more specifically, deep convolutional neural networks. This allows the software developer to understand the elements included in a deep learning framework.

A deep learning framework is a software library of classes and functions particularly suited/optimized for the development, training and testing of deep neural networks, and other machine learning algorithms. There are several such frameworks, for example, TensorFlow, Pytorch, Keras, Swift ML, and MATLAB deep learning toolbox. Two of the most popular frameworks are TensorFlow (by Google) and Keras, a Python-based framework. Keras is such an easy library to use, that TensorFlow is now shipped with Keras included. TensorFlow may be used with Python, C++ or even JavaScript. Section 5.5 provides a brief overview of the use of TensorFlow with Keras. This overview is not meant to be exhaustive, as the laboratories presented in the appendix.

As aforementioned a deep learning software developer should understand the theory associated with the components used in a framework. Therefore this section ends with a breakdown of how to set up a deep learning project and prepare the data, regularization methods such as data augmentation, normalization of data, and other methods used to accelerate training.

5.3.2 Setting up a deep learning application

To train a neural network, the first step is to split the dataset into three parts: train-set, dev-set, and test-set, that is, train | test | split. The train dataset provides the examples from which the network can learn, while dev-set is used to rank trained models to choose the best model. The test-set is used to evaluate a chosen model to determine its accuracy. If the dataset is large, such as 1,000,000, the split can be similar to 98% | 1% | 1%. Otherwise, one rule of thumb may be to use a split such as 70% | 15% | 15%. Generally the test-set is not an absolute necessity, but the dev and test-sets must come from the same distribution.

When evaluating the model, we can compare its performance with Bayes error, which is the lowest possible error rate for any classifier. In the case of image classification for example, we can assume that human error (eye test) is Bayes error. Then, assume that a classification network is used to classify cancer images versus noncancer images. If a human doctor generally is wrong approximately 1% of the time, then we can say Bayes error is 1% for this task. Now, if the training set error = 7% and dev-set error = 11%, then, there is a bias as measured by the gap between Bayes error and the training error. Therefore the focus should be on trying to reduce the bias. However, if Bayes error is 6% and the training set error is 6.7%, while the dev-set error is 9.5%, then there is a variance as measured by the gap between the training and dev-set errors. The focus should therefore be on trying to reduce the variance.

5.3.3 Bias versus variance

In the previous section, we discussed how to determine whether we have an avoidable bias issue with our datasets or a variance issue. If any of these two problems are identified, the aim should be to reduce or eliminate the problem. As a result the first step is to compare our Bayes error with our training set. Any disparity between the two is an indication of the presence of avoidable bias. We also compare the dev and test-sets to determine the level of variance. More specifically, if the error of the model on the training set is high, there is high bias, and if the error on the dev-set is much higher than the error on the training set, there is high variance (overfitting) How are these problems solved?

In the case of high bias, try one of the following:

- Use a bigger neural network.
- Increase the training time.
- Try a different neural network architecture.

In the case of high variance, try one of the following:

- Add more data.
- Regularization; see Section 5.3.4.
- Maybe try different neural network architecture.

Undergoing this process successfully results in a reduction of bias-variance tradeoff, hence increases the effectiveness of the model.

5.3.4 Regularization

As indicated in the Section 5.3.3, to combat the high variance issue (or overfitting), regularization may be employed. Regularization, in deep learning, is a technique used to modify the learning algorithm so that it generalizes better. There are several regularization methods used in deep learning. The succeeding text is a discussion of a few.

5.3.4.1 L_2 regularization

Firstly, let $\lambda = \textit{regularization parameter}$.

Then the L_2 norm of w is given as

$$L_2 - \text{norm} = \|w\|_2^2 = \sqrt{\sum_{j=1}^{n_x} w_j^2} \tag{5.33}$$

So,

$$(L_2\,\text{norm})^2 = \|w\|_2^2 = \sum_{j=1}^{n_x} w_j^2 = w^T w \tag{5.34}$$

Now recall that for logistic regression, the cost function is

$$J(w,b) = \frac{1}{m}\sum_{i=1}^{m} L\left(\acute{y}^{(i)}, y^{(i)}\right) \tag{5.35}$$

Finally, combining Eq. (5.34) with this cost function and the regularization parameter results in

$$J(w,b) = \frac{1}{m}\sum_{i=1}^{m} L\left(\acute{y}^{(i)}, y^{(i)}\right) + \frac{\lambda}{2m}\|w\|_2^2 \tag{5.36}$$

Eq. (5.36) represents L2 regularization applied to a logistic regression model.

5.3.4.2 Dropout regularization

Dropout regularization reduces the size of the neural network. A probability vector is used to randomly eliminate nodes in a hidden layer of the neural network. The algorithms works like this:

- Choose a probability value k_p such that $0 < k_p < 1$.
- For a hidden layer n in the network, create a new vector p with the same dimensions as the layer.
- Populate this new vector with 0's and 1's only, where each entry is chosen based on k_p, that is, generate 0 or 1 randomly with probability $= k_p$.
- Finally, perform an element-wise multiplication between the layer and this new vector p. This will result in some nodes in the layer being eliminated and some remaining.

Dropout should be used only on the training set, not on the test set. This is due to the fact that the test set is used as a proxy for a previously unseen dataset for the purposes of evaluating the trained network. Dropout should be applied in both forward and backward propagation.

5.3.5 Data augmentation

Data augmentation is most useful in situations where there is a shortage of data. If there are no enough data, the dataset can be increased by flipping images horizontally and vertically, skewing, scaling, changing contrast, and shifting horizontally and vertically. Data augmentation is especially critical when working with medical image data such as X-ray and MRI images since there are risks involved in obtaining such data.

5.3.6 Normalizing data input

Normalizing input data helps to accelerate training. The main reason is due to the fact that a three-dimensional plot of a cost function would result in a bowl-like symmetrical shape, rather than a cost function slightly skewed along one of the axes. This helps to speed up gradient descent, hence learning by the neural network. To normalize the data the input X can be replaced by

$$X = \frac{X - \mu}{\sigma^2} \tag{5.37}$$

where

$$\mu = \frac{1}{m}\sum_{i=1}^{m} X_i, \text{ is the mean and} \tag{5.38}$$

$$\sigma^2 = \sqrt{\frac{1}{m}\sum_{i=1}^{m} (x_i - \mu)^2}, \text{ is the variance} \tag{5.39}$$

This preprocessing step is applied to both the training and testing dataset.

5.4 Data collection workflow (step-by-step) with a BCI device

Section 5.3.2 discusses that the dataset used in a neural network is split into training and testing or training/validation/testing. Before this is done, however, the original data must be obtained. In the case of EEG data, a BCI device is necessary as discussed in Section 5.2. There are some challenges involved, particularly with obtaining real-time data for testing or deploying a trained neural network. This would be expounded on in Section 5.7; however, for training a neural network, obtaining the data is much less of a challenge.

Clearly the first step in obtaining EEG data is to use a BCI device. Many such devices are commercially available. In the tutorials section of the appendix and the online component of this chapter, we use the Emotiv Epoc+ BCI headset. In the case of the Emotiv Epoc+ and generally for all commercially available BCI devices, the EEG data may be downloaded as tabular data in excel, csv or similar format. In the tutorials, we demonstrate how to use the python library called Pandas to open such file types and extract data directly into useful data formats for easy graphical analysis and implementation in TensorFlow and Keras.

Here is a code snippet shown in Fig. 5.22.

To declare our intension to use the various python libraries, we use the keyword "import" as seen in Fig. 5.22. The *os* library allows us to manipulate the file/folder structure to perform such operations as listing folders and files. As aforementioned, *Pandas* is imported for easily accessing tabular data in excel, csv files, zip, JSON, txt,

```
%matplotlib inline

import os

import pandas as pd

import numpy as pd
```

FIG. 5.22

Python imports.

html, images, etc. The *Numpy* library is extremely critical as it allows for easy implementation of the numerous linear algebra functions useful with matrix-like data.

The last line in the code snippet in Fig. 5.23 creates a list (array) of all the files in the "Forward" folder. This list is called "flocation."

```
#paths for original data

location = "NEW DATA/Forward"

locationl = "NEW DATA/left"

locationr = "NEW DATA/right"

locations = "NEW DATA/stop"

flocation = os.listdir("NEW DATA/Forward")
```

FIG. 5.23

Location data lists in Python.

The code snippet in Fig. 5.24 opens the excel/csv file at the beginning of the list. These data are immediately in a format easily manipulated with *Numpy*.

```
data1 = pd.read_csv(os.path.join(locationf, flocation[0]))
```

FIG. 5.24

Opening CSV data file in Python.

There are two different modes of data extraction from a commercial BCI device, depending on the policies or licenses of the supplying company. These two modes are "raw EEG data" and "fast Fourier transform (FFT) data."

The tutorials show how to transform the former raw data into FFT data with Python in situations where only raw data are available. Before doing so, however, the following discussion demonstrates the issues with attempting to use raw EEG data in deep learning. At this point the data collection workflow is complete.

5.5 Preprocessing and training using tensorflow and keras

After training data are collected, there are usually some preprocessing steps done before final input into a neural network. The tutorials provide detailed steps to implement preprocessing on the input EEG data. The initial tabular data are similar to the data in Fig. 5.25.

Firstly the data are split into groups of equal rows, where each member of the group represents t seconds of input data. This depends on the sampling rate of the BCI device. In the previous data snippet shown in Fig. 5.25, for example, eight rows of data represented 1s of data. The detailed procedure to determine this is shown in the tutorials section of the appendix. Each eight rows of data now becomes a new data example X_i and is implemented as an two-dimensional array using the *OpenCV* library or any other image data processing library such as *Matplotlib*. Each 2-D array therefore has dimensions of 8×65, as there are 65 columns in the input data.

The next step is to normalize the data using Eq. (5.37). As explained, this speeds up training as the cost function $J(w, b)$ is more symmetrical.

The typical next step is to choose only one channel of the 2-D data, which is in RGB format. Typically, this is done with a code snippet such as shown in Fig. 5.26.

This is not an absolute necessity if computational resources are readily available. In the tutorials, we will test the effects of both of these strategies in the case of EEG data.

Now that the data is ready for training, we implement a split into training and testing data. This may be done using another Python library known as *scikit-learn*, and the following sample code snippet is shown in Fig. 5.27.

In the first line the labels and input data are coupled as tuples, which is an immutable data type in python similar to the coordinate system used in the Cartesian system. The function *train_test_split* is a function used to split the data while maintaining high data integrity. In this example the split is 80% training data and 20% test/validation data, using the parameter and value, *test_size = 0.2*. At this point the data are ready for training. The code, shown in Fig. 5.28, implements the training of the neural network.

The function call model.fit is used, where the training data, correct labels, batch size, number of epochs, and the testing/validation data are the input parameters. The *batch-size* is simply the amount of input data that should be passed through the network at a time. The *epochs* variable is an indication of how many iterations of complete training should be done. We will investigate the effects of this in the tutorials.

	AF3	F7	F3	FC5	T7	P7	O1	O2	P8	T8	FC6	
0	4412.307617	4411.281738	4391.281738	4408.717773	4191.764922	4175.384277	4403.076660	4179.487305	4181.025391	4183.589844	4433.333008	4457.9
1	4397.948730	4413.846191	4382.051270	4401.538574	4192.307617	4173.333008	4388.717773	4174.358887	4180.512695	4183.589844	4406.666504	4449.2
2	4391.794922	4403.076650	4385.127930	4397.948730	4195.384277	4178.461426	4377.435547	4177.948730	4178.974121	4183.589844	4423.076660	4450.7
3	4395.897461	4403.076650	4383.589844	4398.974121	4194.358887	4178.974121	4368.717773	4173.333008	4180.000000	4183.589844	4424.102539	4449.7
4	4397.948730	4404.615234	4384.615234	4393.333008	4195.897461	4184.615234	4371.281738	4175.897451	4182.563955	4183.589844	4387.179199	4446.6
5	4403.076560	4396.922852	4384.615234	4389.743652	4194.871582	4177.948730	4390.769043	4177.436035	4181.538574	4183.589844	4407.179199	4448.2
6	4404.615234	4392.307617	4385.641113	4391.794922	4194.358887	4175.384277	4381.538574	1475.384277	4180.512695	4183.589844	4442.051270	4447.1
7	4396.922852	4998.974121	4386.153809	4400.512695	4194.358887	4181.538574	4360.000000	4178.461426	4182.051270	4183.589844	4433.846191	4443.5
8	4391.281738	4401.025391	4377.948730	4403.076660	4192.307617	4177.436035	4376.410156	4173.333008	4180.000000	4183.589844	4411.794922	4443.5
9	4391.794922	4391.794922	4380.000000	4389.230469	4197.435035	4182.051270	4391.794922	4177.436035	4180.512695	4183.589844	4388.205078	4446.1

FIG. 5.25

Sample EEG data.

```
X = X[:, :, 0]
```

FIG. 5.26

Choosing one channel of data.

```
(X, y) = (train_data[0], train_data[1])

x_train, x_test, y_train, y_test = train_test_split(X, y, test_size = 0.2, random_state =4)
```

FIG. 5.27

Train_test_split function in Python with scikit-learn.

```
model.fit(x_train, y_train,

          batch_size = batch_size,

          epochs = epochs,

          verbose = 1,

          validation_data = (x_test, y_test))

score = model.evaluate(x_test, y_test, verbose = 0)

print('Test loss: ', score[0])

print('Test Accuracy: ', score[1])
```

FIG. 5.28

Code to begin training of neural network.

5.6 Deployment and real-time applications with embedded systems

In Section 5.5, we discussed preprocessing and training. At this point, when training is complete, we need to utilize the neural network in an application. In the tutorials, we discuss in detail the process of applying a deep convolutional neural network to EEG data and applying this network to control a model robot wheelchair.

To use a trained neural network, we need to be able to save the created model (including the model architecture) and the updated final weights. The code snippet in Fig. 5.29 is an example of how to save a model and its weights using Python, TensorFlow and Keras.

```
save_model_path = 'weights.hdf5'

cp = tf.keras.callbacks.ModelCheckpoint(filepath = save_model_path, monitor='val_dice_loss',

save_best_only=True, verbose=1)
```

FIG. 5.29

Saving trained model and associated weights.

The code snippet in Fig. 5.30 can then be used to load the saved model and weights in a new environment.

```
#Alternatively, load the weights directly: model.load_weights(save_model_path)

model = models.load_model(save_model_path, custom_objects = {'bce_dice_loss': bce_dice_loss, 'dice_loss':

dice_loss})
```

FIG. 5.30

Loading previously saved models.

We demonstrate this in the tutorials, where we load the saved weights in Ubuntu Mate and/or Raspbian OS running on a Raspberry Pi 3B+ quad core board. The output of the neural network will be used as input to an Arduino Mega microcontroller that in turn will control the DC motors onboard the wheel chair. The communication between the Raspberry Pi computer and the Arduino Board will be in real time using the Robot Operating Systems (ROS). A brief introduction to ROS will be provided in the tutorial section.

5.7 Conclusion, challenges and future research

Brain-computer interface (BCI) devices are communication systems that provide a direct communication pathway between brain activity signals and an external computer or other devices. This chapter introduced the fundamentals of deep convolutional neural networks (DCNNs) and the deployment of TensorFlow and Keras. This chapter investigated the process of obtaining electroencephalogram (EEG) data in real time using a BCI device. The data are already converted into the frequency domain using the fast Fourier transform (FFT) algorithm. The python programming language and some of its associated scientific and numeric libraries are then used to preprocess the data. The popular TensorFlow and Keras machine learning libraries are used to train a convolutional neural network to classify the EEG data into four different commands: forward, left, right, and stop. Finally the trained neural network is used with embedded systems to control a robotic car/wheelchair. The use of BCI devices to control robotic systems has excellent potential in improving living conditions for paraplegics using wheel chairs; there are many other situations in which this technology would be applicable in an advantageous manner. Despite this, there are challenges involved with using these devices in applications. The main problem is the lack of access to open source, reliable BCI devices. The device used in the tutorials, for instance, is a commercial device whose API is not freely available. This greatly limits the rate of development and scientific research. There is therefore a great need for development of BCI devices with open source, easy to use APIs.

Another problem that is somewhat linked to the first problem is the extent to which an application can be considered real time. Consider the situation where EEG signals from the brain are processed using a neural network and used to make the next decision in driving a car. If the car is moving at a high speed, it is necessary to process every 1 s piece of data in microsecond or milliseconds so as to have effective control of the vehicle. This is extremely difficult with proprietary, complex APIs, and computational power available to most developers and researchers.

Appendix A. Working with Pandas

Pandas is a Python library that facilitates data manipulation, including reading and writing excel/csv files. This chapter deals with EEG data collected and stored from a BCI device. These data are in .csv format. Using pandas the data can easily be opened and manipulated as shown in Fig. A.1.

```
import pandas as pd

#paths for original data locationf = "NEW DATA/Forward"

data1 = pd.read_csv(os.path.join(locationf,flocation[0]))
```

FIG. A.1

Reading csv file with python Pandas.

When working with EEG data, all the columns of the data may not be required. In such a case, Pandas simplifies the process of dropping columns thud creating a new table. In Fig. A.2 below the columns to be dropped are inserted into a python list.

```
dropbpColumns = ["T8_THETA","T8_ALPHA","T8_LOW_BETA","T8_HIGH_BETA","T8_GA
MMA","CQ_AF3","CQ_F7","CQ_F3","CQ_FC5","CQ_T7",
             "CQ_P7","CQ_O1","CQ_O2","CQ_P8","CQ_T8","CQ_FC6","CQ_F4","CQ
_F8","CQ_AF4"]
```

FIG. A.2

Dropping specific columns from Pandas dataframe.

In Fig. A.3 a path to save the csv file after columns has been dropped is specified. In the following line the csv file is opened.

```
#path to store .bp files
fbpPath = "NEW DATA/bp/forward"

#forward bp files
for file in flocation:
    if '.bp' in file:
        temp = pd.read_csv(os.path.join(locationf,file))
        temp = temp.drop(axis = 1,labels=dropbpColumns)
        pd.DataFrame.to_csv(temp,path_or_buf=os.path.join(fbpPath,file))
```

FIG. A.3

Saving csv file with Pandas.

In Fig. A.4, empty python lists are created to store the previously saved data (after columns were dropped) into forward, left, right, and stop lists. The forward data, for example, were created by a user wearing an EEG headset and looking and concentrating on a video or model of a car driving forward. When the car comes at a corner where it begins to turn left, the user concentrates on the idea that the vehicle needs to turn left.

```
temp = pd.read_csv(os.path.join(locationf, file)).
```

The columns to be dropped is then provided to the pandas drop function

```
temp = temp.drop(axis = 1,labels=dropbpColumns).
```

Finally, the new data is saved to a file:

```
pd.DataFrame.to_csv(temp,path_or_buf=os.path.join(fbpPath,file)).
```

```
#collecting the stored .bp files into list of pandas dataframes
forward = []
left = []
right = []
stop = []
```

FIG. A.4

Creating empty lists.

In Fig. A.5 the files are stored in the correct python lists.

```
#forward
for file in os.listdir(fbpPath):
    data = pd.read_csv(os.path.join(fbpPath,file))
    forward.append(data)
    #left
for file in os.listdir(lbpPath):
    data = pd.read_csv(os.path.join(lbpPath,file))
    left.append(data)

#right
for file in os.listdir(rbpPath):
    data = pd.read_csv(os.path.join(rbpPath,file))
    right.append(data)
#stop
for file in os.listdir(sbpPath):
    data = pd.read_csv(os.path.join(sbpPath,file))
    stop.append(data)
```

FIG. A.5

Appending files to appropriate python lists.

The code in Fig. A.6 is used to plot a 1 s sample of data from each category (forward, stop, etc.) to see if there are any discernable differences. The plots are displayed in Fig. A.7.

```
yf = []
jf = random.randrange(lf)
yl = []
jl = random.randrange(ll)
yr = []
jr = random.randrange(lr)
ys = []
js = random.randrange(ls)

for i in range(2,len(forward[jf].iloc[2])):
   temp = forward[jf].iloc[0:,i]
   yf.append(temp)

for i in range(2,len(left[jl].iloc[2])):
   temp = left[jl].iloc[0:,i]
   yl.append(temp)

for i in range(2,len(right[jr].iloc[2])):
   temp = right[jr].iloc[0:,i]
   yr.append(temp)
```

```
for i in range(2,len(stop[js].iloc[2])):
   temp = stop[js].iloc[0:,i]
   ys.append(temp)

 fg = plt.figure(1,figsize=(12,4))
a = random.randrange(len(yf))
print(a)
start = a
end = a+8
t = (end-start)/8
plt.subplot(1,4,1), plt.title("Forward #"+str(jf)+" t = "+str(t)+"s")
for i in range(0, len(yf)):
   plt.plot(yf[i][start:end+1])

plt.subplot(1,4,2), plt.title("Left"+str(jl)+" t = "+str(t)+"s")
for i in range(0, len(yl)):
   plt.plot(yl[i][start:end+1])

plt.subplot(1,4,3), plt.title("Right"+str(jr)+" t = "+str(t)+"s")
for i in range(0, len(yr)):
   plt.plot(yr[i][start:end+1])

plt.subplot(1,4,4), plt.title("Stop"+str(js)+" t = "+str(t)+"s")
for i in range(0, len(ys)):
   plt.plot(ys[i][start:end+1])
plt.subplots_adjust(top=0.92, bottom=0.08, left=0.0, right=1.0, hspace=0.25, wspace=0.35)
```

FIG. A.6

Collecting 1 s sample of EEG data collected.

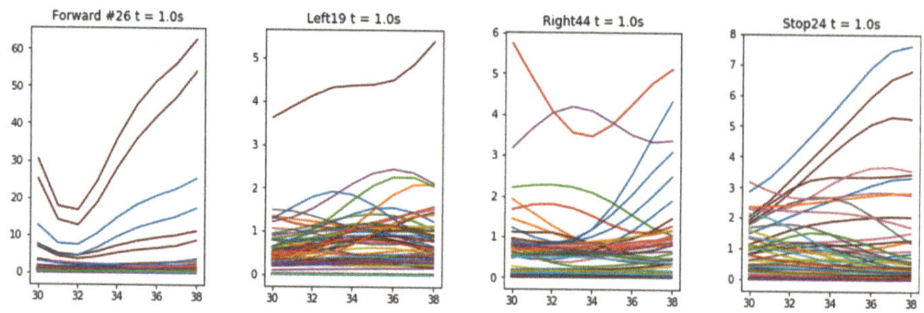

FIG. A.7

One second sample of EEG data collected.

In Fig. A.8 the data for *forward* classification are stored in a new list in 1s snippets. Each eight rows of the Pandas EEG data represented 1 second; hence the data were inserted eight rows at a time as shown in the figure. This is repeated for the other three classifications in Fig. A.9.

```
fdata = []

ldata = []

rdata = []

sdata = []

#collecting 1s samples from forward data

for data in forward:
    f = data
    for a in range(0,len(f)-4,4):
        temp = f.iloc[a:a+8,2:]
        if(len(temp) == 8):
            fdata.append(temp)
```

FIG. A.8

Storing data classified as *forward* in new list.

In Fig. A.10 the forward and stop data are appended for binary classification as a convolutional neural network may be used to learn *forward* and *stop* classes.

The code in Fig. A.11 shows a sample of the data. This table is displayed in Fig. A.12.

The code in Fig. A.13 converts each sample of data from the xdata list into a numpy array, which can be easily fed into a Keras neural network. The new list of numpy data is labeled *npData* as shown in the figure.

The code in Fig. A.14 further prepares the data for the convolutional neural network. The numpy data array is flattened (a requirement for input into a neural network). The labels are created using 0 for forward and 1 for stop. The data are then shuffled as this helps minimize the chances of over training.

```
#collecting 1s samples from left data

for data in left:
    l = data
    for a in range(0,len(l)-4,4):
        temp =l.iloc[a:a+8,2:]
        if(len(temp) == 8):
            ldata.append(temp)

#collecting 1s samples from right data

for data in right:

  r = data

  for a in range(0,len(r)-4,4):

    temp = r.iloc[a:a+8,2:]

    if(len(temp) == 8):

      rdata.append(temp)


      #collecting 1s samples from stop data


      for data in stop:

        s = data

        for a in range(0,len(s)-4,4):

          temp = s.iloc[a:a+8,2:]

          if(len(temp) == 8):

            sdata.append(temp)
```

FIG. A.9

Saving data classified as *right*, *stop*, and *left* data in new list.

```
xdata = fdata+sdata
```

FIG. A.10

Appending *forward* and *stop* data for binary classification.

```
xdata[121]
```

FIG. A.11

Displaying sample data.

	AF3_THETA	AF3_ALPHA	AF3_LOW_BETA	AF3_HIGH_BETA	AF3_GAMMA	F7_THETA	F7_ALPHA	F7_LOW_BETA
0	2.122388	1.720011	1.036150	0.628207	0.304777	3.710562	1.296798	0.417838
1	2.466173	1.598770	0.992723	0.550330	0.334459	3.628745	1.172976	0.361870
2	2.748952	1.406699	0.961172	0.511466	0.384003	3.292173	0.934057	0.320051
3	2.880186	1.189675	0.952837	0.501126	0.445005	2.821198	0.660766	0.299580
4	2.805623	1.004101	0.986912	0.501655	0.501750	2.443549	0.444541	0.314344
5	2.492952	0.878680	1.097172	0.507607	0.537548	2.241423	0.346211	0.386926
6	2.067002	0.825647	1.298613	0.527927	0.541919	2.293460	0.390241	0.530021
7	1.929955	0.845518	1.570341	0.570294	0.516499	2.508449	0.565567	0.741838

FIG. A.12

Sample 1 s data

```
import numpy as np

length = 8
num_samples = len(xdata)
print(num_samples)

img_rows = length
img_cols = 65


npData = []
i = 0
for data in xdata:
    temp = np.array(data)
    temp = temp.reshape(img_rows,img_cols,1)
    npData.append(temp)
    i = i + 1
```

FIG. A.13

Converting data to numpy array for neural network.

```
m,n = npData[0].shape[0:2]
imnbr = len(xdata)

immatrix=array([array(im2).flatten() for im2 in npData],'f')


labels = np.ones((num_samples,),dtype = int)

labels[0:len(fdata)] = 0  #forward
labels[len(fdata):] = 1 #stop


data,Label = shuffle(immatrix,labels,random_state = 2)
train_data = [data,Label]
```

FIG. A.14

Preprocessing data for neural network.

In Fig. A.15 the data are split into two parts, 80% for training and 20% for testing. The code in Fig. A.16 is used to reshape the input data for Keras. It must be stated that at the time this code was created and tested, Keras was used. However, TensorFlow 2.0 provides a better alternative as will be presented on the website version of the tutorials.

```
from sklearn.utils import shuffle
from sklearn.model_selection import train_test_split

(X,y) = (train_data[0],train_data[1])
x_train,x_test,y_train,y_test = train_test_split(X,y,test_size = 0.2,rando
m_state = 4)
```

FIG. A.15

Splitting data into 80% train and 20% test data.

```
if K.image_data_format() == 'channels_first':
  x_train = x_train.reshape(x_train.shape[0], 1, img_rows, img_cols)
  x_test = x_test.reshape(x_test.shape[0], 1, img_rows, img_cols)
  input_shape = (1, img_rows, img_cols)
else:
  x_train = x_train.reshape(x_train.shape[0], img_rows, img_cols, 1)
  x_test = x_test.reshape(x_test.shape[0], img_rows, img_cols, 1)
  input_shape = (img_rows, img_cols, 1)

x_train = x_train.astype('float32')
x_test = x_test.astype('float32')
```

FIG. A.16

Reshaping dataset for Keras library.

The code in Fig. A.17 is used to set some hyperparameters and to convert the labels to a binary class matrices (essentially one-hot encoding).

```
batch_size = 32
num_classes = 2
epochs = 10

# convert class vectors to binary class matrices
y_train = keras.utils.to_categorical(y_train, num_classes)
y_test = keras.utils.to_categorical(y_test, num_classes)
```

FIG. A.17

One-hot encoding of target/label data.

The code in Fig. A.18 generates the neural network as a series of layer additions to a sequence. Here the Softmax activation function was used since the original experiment was to classify four different classes: forward, stop, left, and right. However, an updated version on the website uses the *sigmoid* function for binary classification in the case of two classes, that is, forward/stop or left/right.

```
model = Sequential()
model.add(Conv2D(32, kernel_size=(3, 3),
                 activation='relu',
                 input_shape=input_shape))
model.add(Conv2D(64, (3, 3), activation='relu'))
model.add(MaxPooling2D(pool_size=(2, 2)))
model.add(Dropout(0.25))
model.add(Flatten())
model.add(Dense(128, activation='relu'))
model.add(Dropout(0.5))

model.add(Dense(num_classes, activation='softmax'))

model.compile(loss=keras.losses.categorical_crossentropy,
              optimizer=keras.optimizers.Adadelta(),
              metrics=['accuracy'])

model.fit(x_train, y_train,
          batch_size=batch_size,
          epochs=epochs,
          verbose=1,
          validation_data=(x_test, y_test))
score = model.evaluate(x_test, y_test, verbose=0)
print('Test loss:', score[0])
print('Test accuracy:', score[1])
```

FIG. A.18

Sequential CNN generation with Keras.

The output of the training of the network is shown in Fig. A.19.

The code in Fig. A.20 is used to save the model and weights used in a future case.

The code in Fig. A.21 is used to load a previously saved model.

The code in Fig. A.22 creates a simple list to translate the output of the loaded network when applied to previously unseen data. If the network outputs 0, then "forward" is displayed, and if the output is 1, "stop" is displayed.

The code in Fig. A.23 is used to make predictions from EEG data in a csv file. The prediction here is not real time; however, the aim of the work is to make real-time predictions to control a robot in real time.

```
Train on 9594 samples, validate on 2399 samples Epoch 1/10 9594/9594
[==============================] - 11s 1ms/step - loss: 0.5877 - acc:
0.7456 - val_loss: 0.3075 - val_acc: 0.9004 Epoch 2/10 9594/9594
[==============================] - 2s 191us/step - loss: 0.3128 - acc:
0.8868 - val_loss: 0.1798 - val_acc: 0.9425 Epoch 3/10 9594/9594
[==============================] - 2s 191us/step - loss: 0.2374 - acc:
0.9198 - val_loss: 0.1841 - val_acc: 0.9300 Epoch 4/10 9594/9594
[==============================] - 2s 191us/step - loss: 0.2229 - acc:
0.9242 - val_loss: 0.1540 - val_acc: 0.9458 Epoch 5/10 9594/9594
[==============================] - 2s 192us/step - loss: 0.2000 - acc:
0.9333 - val_loss: 0.1487 - val_acc: 0.9491 Epoch 6/10 9594/9594
[==============================] - 2s 191us/step - loss: 0.1931 - acc:
0.9379 - val_loss: 0.1388 - val_acc: 0.9541 Epoch 7/10 9594/9594
[==============================] - 2s 189us/step - loss: 0.1832 - acc:
0.9395 - val_loss: 0.1305 - val_acc: 0.9566 Epoch 8/10 9594/9594
[==============================] - 2s 189us/step - loss: 0.1716 - acc:
0.9435 - val_loss: 0.1374 - val_acc: 0.9550 Epoch 9/10 9594/9594
[==============================] - 2s 190us/step - loss: 0.1690 - acc:
0.9465 - val_loss: 0.1330 - val_acc: 0.9633 Epoch 10/10 9594/9594
[==============================] - 2s 192us/step - loss: 0.1677 - acc:
0.9503 - val_loss: 0.1255 - val_acc: 0.9629 Test loss: 0.1254883209098225
Test accuracy: 0.9629012084891767
```

FIG. A.19

Verbose training output.

```
i = 1
# serialize model to JSON
model_json = model.to_json()
with open("models/eegbp"+str(i)+".json", "w") as json_file:
    json_file.write(model_json)
# serialize weights to HDF5
model.save_weights("weights/eegbp"+str(i)+".h5")
print("Saved model to disk")
```

FIG. A.20

Saving a trained Keras-based neural network.

```
i = 1
# later...
from keras.models import model_from_json
import time

# load json and create model
json_file = open('models/eegbp'+str(i)+'.json', 'r')
loaded_model_json = json_file.read()
json_file.close()
loaded_model = model_from_json(loaded_model_json)
# load weights into new model
loaded_model.load_weights("weights/eegbp"+str(i)+".h5")
print(".....Loaded model from disk")
```

FIG. A.21

Loaded a previously saved model.

```
yy = ["forward","stop"]
```

FIG. A.22

Proving class labels for output layer.

```
length = 8

i = random.randint(2)

pathf = "NEW DATA/bp/testData/testforward"
paths = "NEW DATA/bp/testData/teststop"

#print("length of forwards: "+str(len(os.listdir(pathf))))
#print("length of stops: "+str(len(os.listdir(paths))))
print(" i = "+str(i))

if i == 0:
    #forward
    r = random.randint(0,len(os.listdir(pathf)))
    data = pd.read_csv(os.path.join(pathf,os.listdir(pathf)[r]))
    a = random.randint(0,len(data)-8)
    data = data.iloc[a:a+8,2:]
    print("forward"+str(r))
    #print(data)


else:
    #stop
    r = random.randint(0,len(os.listdir(paths)))
    data = pd.read_csv(os.path.join(paths,os.listdir(paths)[r]))
    a = random.randint(0,len(data)-8)
    data = data.iloc[a:a+8,2:]
    print("stop"+str(r))
    #print(data)


size1 = length
size2 = 65

test = np.array(data)
print(test.shape)


x = test.reshape(1,size1,size2,1)
predictions = loaded_model.predict(x)
prediction = np.argmax(predictions)
print("I predicted: "+(yy[prediction]))
print("predictions = "+str(predictions))
```

FIG. A.23

Predicted new data from csv file using pretrained model.

References

[1] Tri, Tri, n.d. "The 5 Different Brainwave Frequencies and What They Mean", Examined Existence. https://examinedexistence.com/5-different-brainwave-frequencies-mean/. *Tri, "The 5 Different Brainwave Frequencies and What They Mean", Examined Existence. https://examinedexistence.com/5-different-brainwave-frequencies-mean/.* [Online]

[2] BCI2000, A general-purpose brain-computer interface (BCI) system, G. Schalk, D. J. McFarland, T. Hinterberger, N. Birbaumer, and J.R. Wolpaw. s.l.: I.E.E.E. Trans. Biomed. Eng., 2004. Vol. 51, pp. 1034–1043. 1300799.

[3] L.V. Fausett, Fundamentals of Neural Networks Architectures, Algorithms and Applications, (1994).

[4] H. Marting, Neural Network Design, second ed., (2014).

[5] G. Ian, C. Aaraon, Deep Learning.

[6] Convolutional Neural Networks (Convnets), Stanford University. [Online], http://cs231n.github.io/convolutional-networks/.

[7] On Vectorization of Deep Convolutional Neural Networks for Vision Tasks, AAAI. R. Jimmy, and X. Liu. 2015. AAAI.

[8] Generating Sequences with Recurrent Neural Networks. Alex, G. Toronto: s.n., 2014.

[9] R. Sebastian, An overview of gradient descent optimization algorithms, Dublin: s.n. June 2017.

CHAPTER

Fuzzy logic in medicine

6

Dr. Dilber Uzun Ozsahin[a,b], Dr. Berna Uzun[b,c], Dr. Ilker Ozsahin[a,b], Mubarak Taiwo Mustapha[a,b], and Musa Sani Musa[a]

[a]*Department of Biomedical Engineering, Faculty of Engineering, Near East University, Nicosia, Northern Cyprus, Turkey* [b]*DESAM Institute, Near East University, Nicosia, Northern Cyprus, Turkey* [c]*Department of Mathematics, Near East University, Nicosia, Northern Cyprus, Turkey*

6.1 Introduction to fuzzy logic

Fuzzy logic is a technique that studies reasoning systems in which the notions of truth and falsehood are considered in a graded fashion. Fuzzy logic analyzes the vagueness in natural language and several other application domains. Fuzzy logic is a soft-computing technique that tolerates suboptimality and vagueness, thereby producing very good solutions [1]. It was originally introduced by a professor of computer science named Lotfi A. Zadeh [2–4]. Essentially, fuzzy logic enables transitional values to be characterized between evaluations such as high or low, yes or no, and true or false. Ideas such as very quick or relatively tall can be handled by computers and defined mathematically so as to implement an increasing humanlike perspective in the programming of PCs [5].

Conventional thoughts of set membership that have their origin in the ancient Greek way of thinking are in contrast to fuzzy logic. In an attempt by Aristotle and other philosophers who came before him, a concise theory of logic and later mathematics was postulated called the "laws of thought" [6]. The "law of excluded middle" expresses that each suggestion should be either true or false. Parmenides suggested the original interpretation of this law (about 400 BC), but philosophers like Heraclitus and Plato protested against the law. Heraclitus suggested that things could be either true or not true. The framework that is now called fuzzy logic was established by Plato. Although other recent philosophers such as Hegel, Marx, and Engels objected to that, fuzzy logic is a Boolean logic extension. It is based on the mathematical theory of fuzzy sets.

Advantages of fuzzy logic systems [7]:

- Simple in structure and easily understandable.
- Have broad applications in commercial and practical use.
- Present the only acceptable reasoning.
- Solve uncertainty problems in various fields of study.

Biomedical Signal Processing and Artificial Intelligence in Healthcare. https://doi.org/10.1016/B978-0-12-818946-7.00006-8

- No specific input is needed.
- Modification and adjustment are possible.
- It gives the best answer to a complex problem.

Disadvantages [7]:

- May not be widely accepted due to certain inaccuracies in the system that requires assumption in obtaining the final results.
- Lack capacity when compared with machine learning.
- Extensive testing and hardware are required for validation and verification of the system.
- Some tasks may be difficult.

6.2 Fuzzy sets

A fuzzy set is an expansion of standard sets and can be comprehended as a membership degree of the set. It permits differential membership in the set [2]. This is possible because it contains an element with varying degrees of set membership. Standard sets incorporate values of 0 or 1, whereas a fuzzy set incorporates value in the range of 0–1.

6.2.1 The mathematical definition of fuzzy sets

A fuzzy set $\tilde{A}$ in IR is a set of ordered pairs:

$$\tilde{A} = \{(x, \mu_{\tilde{A}}(x)) \mid x \in IR\} \tag{6.1}$$

where $\mu_{\tilde{A}} : IR \rightarrow [0, 1]$ and $\mu_{\tilde{A}}(x)$ is called the membership function for the fuzzy set [8].

6.2.2 Representation of fuzzy sets

The fuzzy set can be described in discrete and continuous cases:

➢ *First Case*

where "U" is discrete and finite:

$$\tilde{A} = \left\{ \frac{\mu_{\tilde{A}}(x_1)}{x_1} + \frac{\mu_{\tilde{A}}(x_2)}{x_2} + \frac{\mu_{\tilde{A}}(x_3)}{x_3} + \ldots \right\} = \sum_{i=1}^{n} \frac{\mu_{\tilde{A}}(x_i)}{x_i} \tag{6.2}$$

➢ *Second Case*

where "U" is continuous and infinite:

$$\tilde{A} = \left\{ \int \frac{\mu_{\tilde{A}}(x)}{x} \right\} \tag{6.3}$$

As shown earlier the collection of each element is represented by the summation of the symbol, where U is the universe of information.

6.2.3 Basic operations on fuzzy sets

The following relations express the union, intersection, and complement operation on fuzzy sets.

(a) Union:

$$\mu_{\tilde{A}\cup\tilde{B}}(x)=\mu_{\tilde{A}}\vee\mu_{\tilde{B}},\forall x\in U \tag{6.4}$$

$\vee$ denotes the "max" operation (Fig. 6.1).

➢ Intersection:

$$\mu_{\tilde{A}\cap\tilde{B}}(x)=\mu_{\tilde{A}}\wedge\mu_{\tilde{B}},\forall x\in U \tag{6.5}$$

$\wedge$ denotes the "min" operation (Fig. 6.2).

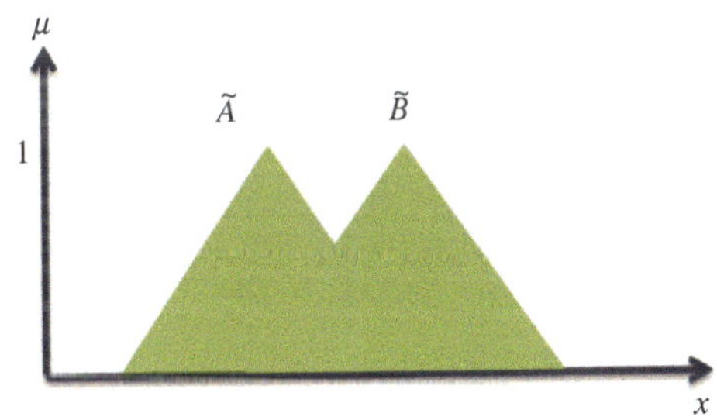

FIG. 6.1

The union of the fuzzy sets.

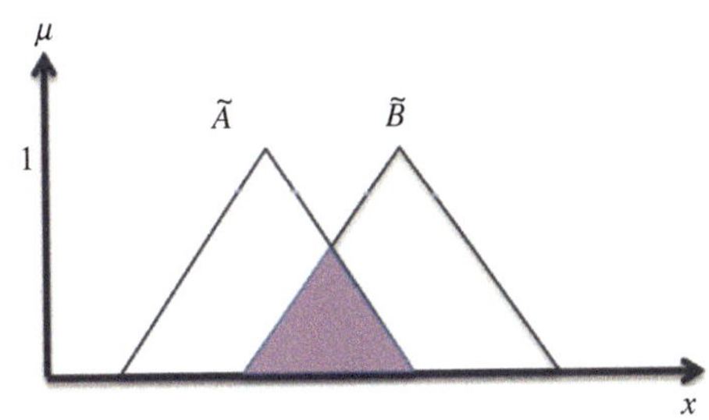

FIG. 6.2

The intersection of the fuzzy sets.

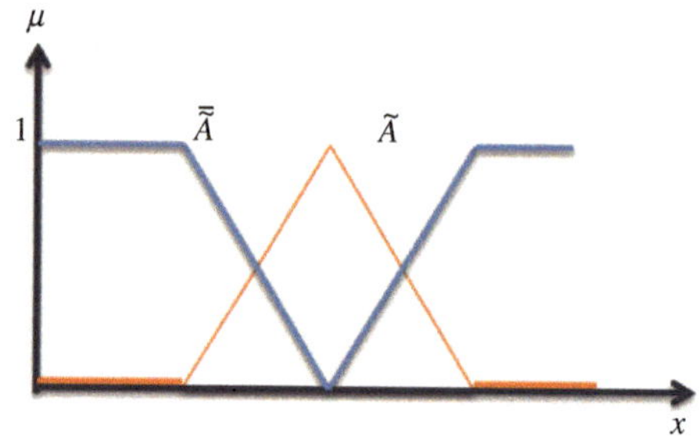

FIG. 6.3

The complement of a fuzzy set.

(b) Complement (Fig. 6.3):

$$\mu'_{(\tilde{A})}(x) = 1 - \mu_{\tilde{A}}(x) \tag{6.6}$$

There may be some cases where

$$\tilde{A} \cap \tilde{A}' \neq 0 \tag{6.7}$$

6.2.4 Properties of fuzzy sets

The main properties of the fuzzy set can be described as follows:

(a) Commutative property: This involves fuzzy set $\tilde{A}$ and $\tilde{B}$ and states that

$$\tilde{A} \cup \tilde{B} = \tilde{B} \cup \tilde{A} \tag{6.8}$$

$$\tilde{A} \cap \tilde{B} = \tilde{B} \cap \tilde{A} \tag{6.9}$$

(b) Associative property: This involves fuzzy sets $\tilde{A}$, $\tilde{B}$, and $\tilde{C}$ and states that

$$\tilde{A} \cup \left(\tilde{B} \cup \tilde{C}\right) = \left(\tilde{A} \cup \tilde{B}\right) \cup \tilde{C} \tag{6.10}$$

$$\tilde{A} \cap \left(\tilde{B} \cap \tilde{C}\right) = \left(\tilde{A} \cap \tilde{B}\right) \cap \tilde{C} \tag{6.11}$$

(c) Distributive property: This involves fuzzy sets $\tilde{A}$, $\tilde{B}$, and $\tilde{C}$ and states that

$$\tilde{A} \cup \left(\tilde{B} \cap \tilde{C}\right) = \left(\tilde{A} \cup \tilde{B}\right) \cap \left(\tilde{A} \cup \tilde{C}\right) \tag{6.12}$$

$$\tilde{A} \cap \left(\tilde{B} \cup \tilde{C}\right) = \left(\tilde{A} \cap \tilde{B}\right) \cup \left(\tilde{A} \cap \tilde{C}\right) \tag{6.13}$$

(d) Idempotent property: Provided there is a given fuzzy set $\tilde{A}$, it can be stated that

$$\tilde{A} \cup \tilde{A} = \tilde{A} \tag{6.14}$$

$$\tilde{A} = \tilde{A} \cap \tilde{A} \tag{6.15}$$

(e) Identity property: For a given fuzzy set $\tilde{A}$ and a universal set U, it can be stated that:

$$\tilde{A} = \tilde{A} \cup \emptyset \tag{6.16}$$

$$\emptyset = \tilde{A} \cap \emptyset \tag{6.17}$$

$$A = \tilde{A} \cap \mathrm{U} \tag{6.18}$$

$$\mathrm{U} = \tilde{A} \cup \mathrm{U} \tag{6.19}$$

(f) Transitive property: Provided there are fuzzy sets $\tilde{A}$, $\tilde{B}$, and $\tilde{C}$, the property states that

$$\text{If } \tilde{A} \subseteq \tilde{B} \text{ and } \tilde{B} \subseteq \tilde{C} \text{ then } \tilde{A} \subseteq \tilde{C} \tag{6.20}$$

(g) Involution property: Provided there is a fuzzy set $\tilde{A}$, it can be stated that

$$\overline{\overline{\tilde{A}}} = \tilde{A} \tag{6.21}$$

(h) De Morgan's law: This law plays a significant role in demonstrating redundancies and logical inconsistency. It states that

$$\overline{\tilde{A} \cup \tilde{B}} = \overline{\tilde{A}} \cap \overline{\tilde{B}} \tag{6.22}$$

$$\overline{\tilde{A} \cap \tilde{B}} = \overline{\tilde{A}} \cup \overline{\tilde{B}} \tag{6.23}$$

6.2.5 Membership function

It has been demonstrated that fuzzy logic is not a logic that is fuzzy but logic (rational) that is used to describe fuzziness. This fuzziness is best characterized by its membership function (Fig. 6.4).

Lotfi A. Zadeh defined the membership function in his first research paper called "fuzzy sets." Important membership function characteristics include the following:

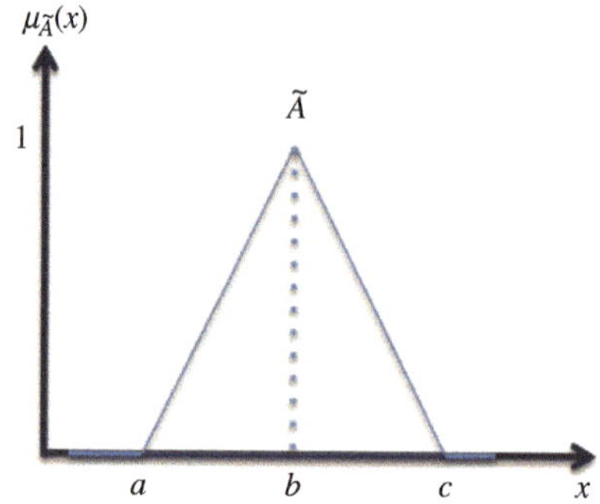

FIG. 6.4

An example of a triangular fuzzy set.

- They distinguish fuzziness.
- They resolve real-life problems based on occurrences rather than knowledge.
- They are usually represented in a graph.

The features of membership functions are as follows:

(a) Core—the core equation in the succeeding text defines the core of the fuzzy set $\underset{\sim}{A}$ in the universe:

$$\mu_{\underset{\sim}{A}}(x) = 1 \tag{6.24}$$

(b) Support—the support equation in the succeeding text defines the core of the fuzzy set $\underset{\sim}{A}$ in the universe:

$$\mu_{\underset{\sim}{A}}(x) > 0 \tag{6.25}$$

(c) Boundary—the boundary equation in the succeeding text defines the core of the fuzzy set $\underset{\sim}{A}$ in the universe (Fig. 6.5):

$$1 > \mu_{\underset{\sim}{A}}(x) > 0 \tag{6.26}$$

A fuzzy number is a fuzzy set on the real line that satisfies the conditions of normality and convexity.

6.2.6 Fuzzification

Fuzzification can be defined as the conversion of a fuzzy set to a fuzzier set or crisp sets to a fuzzy set. There are two distinct methods of fuzzification:

(1) Support fuzzification (s-fuzzification) method:

$$\tilde{A} = \mu_1 Q(x_1) + \mu_2 Q(x_2) + \ldots + \mu_n Q(x_n) \tag{6.27}$$

where $Q(x_i)$ is referred to as the Kernel of fuzzification.

(2) Grade fuzzification (g-fuzzification) method:
where x_i is constant and μ_i is expressed as a fuzzy set.

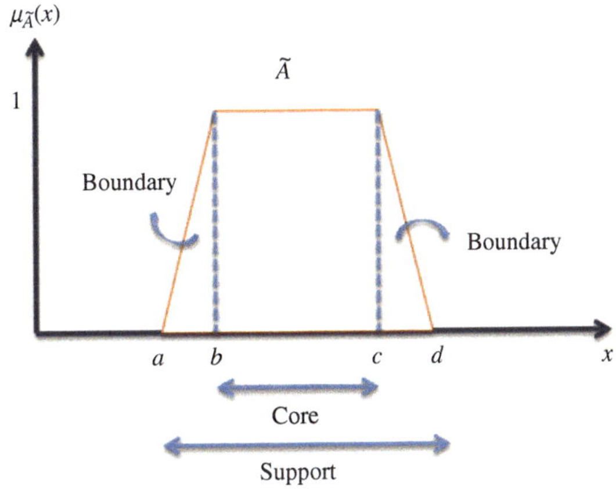

FIG. 6.5

Membership function features.

6.2.7 Defuzzification

This process converts the fuzzy member into crisp data. It can also be defined as the reduction of a fuzzy set into a crisp set. Defuzzification of the result is important in engineering applications. The term defuzzification is sometimes referred to as "rounding it off." To defuzzify a result, the following methods could be used:

(a) Max membership method: The method is restricted to peak output functions. Sometimes, it is referred to as the height method. It is mathematically represented as

$$\mu_{\tilde{A}}(x^*) > \mu_{\tilde{A}}(x), \forall x \epsilon X \tag{6.28}$$

where x^* is the defuzzified output.

(b) Centroid method: This determines the center corresponding crisp value. It is represented as

$$x^* = \frac{\int \mu_{\tilde{A}}(x).xdx}{\int \mu_{\tilde{A}}(x).dx} \tag{6.29}$$

(c) Weighted average method: In this method the membership function is weighted based on its maximum membership value. This is represented by

$$x^* = \frac{\sum \mu_{\tilde{A}}(\overline{x_i}).(\overline{x_i})}{\sum \mu_{\tilde{A}}(\overline{x_i})} \tag{6.30}$$

(d) Mean max membership: It can be represented as

$$x^* = \frac{\sum_{i=1}^{n} \overline{x_i}}{n} \tag{6.31}$$

6.2.8 An overview of the algebraic operations for fuzzy sets

Here, we give some necessary definitions about the operation of the fuzzy set theory:

$$\text{(a) Algebraic product: } \tilde{A}\,.\,\tilde{B} \Leftrightarrow \mu_{\tilde{A}.\tilde{B}} = \mu_{\tilde{A}} \cdot \mu_{\tilde{B}} \tag{6.32}$$

$$\text{(b) Algebraic sum :} \tilde{A} + \tilde{B} \Leftrightarrow \mu_{\tilde{A}+\tilde{B}} = \mu_{\tilde{A}} + \mu_{\tilde{B}} - \mu_{\tilde{A}} \cdot \mu_{\tilde{B}} \tag{6.33}$$

$$\text{(c) Bounded sum :} \tilde{A} \oplus \tilde{B} \Leftrightarrow \mu_{\tilde{A}\oplus\tilde{B}} = 1 \wedge \left(\mu_{\tilde{A}} + \mu_{\tilde{B}}\right) \tag{6.34}$$

$$\text{(d) Bounded difference: } \tilde{A} \ominus \tilde{B} \Leftrightarrow \mu_{\tilde{A}\ominus\tilde{B}} = 0 \vee \left(\mu_{\tilde{A}} - \mu_{\tilde{B}}\right) \tag{6.35}$$

$$\text{(e) Bounded product :} \tilde{A} \odot \tilde{B} \Leftrightarrow \mu_{\tilde{A}\odot\tilde{B}} = 0 \vee \left(\mu_{\tilde{A}} + \mu_{\tilde{B}} - 1\right) \tag{6.36}$$

where the operations of $\vee$, Λ, $+$, and $-$ denote the max, min, arithmetic sum, and arithmetic difference, respectively.

6.3 Application of fuzzy logic in medicine

In medicine the procedure of disease diagnosis encompasses various uncertainties and imprecisions. An example is that of a particular disease that behaves differently among different patients. Also, two different diseases may present with similar symptoms, which present certain difficulties when it comes to the treatment of such diseases. These uncertainty issues have led to the inclusion of fuzzy logic to the medicine field. Fuzzy logic is very suitable for developing knowledge-based systems in medicine and also in tasks such as diagnosis of diseases, selection of medical treatments, and real-time monitoring of patients' data. Fuzzy expert systems have been used in numerous studies to diagnose diseases affecting the lungs, syndrome differentiation, disease classification, and so on. These systems were developed and tested at hospitals.

In recent years, there has been an increase in the application to optimize techniques for the study of the medical problems and the delivery of healthcare. Due to the increase in uncertainty and imprecision in medicine, fuzzy logic was introduced to the field to address some of these problems. The field of medicine has such a level of complexity that it has become inappropriate to employ conventional analysis techniques. Some of the sources of these uncertainties include but are not limited to the following:

- Patient's medical history, which is often subjective.
- Objective information derived from only physically examining the patient. Sometimes the difference between normal and abnormal health state is not clear.
- A diagnostic test may sometimes contain errors, or patient's activity before conducting the test may lead to some errors in the test results.

Fuzzy logic plays an important role in medicine; for example, some of the published studies that have used fuzzy logic include the following:

In 2008 Caetano et al. [9] discussed optimal medication in HIV-seropositive patient treatment using a fuzzy cost function. In 2013 Persi Pamela et al. [10] proposed a fuzzy optimization technique for the prediction of coronary heart disease using a decision tree. In 2010 Zhao Jingwei [11] discussed the fuzzy multi-objective routing inventory problem in the context of recycling infectious medical waste. In 2012 Mason et al. [12] developed optimization model for optimizing strain treatment decisions for diabetes patients in the presence of uncertain future adherence.

Other studies were conducted to calculate volumes of brain tissue from magnetic resonance imaging (MRI) [13]; to analyze functional MRI data [14]; to improve decision-making in radiation therapy [15]; to detect breast cancer [16, 17], lung cancer [18], and prostate cancer [17]; to assist the diagnosis of central nervous systems tumors (astrocytic tumors) [19]; to discriminate benign skin lesions from malignant melanomas [20]; to visualize nerve fibers in the human brain [21]; to study fuzzy epidemics [22]; and to make decisions in nursing [23].

6.3.1 Fuzzy linear programming in medicine

Also known as linear optimization, this is a technique in which under a given circumstance, an optimum result can be achieved in a mathematical model. In various specializations, professionals have to make decisions, which are either to minimize effort or to maximize benefit. Mathematically, linear programming (LP) is an optimization technique of linear objective functions, subject to linear equality and inequality constraints.

Determining the parameters in real life may not always be possible. This is due to a lack of experience, knowledge, or information as well as expensive and time-consuming data collection processes. However, fuzzy optimization techniques are employed to overcome these problems and deal with more realistic situations (where data are imprecise). Fuzzy quantities are distinguished by some specific functions called membership functions. These techniques are more practical and easier to apply than the classical crisp programming techniques.

Various different optimization methods that have been developed and applied successfully for optimizing problems in many fields such as economics, computer sciences, information technology, engineering and, recently, medicine. For different types of optimization problems, different modeling techniques are created depending on the requirements of the problems. The main modeling approaches are linear programming, nonlinear programming, geometric programming, dynamic programming, integer programming, etc. Recently, this approach has been combined with fuzzy logic to create an optimum point for more fuzzy data. This gives a more flexible option for the decision-maker.

Fuzzy linear programming is another aspect of fuzzy logic that has recently been applied to medicine. It has several modeling approaches such as linear programming, nonlinear programming, geometric programming, dynamic programming, and integer programming. These approaches are combined with fuzzy logic to create an optimum point under vague conditions, which provides more flexible options for decision-makers. Several works have been published related to the application of fuzzy linear programming in medicine, including one study that aimed to distribute several treatments to different disease populations to minimize human productivity loss.

In medicine, several studies have been conducted in relation to the application of fuzzy linear programming. They include studies conducted by Venkatesh et al. [24], which aimed to "minimize the human productivity loss by distributing various treatments to different disease population." Another study is that of M. Mamat et al. [25], which used fuzzy linear programming in balanced diet planning for eating disorder and disease-related lifestyles. The technique was used to obtain the optimum amount of nutrients in food consumed and to estimate the nutritional requirements for the human body in a daily routine. Lastly, based on this outcome, a balanced diet plan was obtained. The general form of a mathematical model of the fuzzy linear programming is shown in the succeeding text:

$$Max\,Z\,or\,Min\,Z = \sum_{J=1}^{n} \tilde{c}_j \tilde{x}_j \tag{6.37}$$

$$\sum_{J=1}^{n} \tilde{a}_{ij} x_j \leq, =, \geq \tilde{b}_i, i = 1,2,\ldots,m$$

$$x_j \geq 0, j = 1,2,\ldots,n$$

where $\tilde{a}_{ij}$, $\tilde{b}_i$, $\tilde{c}_j$, are fuzzy numbers.

6.3.1.1 Fuzzy linear programming models

There are different types of fuzzy linear programming models according to how the fuzzy inputs occur in the problem. In the literature, there are four commonly used models:

1. linear programming with fuzzy constraint problems,
2. linear programming problem with fuzzy objective function and fuzzy constraints,
3. linear programming with fuzzy objective coefficient problem,
4. linear programming problem with fuzzy parameters.

Zimmermann [26], Werners [27], Carlsson and Korhonen [28], and many others have suggested different kinds of solutions for different types of fuzzy linear programming models. Another approach to fuzzy linear programming is known as the multiobjective approach. This is usually employed in situations where some of the objective coefficients are uncertain. Problems related to multiobjective linear programming (MLP) can be found in different research fields including healthcare. An article published by M. Mamat et al. [25] is among those that used the MLP approach in healthcare.

In this chapter, we will only discuss the Zimmerman method, which has been commonly and successfully applied by many researchers to linear programming problems that have fuzzy constraints or fuzzy aim functions.

➢ Zimmermann method

Zimmermann defined the fuzzy inequality and objective function as follows [26]:

$$C^T x \tilde{\geq} b_0 \tag{6.38}$$

$$C^T x \tilde{\leq} b_i \tag{6.39}$$

where $x \geq 0$ and $i = 1, 2, \ldots, n$.

Inequality is a symmetrical model. In this the objective function becomes one constraint. It is represented as follows [26]:

$$-C^T x \sim -b_0 \tag{6.40}$$

where

$$B = \begin{bmatrix} -C \\ A_i \end{bmatrix} b = \begin{bmatrix} -b_0 \\ b_i \end{bmatrix} \tag{6.41}$$

The inequalities of the constraint can be allowed to violate the right-hand side by adding some value. The degree of violation is shown by the membership function as [26]

$$\mu_0(x) = \begin{cases} 0 & if\ Cx \leq b_0 - d_0 \\ 1 - \dfrac{b_0 - Cx}{d_0} & b_0 - d_0 \leq Cx \leq b_0 \\ 1 & if\ Cx \leq b_0 \end{cases} \tag{6.42}$$

$$\mu_i(x) = \begin{cases} 0 & if\,(Ax)_i \geq b_i + d_i \\ 1 - \dfrac{(Ax)_i - b_i}{d_i} & b_i \leq (Ax)_i \leq b_i + d_i \\ 1 & if\,(Ax)_i \leq b_i \end{cases} \tag{6.43}$$

where d is a matrix of the admissible violation. The auxiliary variable λ can be used to transform the problem as follows:

$$\mu_0(x) \geq \lambda \tag{6.44}$$

$$\mu_i(x) \geq \lambda \tag{6.45}$$

$$\lambda \in [0, 1](5.1) \tag{6.46}$$

A linear programming problem can be shown as

$$\text{Max } \lambda \tag{6.47}$$

such that

$$\mu_0(x) \geq \lambda$$

$$\mu_i(x) \geq \lambda$$

$$\lambda \in [0, 1]$$

It can further be shown with the membership functions of the fuzzy objective function and fuzzy constraints as follows:

$$1 - \frac{b_0 - Cx}{d_0} \geq \lambda \tag{6.48}$$

$$1 - \frac{(Ax)_i - b_i}{d_i} \geq \lambda, \forall i \tag{6.49}$$

$$\lambda \in [0, 1]$$

$$x \geq 0$$

After simplification the fuzzy linear programming model can be given as

$$\text{Max } \lambda \tag{6.50}$$

such that

$$C^T x - \lambda d_0 \geq b_0 - d_0 \tag{6.51}$$

$$(Ax)_i + \lambda d_i \leq b_i + d_i, \forall i \tag{6.52}$$

$$\lambda \in [0, 1]$$

$$x \geq 0$$

Example 1 Solve the fuzzy linear programming problem shown in the succeeding text by using the Zimmerman method with a tolerance level $p_0 = 15$ and aspiration level $b_0 = 50$ of the aim function. The tolerance levels for the constraints are 8, 12, and 15 sequentially.

Aim function:

$$\text{MaksZ} \cong 2X_1 + 4X_2 + 6X_3 + 2X_4 \tag{6.53}$$

Constraints:

$$8X_1 + 6X_2 + 4X_3 \sim 20 \tag{6.54}$$

$$2X_1 - 2X_2 + 2X_3 \sim 13 \tag{6.55}$$

$$3X_1 + 3X_2 + 3X_3 + 3X_4 \sim 25 \tag{6.56}$$

$$X_1, X_2, X_3, X_4 \tilde{\geq} 0 \tag{6.57}$$

Based on this information the membership functions of the aim function and the membership functions of the constraints can be arranged as

$$\mu_Z(x) = \begin{cases} 1, & \text{if } 2X_1 + 4X_2 + 6X_3 + 2X_4 \geq 50 \\ 1 - \dfrac{50 - (2X_1 + 4X_2 + 6X_3 + 2X_4)}{15}), & \text{if } 35 \leq 2X_1 + 4X_2 + 6X_3 + 2X_4 \leq 50 \\ 0, & \text{if } 2X_1 + 4X_2 + 6X_3 + 2X_4 \leq 50 \end{cases} \tag{6.58}$$

$$\mu_1(x) = \begin{cases} 1, & \text{if } 8X_1 + 6X_2 + 4X_3 \leq 20 \\ 1 - \dfrac{(8X_1 + 6X_2 + 4X_3) - 20}{8}), & \text{if } 20 \leq 8X_1 + 6X_2 + 4X_3 \leq 28 \\ 0, & \text{if } 8X_1 + 6X_2 + 4X_3 \geq 20 \end{cases} \tag{6.59}$$

$$\mu_2(x) = \begin{cases} 1, & \text{if } 2X_1 - 2X_2 + 2X_3 \leq 13 \\ 1 - \dfrac{(2X_1 - 2X_2 + 2X_3) - 13}{12}), & \text{if } 13 \leq 2X_1 - 2X_2 + 2X_3 \leq 25 \\ 0, & \text{if } 2X_1 - 2X_2 + 2X_3 \geq 25 \end{cases} \tag{6.60}$$

$$\mu_3(x) = \begin{cases} 1, & \text{if } 3X_1 + 3X_2 + 3X_3 + 3X_4 \leq 25 \\ 1 - \frac{(3X_1 + 3X_2 + 3X_3 + 3X_4) - 25}{15}), & \text{if } 25 \leq 3X_1 + 3X_2 + 3X_3 + 3X_4 \leq 40 \\ 0, & \text{if } 3X_1 + 3X_2 + 3X_3 + 3X_4 \geq 40 \end{cases} \quad (6.61)$$

By adding variable λ to the membership function, we can convert the fuzzy linear programming problem to a classical linear programming problem, as shown in the succeeding text:

Aim function:

$$\text{Maks}\, Z = \lambda \quad (6.62)$$

Constraints:

$$2X_1 + 4X_2 + 6X_3 + 2X_4 \geq 50 - 15(1 - \lambda) \quad (6.63)$$

$$8X_1 + 6X_2 + 4X_3 \leq 20 + 8(1 - \lambda) \quad (6.64)$$

$$2X_1 - 2X_2 + 2X_3 \leq 13 + 12(1 - \lambda) \quad (6.65)$$

$$3X_1 + 3X_2 + 3X_3 + 3X_4 \leq 25 + 15(1 - \lambda) \quad (6.66)$$

$$X_1, X_2, X_3, X_4 \geq 0$$

$$\alpha \in [0, 1]$$

When we solve this problem using the Excel solver function where $\lambda = 0$, the decision variables are $X_1 = 0$, $X_2 = 0$, $X_3 = 7.00$, and $X_4 = 6.33$. Based on these results the value of the aim function is calculated as $Z = 54.66$.

6.3.2 Fuzzy multiple-criteria decision analysis in medicine

Multiple-criteria decision analysis (MCDA) is an important aspect of operational research, which evaluates alternatives with multiple conflicting criteria in various fields such as economics medicine, government, and engineering. A classic example is a situation in which an individual wants to purchase a car, where criteria like cost, fuel economy, comfort, emissions, and engine size are taken into account. It is difficult to choose the best option considering the various criteria available. An easy way to solve this is by employing the MCDA technique. It can also be applied in a similar manner in the field of medicine and healthcare, where we deal with multiple criteria regarding the alternatives in every case. There are various diagnostic and treatment devices in addition to different patient conditions. MCDA has been tested since 2011 in this field, and it has proved to be an efficient application.

In medicine, decision-making is a complex task, which involves trade-offs between multiple, often conflicting, objectives. The quality of decision-making can be improved by using a systemic, well-structured approach to alternatives with multiple criteria. MCDA techniques are very suitable for this purpose.

Fuzzy multiple-criteria decision analysis (MCDA) is another important aspect of operational research, which has been employed in medicine because of its efficiency and effectiveness at evaluating alternatives with multiple conflicting criteria. In medicine and healthcare, there are various diagnostic and treatment devices, which need to be evaluated according to their properties and the needs of the hospital or patient. These methods support the decision-maker to obtain the best option among the alternatives.

The MCDA technique has only recently been used in medical applications, even though it first emerged in the 1980s. There are different MCDA methods available, but choosing the most appropriate to use depends on the nature of the data and the aims of the decision-maker. The most used are analytic hierarchy process (AHP), technique for order of preference by similarity to ideal solution (TOPSIS), and the preference ranking organization method for enrichment of evaluations (PROMETHEE). Recently the MCDA methods have been combined with fuzzy logic to make good decisions under fuzzy conditions. This hybridization makes it easier for the decision-maker to use linguistic data or bounded continuous data. Detailed explanations of the previously listed MCDA techniques are given in the succeeding text. The multicriteria programming model for medical diagnosis and treatment was developed by Crina Grosan et al. [29].

There is a diverse application of MCDA fused with fuzzy logic in the medical field. Several studies conducted using fuzzy logic and MCDA include the analysis of colon cancer [30], liver cancer [31], leukemia [32], pancreatic cancer [33], lung cancer [34], and breast cancer [35] and the evaluation of drug alternatives for HIV therapy [36]. This technique has also been successfully used to analyze alternative nuclear medicine imaging devices [37], X-ray-based medical imaging devices [38], algorithms of image reconstruction in nuclear medicine [39], solid-state detectors in medical imaging [40], and sterilization methods for medical devices [41].

However, other studies have utilized only one MCDA tool, and they include analysis in oncology [42], in health-care decision-making [43], and in frameworks for orphan drugs [44].

6.3.2.1 Preference ranking organization method for enrichment evaluations (PROMETHEE)

PROMETHEE is a multicriteria decision-making tool that allows a user to analyze and rank available alternatives based on the criteria of each alternative and the importance weight of the alternatives. PROMETHEE compares the available alternatives based on the selected criteria. PROMETHEE is preferred over other multicriteria decision methods for reasons that include the following:

- PROMETHEE can be used to handle qualitative and quantitative criteria simultaneously.
- PROMETHEE deals with fuzzy relations, vagueness, and uncertainties.
- PROMETHEE is easy to handle and provides the user with maximum control over the weights of the criteria.

Using PROMETHEE requires only two types of information from the decision-maker: information regarding the weights of the selected criteria and the preference function to be used in comparing the alternatives' contribution in regard to each criterion [34]. Different preference functions (P_j) are available on PROMETHEE. This makes the model unique giving control to the decision-maker on defining the preference value to the alternatives for each criterion differently. The discrepancy between two alternatives (a and a_t) in relation to a specific criterion and a preference degree ranging between 0 and 1 is referred to as the preference function. The preference functions for practical purposes include Gaussian function, V-shape function, linear function, usual function, level function, and U-shaped function. A detailed description of the preference functions used, their ranking, and how to make a decision on which function best suits a scenario was discussed by Brans et al. [45]. Generally, type III (V-shape) and type V (linear) preference functions are mostly used for data with quantitative measures, while type I (usual shape) and type IV (level) preference functions are mostly used for qualitative data (Fig. 6.6). The definitions of the parameters are as follows:

- q indicates a threshold of indifference.
- p is a threshold that indicates a strict preference.
- σ is an intermediate point between q and p.

The basic steps involved in the PROMETHEE method are as follows [45]:

The creators of the technique (2) have discussed the complete steps of the PROMETHEE method, and this method has not been altered in any way for this research.

1. Define a specific preference function$p_j(d)$ for each criterion j.
2. Determine the weight of each criterion $w = (w_1, w_2, \ldots, w_k)$. Normalization of weights or equality of weights can be decided at the discretion of the decision-maker based on the application.
3. For every alternativea_t, $a_{t'} \in A$, determine the outranking relation π.

$$\pi(a_t, a_{t'}) = \sum_{k=1}^{K} w_k.[p_k(f_k(a_t) - f_k(a_{t'}))], AXA \rightarrow [0, 1] \tag{6.67}$$

4. Determine the positive and negative outranking flows:
   - Positive outranking flow for a_t:

$$\Phi^+(a_t) = \frac{1}{n-1} \sum_{\substack{t'=1 \\ t' \neq t}}^{n} \pi(a_t, a_{t'}) \tag{6.68}$$

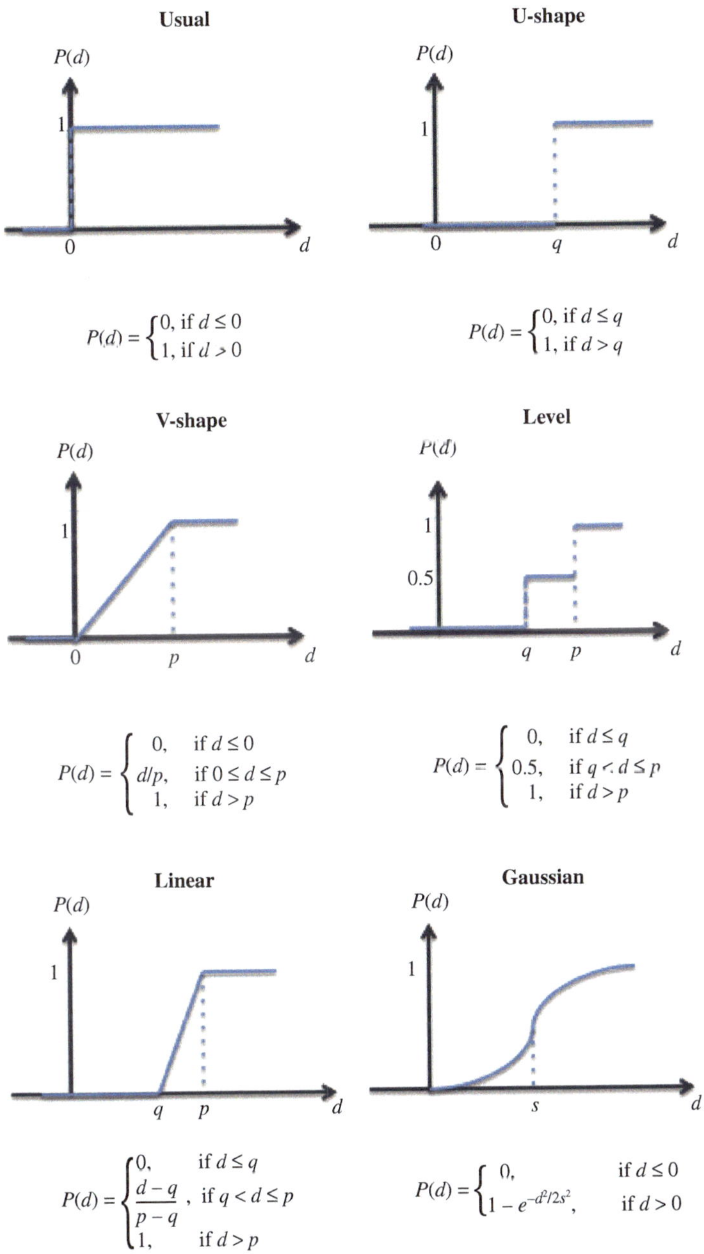

FIG. 6.6

Types of the preference functions of the PROMETHEE method [46].

- Negative outranking flow for a_t:

$$\Phi^-(a_t) = \frac{1}{n-1} \sum_{\substack{t'=1 \\ t' \neq t}}^{n} \pi(a_{t'}, a_t) \tag{6.69}$$

where n indicates the number of alternatives and every alternative is compared with an $(n - 1)$ other alternatives.

The positive outranking flow is an expression of how a particular alternative beats the other alternatives. The higher the positive outranking value of a particular alternative, the better the alternative.

The negative outranking flows are an expression of how a particular alternative is beaten by other alternatives. The lower the negative outranking value, the better the alternative.

5. Define the partial preorder on the alternatives of A. $a_t$is desirable to $a_{t'}$ $(a_t P a_{t'})$in PROMETHEE in any of the following scenarios:

$$\begin{cases} \Phi^+(a_t) > \Phi^+(a_{t'}) \; and \; \Phi^-(a_t) < \Phi^-(a_{t'}) \\ \Phi^+(a_t) > \Phi^+(a_{t'}) \; and \; \Phi^-(a_t) = \Phi^-(a_{t'}) \\ \Phi^+(a_t) = \Phi^+(a_{t'}) \; and \; \Phi^-(a_t) < \Phi^-(a_{t,} a_{t'}) \end{cases} \tag{6.70}$$

If there are two alternatives (a_t and $a_{t'}$) with similar or equal leaving and entering flows, a_t is indifferent to $a_{t'}$ ($a_t I a_{t'}$) if

$$\Phi^+(a_t) = \Phi^+(a_{t'}) \; and \; \Phi^-(a_t) = \Phi^-(a_{t'}) \tag{6.71}$$

a_t is in comparable with $a_{t'}(a_t R a_{t'}$) if

$$\begin{cases} \Phi^+(a_t) > \Phi^+(a_{t'}) \; and \; \Phi^-(a_t) > \Phi^-(a_{t'}) \\ \Phi^+(a_t) < \Phi^+(a_{t'}) \; and \; \Phi^-(a_t) < \Phi^-(a_{t'}) \end{cases} \tag{6.72}$$

6. Determine the net outranking flow for each alternative:

$$\Phi^{net}(a_t) = \Phi^+(a_t) - \Phi^-(a_t) \tag{6.73}$$

A complete preorder could be derived from the net flow and given as

$$a_t \; is \; \text{preferred to} \; a_{t'} \; (a_t P a_{t'}) \; \text{if} \; \Phi^{net}(a_t) > \Phi^{net}(a_{t'}) \tag{6.74}$$

$$\text{a is indifferent to} \; a_{t'} \; (a_t I a_{t'}) \; \text{if} \; \Phi^{net}(a_t) = \Phi^{net}(a_{t'}) \tag{6.75}$$

6.3.2.2 Fuzzy PROMETHEE (F-PROMETHEE)

Recently, various researchers have used the fuzzy PROMETHEE method in the field of health and medicine [30–41]. This technique is a combination of fuzzy logic and the PROMETHEE technique. This method aims to define the problem under vague conditions and make decisions where there is insufficient information about the alternatives' properties. The fuzzy PROMETHEE technique was designed for the evaluation of the difference between two fuzzy sets. Yager defined an index, which depends on the center of weight of the surface of the triangular membership function for comparing the fuzzy numbers. The magnitude of a triangular fuzzy number $\tilde{F} = (N, a, b)$ was defined by Yager, which is equivalent to $\tilde{F} = (N - a, N, N + b)$, corresponding to the center of the triangle with the $YI = (3N - a + b)/3$ formula. In this chapter, we applied the triangular linguistic fuzzy scale, which has been shown in the succeeding text for defining the fuzzy data of the problems and the importance weights of each criterion of the alternatives (Table 6.1).

Table 6.1 Linguistic triangular fuzzy scale.

Linguistic scale for evaluation	Triangular fuzzy scale
Very high (VH)	(0.75, 1, 1)
Important (H)	(0.50, 0.75, 1)
Medium (M)	(0.25, 0.50, 0.75)
Low (L)	(0, 0.25, 0.50)
Very low (VL)	(0, 0, 0.25)

Example 2 Assume that there is a decision-making problem for three alternative biomedical devices (A_1, A_2, A_3) that works for the same specific aim and each alternative has four different properties, which are the cost (c_1), life length (c_2), practicability (c_3), and efficiency (c_4). The decision-maker composes the weight of the criteria ($w_i, i = 1,2,3,4$), and the decision matrix A is shown in Table 6.2.

Firstly the linguistic fuzzy data have been converted to numerical data by using the Yager index. Then the raw data are rearranged as shown in Table 6.3.

We used the Gaussian preference function for each criterion to calculate the outranking relation π using the formula in the succeeding text:

$$P(d) = \begin{cases} 0, & d \leq 0 \\ 1 - e^{\frac{d^2}{2s^2}} & d > 0 \end{cases}$$

Table 6.2 The decision matrix *A*.

	High	Medium	Low	Very high
Importance weight	**c_1 ($)**	**c_2 (year)**	**c_3**	**c_4 (%)**
Aim	**Min**	**Max**	**Max**	**Max**
A_1	5000	12	High	95
A_2	1800	10	Very high	70
A_3	3000	15	Medium	60

Table 6.3 Rearranged raw data.

Importance of weight	High (0.75)	Medium (0.50)	Low (0.25)	Very high (0.92)
	c_1 ($)	c_2 (year)	c_3	c_4 (%)
Aim	*Min*	*Max*	*Max*	*Max*
A_1	5000	12	0.75	95
A_2	1800	10	0.92	70
A_3	3000	15	0.50	60

where d is the difference between parameters of the devices in terms of each criterion. Then, we obtained the preference values of the alternatives for each criterion: $P(d)_{c_1}$, $P(d)_{c_2}$, $P(d)_{c_3}$, and $P(d)_{c_4}$ as shown in Tables 6.4–6.7.

The outranking relation (Table 6.8):

Positive and negative outranking flows are calculated using Eqs. (6.68) and (6.69) of step 4 (Table 6.9).

Net ranking flow is calculated by subtracting the negative outranking flow from the positive outranking flow (Table 6.10).

Table 6.4 The preference value $P(d)_{c_1}$.

Alternatives	A1	A2	A3
A1	0	0	0
A2	1	0	1
A3	1	0	0

Table 6.5 The preference value $P(d)_{c_2}$.

Alternatives	A1	A2	A3
A1	0	0.857	0
A2	0	0	0
A3	0.987	0.999	0

Table 6.6 The preference value $P(d)_{c_3}$.

Alternatives	A1	A2	A3
A1	0	0	0.304
A2	0.154	0	0.640
A3	0	0	0

Table 6.7 The preference value $P(d)_{c_4}$.

Alternatives	A1	A2	A3
A1	0	1	1
A2	0	0	0.999
A3	0	0	0

Table 6.8 The outranking relation $\pi(A_i, A_j)$.

Alternatives	A1	A2	A3
A1	0	0.557	0.412
A2	0.326	0	0.756
A3	0.514	0.207	0

Table 6.9 Positive and negative outranking.

Alternatives	Positive outranking flow	Negative outranking flow
A1	0.484	0.420
A2	0.541	0.382
A3	0.360	0.584

Table 6.10 Net ranking flow.

Alternatives	Net ranking flow
A1	0.064
A2	0.159
A3	-0.224

The best alternative is the one with the higher net ranking flow. Therefore A2 is the best alternative, followed by A1, and the last alternative is A3.

6.3.2.3 The technique for order of preference by similarity to ideal solution (TOPSIS)

Originally the TOPSIS method was designed to represent weights and ratings of alternatives by numerical data. As a result a single decision-maker solves a particular problem. Solving the problem may sometimes be complex when there are two or more decision-makers with varying priorities and goals. However, an agreement must be reached by the several interest groups who have difference to enable a preferred and mutual solution. The TOPSIS algorithm for a single decision-maker is described in the succeeding text [47]:

Step 1: Determination of weight criteria and building a decision matrix.
The decision matrix $X = X_{ij}$ and weighing vector W=$[w_1, w_2, \ldots, w_n]$ are chosen, respectively, where $X_{ij} \in R$, $w_j \in R$ and

$$w_1 + w_2 + \ldots + w_n = 1 \tag{6.76}$$

The criteria of the function could be a benefit function (more criteria and a better result) or a cost function (least cost and better results).

Step 2: Calculate the normalized decision matrix.
All dimensional attributes are converted to nondimensional attributes to enable a comparison of the criteria. To do this, each value in the evaluation matrix is reduced to a normalized scale. This normalization is carried out by several standardized formulas. The most frequently used method for calculating the normalized value n_{ij} is

$$n_{ij} = \frac{X_{ij}}{\sqrt{\sum_{i=1}^{m} X_{ij}^2}} \tag{6.77}$$

$$n_{ij} = \frac{X_{ij}}{\max_{(i)} X_{ij}} \tag{6.78}$$

$$n_{ij} = \begin{cases} \dfrac{x_{ij} - \min_{(i)} x_{ij}}{\max_{(i)} x_{ij} - \min_{(i)} x_{ij}} \\ \dfrac{\max_{(i)} x_{ij} - x_{ij}}{\max_{(i)} x_{ij} - \min_{(i)} x_{ij}} \end{cases} \tag{6.79}$$

if C_i is a benefit criterion and C_i is a cost criterion, for $i = 1, \ldots, m$; $j = 1, \ldots, n$.

Step 3: Calculation of weighted normalized decision matrix.
The weighted matrix v_{ij} is calculated by

$$v_{ij} = w_j n_{ij} \quad \text{for } i = 1, \ldots, m; j = 1, \ldots, n. \tag{6.80}$$

where w_j is the weight and j is the criterion:

$$\sum_{j=1}^{n} w_j = 1$$

Step 4: Determine the positive ideal and negative ideal solutions.
Identify positive and negative ideal alternatives.
The positive ideal solution(A^+)is given as

$$A^+ = (v_1^+, v_2^+, \ldots, v_n^+) = \left[\left[\max_{(i)} v_{ij} \mid j \in I\right], \left[\min_{(i)} v_{ij} \mid j \in J\right]\right] \tag{6.81}$$

While the negative ideal solution (A^-) is given as

$$A^- = (v_1^-, v_2^-, \ldots, v_n^-) = \left[\left[\min_{(i)} v_{ij} | j \in I\right], \left[\max_{(i)} v_{ij} | j \in J\right]\right] \quad (6.82)$$

where I denotes benefit criteria and J denotes cost criteria, $i = 1, \ldots, m; j = 1, \ldots, n$.

Step 5: Calculation of separation measures from the positive ideal solution and the negative ideal solution.

The separation of alternatives from the positive ideal solution is represented as

$$d_i^+ - \left(\sum_{j=1}^{n} \left(v_{ij} - v_j^+\right)^p\right)^{1/p} .., \; i = 1,2,\ldots,m. \quad (6.83)$$

The separation of alternatives from the negative ideal solution is represented in the succeeding text:

$$d_i^- = \left(\sum_{j=1}^{n} \left(v_{ij} - v_j^-\right)^p\right)^{1/p}, .. i = 1,2,\ldots,m. \quad (6.84)$$

where $p \geq 1$.For $p = 2$, we have the most used traditional n-dimensional Euclidean metric.

$$d_i^+ = \sqrt{\sum_{j=1}^{n} \left(v_{ij} - v_j^+\right)^2} ., i = 1,2,\ldots\ldots,m, \quad (6.85)$$

$$d_i^- = \sqrt{\sum_{j=1}^{n} \left(v_{ij} - v_j^-\right)^2} ., i = 1,2,\ldots\ldots,m. \quad (6.86)$$

Step 6: Calculation of the relative closeness to the positive ideal solution.

The closeness of A^+ with respect to the ith alternative is represented as

$$R_i = \frac{d_i^-}{d_i^- + d_i^+} \quad (6.87)$$

where $0 \leq R_i \leq 1$, $i = 1, 2, \ldots, m$.

Step 7: Selection of the alternatives closest to 1 or ranking of the preference order.

The alternatives are ranked in descending order of R_i value.

Example 3. In this part the same question presented in Example 2 will be solved by the TOPSIS method: After the decision-maker defuzzifies the linguistic data by using the Yager index, the decision matrix will be obtained as in the succeeding text, which is the same step used in the fuzzy PROMETHEE technique (Table 6.11).

After obtaining the numerical data in the first step, the standardized decision matrix is calculated (Table 6.12).

Table 6.11 The decision matrix.

Importance of weight	High (0.75)	Medium (0.50)	Low (0.25)	Very high (0.92)
	c_1 ($)	c_2 (year)	c_3	c_4 (%)
Aim	*Min*	*Max*	*Max*	*Max*
A_1	5000	12	0.75	95
A_2	1800	10	0.92	70
A_3	3000	15	0.50	60

Table 6.12 The standardized decision matrix.

Importance weight	High (0.31)	Medium (0.21)	Low (0.10)	Very high (0.38)
	c_1 ($)	c_2 (year)	c_3	c_4 (%)
Aim	*Min*	*Max*	*Max*	*Max*
A_1	0.82	0.55	0.58	0.72
A_2	0.29	0.46	0.71	0.53
A_3	0.49	0.69	0.39	0.45

Table 6.13 The weighted standardized decision matrix.

Importance weight	High (0.31)	Medium (0.21)	Low (0.10)	Very high (0.38)
	c_1 ($)	c_2 (year)	c_3	c_4 (%)
Aim	*Min*	*Max*	*Max*	*Max*
A_1	0.25	0.11	0.06	0.27
A_2	0.09	0.10	0.07	0.20
A_3	0.15	0.14	0.04	0.17

In the second step the weighted standardized decision matrix is calculated by multiplying each normalized column with its related normalized weight of the criterion (Table 6.13).

Then the positive and negative ideal solution sets are obtained as

$$A^+ = (minv_{i1}, maxv_{i2}, maxv_{i3}, maxv_{i4}) = (0.09, 0.14, 0.07, 0.27) \tag{6.88}$$

$$A^- = (maxv_{i1}, minv_{i2}, minv_{i3}, minv_{i4}) = (0.25, 0.10, 0.04, 0.17) \tag{6.89}$$

The separation of alternatives from the positive ideal solution is shown in Table 6.14.

Table 6.14 The separation of alternatives from the positive ideal solution.

$A_1 - A^+$	0.16	−0.03	−0.01	0.00
$A_2 - A^+$	0.00	−0.04	0.00	−0.07
$A_3 - A^+$	0.06	0.00	−0.03	−0.10

Table 6.15 The separation of alternatives from the negative ideal solution.

$A_1 - A^-$	0.00	0.01	0.02	0.10
$A_2 - A^-$	−0.16	0.00	0.03	0.03
$A_3 - A^-$	−0.10	0.04	0.00	0.00

Table 6.16 The relative closeness to the positive ideal solution of each alternative.

Alternatives	d_i^+	d_i^-	R_i
A_1	0.25	0.11	0.29
A_2	0.09	0.10	0.80
A_3	0.15	0.14	0.44

The separation of alternatives from the negative ideal solution is shown in Table 6.15.

Lastly, for three decision points, the distance to the positive ideal solution (d_i^+) and the distance to the negative ideal solution (d_i^-) are obtained, and the relative closeness to the positive ideal solution of each alternative (R_i) is calculated, as shown in Table 6.16.

R_i gives the preference order. Since

$$R_{(A_2)} > R_{(A_3)} > R_{(A_1)} \tag{6.90}$$

A_2 should be more preferable than A_3, and A_3 is more preferable than A_1. As can be observed the ranking results of the TOPSIS method validate the ranking results of the PROMETHEE method.

Those methods are the supportive systems that should be considered by the decision-makers and understood well.

6.4 Challenges and opportunities

The operational capacity of the human body is viewed as the complex and profoundly intelligent interplay of its body part and mind. The objective of this determined effort is homeostasis, the stableness of all physiological elements. Fuzzy logic is a solution to complex problems in the field of medicine as it resembles human reasoning and decision-making capability. It looks into all shades of gray and answers uncertainties and ambiguities created by human language where everything cannot be described in precise and discrete terms.

On the other hand, it has a number of challenges too. Firstly, it is tedious to develop fuzzy rules and membership functions, and fuzzy outputs can be interpreted in a number of ways making medical analysis difficult. Secondly, it requires lot of medical data and expertise to develop a fuzzy system used in medicine. Thirdly, it does not give generalizable results, and the program has to be run for each individual patient. Hence, its clinical applicability and utilization are difficult without the availability of preprogrammed software for different pathologies and the basic training of clinicians to use these programs.

For the challenges come several opportunities. First of all, fuzzy model has been shown to be an effective tool for research related to neuroanatomy and has been used for imaging nerve fibers [21, 48]. Secondly, fuzzy logic can be used in the diagnosis, management, and outcome prediction of common neurological diseases such as stroke with considerable success [49, 50]. Thirdly, fuzzy logic can be applied in neurosurgical intensive care units (ICUs) for precise control of different parameters like intracranial pressure (ICP) and blood pressure. Fuzzy logic-based controllers are found to be effective at maintaining stable ICP via varying propofol infusion rates [51–53].

6.5 Future direction

The opportunities provided by fuzzy logic clearly indicate it as promising, sensitive, and specific tool for various clinical problems. Fuzzy logic has the potential of changing medical diagnosis and management completely, and it can be effectively incorporated into routine clinical practice. If focused research is conducted, it is possible that in the future, neurophysiology labs will be reporting EMGs and EEGs with the help of fuzzy logic; ICUs will have fuzzy controllers for controlling blood pressure, ICP, and ventilator settings; MRI scans will be analyzed by fuzzy logic software; and neurosurgeries will be planned by FIS.

6.6 Summary

Fuzzy logic is a technique that studies reasoning systems in which the notions of truth and falsehood are considered in a graded fashion. Fuzzy logic analyzes the vagueness in natural language and several other application domains. Fuzzy logic is a soft-computing technique that tolerates suboptimality and vagueness, thereby producing very good solutions.

In medicine the procedure of disease diagnosis encompasses various uncertainties and imprecisions. An example is that of a particular disease that behaves differently among different patients. Also, two different diseases may present with similar symptoms, which presents certain challenges when it comes to the treatment of the disease. These uncertainty issues have led to the inclusion of fuzzy logic in the field of medicine. Fuzzy logic is very suitable for developing knowledge-based systems in medicine and also in tasks such as diagnosis of diseases, selection of medical treatments, and real-time monitoring of patients' data. Fuzzy expert systems have been used in many studies to diagnose diseases affecting the lungs, syndrome differentiation, disease classification, and so on. These systems were developed and tested at hospitals.

Fuzzy linear programming is another aspect of fuzzy logic that has recently been applied in medicine. It has several modeling approaches such as linear programming, nonlinear programming, geometric programming, dynamic programming, and integer programming. These approaches are combined with fuzzy logic to create an optimum point under vague conditions, which gives a more flexible option to decision-makers. Several works have been published related to the application of fuzzy linear programming in medicine, which includes one study that aimed to distribute several treatments to different disease populations to minimize human productivity loss.

Fuzzy multiple-criteria decision analysis (MCDA) is another important aspect of operational research that has been employed in medicine because of its efficiency and effectiveness at evaluating alternatives with multiple conflicting criteria. In medicine and healthcare, there are various diagnostic and treatment devices that need to be evaluated according to their properties and the needs of the hospital or patient. These methods support the decision-maker in obtaining the best option among the alternatives.

This chapter introduced fuzzy logic and its application in medicine and healthcare systems. It discussed fuzzy-based models such as fuzzy linear programming (FLP) and fuzzy multicriteria decision analysis (MCDA).

References

[1] H. Nguyen, E. Walker, A first course in fuzzy logic, Chapman & Hall, Boca Raton, FL, 2000.

[2] L. Zadeh, Fuzzy sets. Inform. Contr. 8 (3) (1965) 338–353. Available: https://doi.org/10.1016/s0019-9958(65)90241-x.

[3] L. Zadeh, Outline of a new approach to the analysis of complex systems and decision processes. IEEE Trans. Syst. Man Cybern. 3 (1) (1973) 28–44. Available: https://doi.org/10.1109/tsmc.1973.5408575.

[4] L. Zadeh, Fuzzy algorithms. Inform. Contr. 12 (2) (1968) 94–102. Available: https://doi.org/10.1016/s0019-9958(68)90211-8.

[5] L. Zadeh, Making computers think like people [fuzzy set theory]. IEEE Spectrum 21 (8) (1984) 26–32. Available: https://doi.org/10.1109/mspec.1984.6370431.

[6] S. Korner, Laws of thought, in: Encyclopedia of philosophy, 4 MacMillan, New York, 1967, pp. 414–417.

[7] Guru99.com, [Online]. Available: https://www.guru99.com/what-is-fuzzy-logic.html, 2019. Accessed 4 July 2019.

[8] B. Uzun, E. Kıral, Application of Markov chains-fuzzy states to gold price. Proc. Comput. Sci. 120 (2017) 365–371. Available: https://doi.org/10.1016/j.procs.2017.11.251.
[9] M. Caetano, J. de Souza and Takashi Yoneyama, "Optimal medication in HIV seropositive patient treatment using fuzzy cost function", 2008 American Control Conference, 2008. Available: https://doi.org/10.1109/acc.2008.4586823 [Accessed 4 July 2019].
[10] I. Persi Pamela, P. Gayathri, N. Jaisankar, A fuzzy optimization technique for the prediction of coronary heart disease using decision tree, Int. J. Eng. Technol. (IJET) 53 (2013). Available: http://file:///C:/Users/Ben/Downloads/A_Fuzzy_Optimization_Technique_for_the_Prediction_.pdf. Accessed 4 July 2019.
[11] Z. Jingwei and M. Zujun, "Fuzzy multi-objective location-routing-inventory problem in recycling infectious medical waste", 2010 International Conference on E-Business and E-Government, 2010. Available: https://doi.org/10.1109/icee.2010.1021 [Accessed 4 July 2019].
[12] J. Mason, D. England, B. Denton, S. Smith, M. Kurt and N. Shah, "Optimizing statin treatment decisions for diabetes patients in the presence of uncertain future adherence", Med. Decis. Making, vol. 32, no. 1, pp. 154-166, 2011. Available: https://doi.org/10.1177/0272989x11404076 [Accessed 4 July 2019].
[13] M. Brandt, T. Bohant, L. Kramer, J. Fletcher, Estimation of CSF, white and gray matter volumes in hydrocephalic children using fuzzy clustering of Mr Images. Comput. Med. Imaging Graph. 18 (1) (1994) 25–34. Available: https://doi.org/10.1016/0895-6111(94)90058-2.
[14] Y. Lu, T. Jiang, Y. Zang, Region growing method for the analysis of functional MRI data. Neuroimage 20 (1) (2003) 455–465. Available: https://doi.org/10.1016/s1053-8119(03)00352-5.
[15] E. Papageorgiou, C. Stylios, P. Groumpos, An integrated two-level hierarchical system for decision making in radiation therapy based on fuzzy cognitive maps. IEEE Trans. Biomed. Eng. 50 (12) (2003) 1326–1339. Available: https://doi.org/10.1109/tbme.2003.819845.
[16] A. Hassanien, Intelligent data analysis of breast cancer based on rough set theory. Int. J. Artif. Intell. Tools 12 (4) (2003) 465–479. Available: https://doi.org/10.1142/s0218213003001319.
[17] H. Seker, M. Odetayo, D. Petrovic, R. Naguib, A fuzzy logic based-method for prognostic decision making in breast and prostate cancers. IEEE Trans. Inf. Technol. Biomed. 7 (2) (2003) 114–122. Available: https://doi.org/10.1109/titb.2003.811876.
[18] J. Schneider, et al., Fuzzy logic-based tumor marker profiles improved sensitivity of the detection of progression in small-cell lung cancer patients. Clin. Exp. Med. 2 (4) (2003) 185–191. Available: https://doi.org/10.1007/s102380300005.
[19] N. Belacel, M. Boulassel, Multicriteria fuzzy classification procedure PROCFTN: methodology and medical application. Fuzzy Set. Syst. 141 (2) (2004) 203–217. Available: https://doi.org/10.1016/s0165-0114(03)00022-8.
[20] R. Stanley, R. Moss, W. Van Stoecker, C. Aggarwal, A fuzzy-based histogram analysis technique for skin lesion discrimination in dermatology clinical images. Comput. Med. Imaging Graph. 27 (5) (2003) 387–396. Available: https://doi.org/10.1016/s0895-6111(03)00030-2.
[21] H. Axer, J. Jantzen, D. Keyserlingk, G. Berks, The application of fuzzy-based methods to central nerve fiber imaging. Artif. Intell. Med. 29 (3) (2003) 225–239. Available: https://doi.org/10.1016/s0933-3657(02)00071-4.
[22] E. Massad, N. Ortega, C. Struchiner, M. Burattini, Fuzzy epidemics. Artif. Intell. Med. 29 (3) (2003) 241–259. Available: https://doi.org/10.1016/s0933-3657(02)00070-2.

[23] E. Im, W. Chee, Fuzzy logic and nursing. Nurs. Philos. 4 (1) (2003) 53–60. Available: https://doi.org/10.1046/j.1466-769x.2003.00116.x.

[24] A. Venkatesh, G. Sivakumar, On fuzzy optimization modeling in healthcare analysis based on linear programming problem, Int. J. Curr. Res. Mod. Educ. (IJCRME) 2 (2017). Available: http://ijcrme.rdmodernresearch.com/wp-content/uploads/2017/06/166.pdf. (Accessed 4 July 2019).

[25] M. Mamat, N.F. Zulkifli, S.K. Deraman, N.M. Noor, Fuzzy linear programming approach in balance diet planning for eating disorder and disease-related lifestyle, Appl. Math. Sci. 6 (103) (2012) 5109–5118. Available: http://www.m-hikari.com/ams/ams-2012/ams-101-104-2012/mamatAMS101-104-2012.pdf. (Accessed 4 July 2019).

[26] H. Zimmermann, Fuzzy mathematical programming. Comput. Oper. Res. 10 (4) (1983) 291–298. Available: https://doi.org/10.1016/0305-0548(83)90004-7.

[27] B. Werners, An interactive fuzzy programming system. Fuzzy Set. Syst. 23 (1) (1987) 131–147. Available: https://doi.org/10.1016/0165-0114(87)90105-9.

[28] C. Carlsson, P. Korhonen, A parametric approach to fuzzy linear programming. Fuzzy Set. Syst. 20 (1) (1986) 17–30, https://doi.org/10.1016/s0165-0114(86)80028-8.

[29] C. Grosan, A. Abraham and S. Tigan, Multicriteria programming in medical diagnosis and treatments, Appl. Soft Comput., vol. 8, no. 4, pp. 1407-1417, 2008. Available: https://doi.org/10.1016/j.asoc.2007.10.014. [Accessed 4 July 2019].

[30] D. Ozsahin, K. Nyakuwanikwa, T. Wallace and I. Ozsahin, "Evaluation and simulation of colon cancer treatment techniques with fuzzy PROMETHEE", 2019, pp. 1-6.

[31] M. Sani Musa, D. Uzun Ozsahin, I. Ozsahin, A comparison for liver cancer treatment alternatives, in: ASET, 2019. pp. 1–4.

[32] I. Ozsahin, D. Uzun Ozsahin, M. Maisaini, G.S.P. Mok, Fuzzy PROMETHEE analysis of leukemia treatment techniques, in: WCRJ, 2019. Available: https://www.wcrj.net/article/1315. (Accessed 4 July 2019).

[33] I. Ozsahin, D. Uzun Ozsahin, K. Nyakuwanikwa and T. Wallace Simbanegav, "Fuzzy PROMETHEE for ranking pancreatic cancer treatment techniques", IEEE Xplore, 2019. [Accessed 4 July 2019].

[34] M. Maisaini, B. Uzun, I. Ozsahin and D. Uzun, "Evaluating lung cancer treatment techniques using fuzzy PROMETHEE approach", 13th International Conference on Theory and Application of Fuzzy Systems and Soft Computing—ICAFS-2018, pp. 209-215, 2018. Available: https://doi.org/10.1007/978-3-030-04164-9_29. [Accessed 4 July 2019].

[35] D. Uzun Ozsahin and I. Ozsahin, "A fuzzy PROMETHEE approach for breast cancer treatment techniques", Health Sci., pp. 29-32, 2018. [Accessed 4 July 2019].

[36] B. Uzun, F. Sarigul Yildirim, M. Sayan, T. Sanlidag, D. Uzun Ozsahin, The Use of Fuzzy PROMETHEE Technique in Antiretroviral Combination Decision in Pediatric HIV Treatments, (2019).

[37] D. Ozsahin, B. Uzun, M. Musa, N. Şentürk, F. Nurçin and I. Ozsahin, "Evaluating nuclear medicine imaging devices using fuzzy PROMETHEE method", Proc. Comput. Sci., vol. 120, pp. 699-705, 2017. Available: https://doi.org/10.1016/j.procs.2017.11.298.

[38] D. Uzun, B. Uzun, M. Sani and I. Ozsahin, "Evaluating X-ray based medical imaging devices with fuzzy preference ranking organization method for enrichment evaluations", Int. J. Adv. Comput. Sci. Appl., vol. 9, no. 3, 2018. Available: 10.14569/ijacsa.2018.090302. [Accessed 4 July 2019].

[39] D. Ozsahin, N. Isa, B. Uzun, I. Ozsahin, Effective analysis of image reconstruction algorithms in nuclear medicine using fuzzy PROMETHEE, in: 2018 Advances in Science and Engineering Technology International Conferences (ASET), 2019 pp. 1–5.

[40] I. Ozsahin, T. Sharif, D. Ozsahin, B. Uzun, Evaluation of solid-state detectors in medical imaging with fuzzy PROMETHEE. J. Instrum. 14 (01) (2019). Available: https://doi.org/10.1088/1748-0221/14/01/c01019. pp. C01019–C01019.

[41] M. Taiwo Mubarak, I. Ozsahin and D. Uzun Ozsahin, "Evaluation of Sterilization Methods for Medical Devices", 2019, pp. 1–4.

[42] G. Adunlin, V. Diaby, A. Montero and H. Xiao, "Multicriteria decision analysis in oncology", Health Expect., vol. 18, no. 6, pp. 1812-1826, 2014. Available: https://doi.org/10.1111/hex.12178 [Accessed 4 July 2019].

[43] K. Marsh, et al., Multiple criteria decision analysis for health care decision making—emerging good practices: Report 2 of the ISPOR MCDA emerging good practices task force. Value Health 19 (2) (2016) 125–137. Available: https://doi.org/10.1016/j.jval.2015.12.016.

[44] C. Schey, P. Krabbe, M. Postma and M. Connolly, "Multi-criteria decision analysis (MCDA): testing a proposed MCDA framework for orphan drugs", Orphanet J. Rare Dis., vol. 12, no. 1, 2017. Available: https://doi.org/10.1186/s13023-016-0555-3. [Accessed 4 July 2019].

[45] J. Brans, P. Vincke, B. Mareschal, How to select and how to rank projects: The Promethee method. Eur. J. Oper. Res. 24 (2) (1986) 228–238. Available: https://doi.org/10.1016/0377-2217(86)90044-5.

[46] J. Brans and B. Mareschal, "PROMETHEE methods", Cin.ufpe.br, 2019. [Online]. Available: https://www.cin.ufpe.br/~if703/aulas/promethee.pdf. [Accessed 04 October 2019].

[47] H. Shih, H. Shyur, E. Lee, An extension of TOPSIS for group decision making. Math. Comput. Model. 45 (7–8) (2007) 801–813. Available: https://doi.org/10.1016/j.mcm.2006.03.023.

[48] Y. Kilic, A. Konan, K. Yorganci and I. Sayek, "A novel fuzzy-logic inference system for predicting trauma-related mortality: emphasis on the impact of response to resuscitation", Eur. J. Trauma Emerg. Surg., vol. 36, no. 6, pp. 543-550, 2010. Available: https://doi.org/10.1007/s00068-010-0010-4. [Accessed 4 October 2019].

[49] T. Jobe, C. Helgason, A. Kim and B. Roitberg, "Show me the numbers": the application of numbers to medical science, Surg. Neurol., vol. 56, no. 1, pp. 3-7, 2001. Available: https://doi.org/10.1016/s0090-3019(01)00463-3. [Accessed 4 October 2019].

[50] C. Helgason, D. Malik, S. Cheng, T. Jobe and J. Mordeson, Statistical versus fuzzy measures of variable interaction in patients with stroke, Neuroepidemiology, vol. 20, no. 2, pp. 77-84, 2001. Available: https://doi.org/10.1159/000054764. [Accessed 4 October 2019].

[51] S. Huang, J. Shieh, M. Fu, M. Kao, Fuzzy logic control for intracranial pressure via continuous propofol sedation in a neurosurgical intensive care unit, Med. Eng. Phys., vol. 28, no. 7, pp. 639-647, 2006. Available: https://doi.org/10.1016/j.medengphy.2005.10.009. [Accessed 4 October 2019].

[52] B. Cunha, "Clinical approach to fever in the neurosurgical intensive care unit: focus on drug fever", Surg. Neurol. Int., vol. 4, no. 6, p. 318, 2013. Available: https://doi.org/10.4103/2152-7806.111432. [Accessed 4 October 2019].

[53] S. Hemm et al., "Postoperative control in deep brain stimulation of the subthalamic region: the contact membership concept", Int. J. Comput. Assist. Radiol. Surg., vol. 3, no. 1–2, pp. 69-77, 2008. Available: https://doi.org/10.1007/s11548-008-0152-6. [Accessed 4 October 2019].

CHAPTER

Neural network applications in medicine

7

Dr. Ilker Ozsahin[a,b] and Dr. Dilber Uzun Ozsahin[a,b]

[a]*Department of Biomedical Engineering, Faculty of Engineering, Near East University, Nicosia, Northern Cyprus, Turkey,* [b]*DESAM Institute, Near East University, Nicosia, Northern Cyprus, Turkey*

7.1 Introduction to artificial neural networks

An artificial neural network (ANN) is a network of highly computed cells that mimics the physiological capability of the human brain. These cells occur in layers and are often referred to as nodes. The major function of the brain is to send information to the body in the form of signals. As a result the brain is capable of adapting, learning new things, analyzing incomplete and unclear information, and making relevant judgements. A simple analogy is being able to read letters and words written by other people even when the handwriting is not the same as ours or the ability of the human brain to differentiate between a ball and an apple. The human brain is able to carry out numerous tasks involving intelligence, patterns, and object recognition. Although such tasks seem extremely difficult to automate, they can be performed using ANNs. It is for these reasons that any computing system that pursues similar tasks will benefit greatly from understanding how the human brain works and how to imitate the process. This necessitates the study of the neural network. The human central nervous system has billions of neurons with three major functional parts: axon, cell body, and dendrite. The axon transmits signals from one neuron to another, the cell body (soma) incorporates the nucleus that gives support to the cell, while the dendrite obtains signals from the neurons and transmits them to the cell body. Thus the neuron receives signals from other neurons through dendrite. Neurons do not touch each other, and neither do they touch muscles, tissues, or dendrites (except in the case of the electrical synapse); rather, they interact at a contact point, which is usually a gap referred to as a synapse. The gap contains chemicals that transmit impulses from neurons to neurons, muscles, and tissues. These chemicals are called neurotransmitters. Most important neurotransmitters present in the human brain include glutamate, aspartate, gamma-aminobutyric acid, acetylcholine, dopamine, and serotonin, which are also involved in many neurological diseases.

The artificial neural network is inspired by the exceptional capability of the human brain to learn, adapt, and make exceptional judgements in regard to

Biomedical Signal Processing and Artificial Intelligence in Healthcare. https://doi.org/10.1016/B978-0-12-818946-7.00007-X

complex world problems. The first artificial neuron was proposed in 1943 by a neurophysiologist and a mathematician named McCulloch and Pitts. It was proved that the computing model was able to perform a computable function using a finite number and synaptic weight adjustment. Since then, ANNs have found acceptance in several fields including medicine, and they have shown the capacity to solve real-world problems. In an artificial neural network, neurons are connected in identical ways as the biological neural network of the brain. Data are mathematically processed with the results transferred to neurons in the next layer. ANNs are used in modeling parts of the human body and recognizing diseases from various scans, such as magnetic resonance imaging (MRI) and positron emission tomography (PET).

7.1.1 Artificial neural network architectures

The ANN architecture includes the input layer, hidden layer, and output layer. The input layer receives raw input data/value. These values are transmitted to the hidden layer(s) before being transmitted further to the output layer. The hidden layer can be single or multiple. In ANNs, training is based on two main learning methods: supervised and unsupervised learning methods.

Supervised learning methods are attempts to find the connection between input data (training set) and target data. In simple terms, it is learning from example, where the computer program (learner) is first given training data and subsequently tests data. By providing the computer program with labeled training data, it will develop a model to classify or regress the data and identify the same classes of data when provided without labels. In supervised learning, accuracy is very important. As a result, it is recommended that the computer program is trained with large amounts of data of the same class of image with varying degrees of shapes, indentations, and differences. This will ensure that the computer can still identify the image even if the same image is indented or curved. A simple analogy to this is providing a computer program with a set of different fruit images (such as cashews, apples, oranges, and strawberries) where the name of the fruit in each image is given to the learner. Afterward the learner is provided with a set of unlabeled fruit images of the same class as provided early and tested to identify each fruit with high accuracy.

An unsupervised learning method is simply where learning is performed without a teacher but by observation. In unsupervised learning the training set does not include labels. The computer program receives inputs but obtains neither supervised target outputs nor impact from its environment. It does this by building a representation of the inputs, which can be used for predicting future inputs and decision-making. Success in unsupervised learning is determined by whether the network is able to reduce or increase an associated cost function.

7.1.1.1 Multilayer perceptron and neural networks

A multilayer perceptron (MLP) is a class of ANN. A perceptron is the simplest form of an ANN. The perceptron consists of one neuron with two inputs and one output. In MLPs, signals are transmitted from the input to the output without a loop. This means that the neuron is unaffected by the output. This kind of architecture is referred to as feedforward. MLPs usually consist of more than one perceptron. This includes an input layer that receives the signal, a hidden layer(s), an output layer that makes a prediction about the input layer, and a hidden layer(s) that represent the true engine of the MLP (Fig. 7.1). There also exist feedback networks, which can transmit impulses both ways (in both directions). This network is dynamic and is capable of changing its conditions at all times until an equilibrium is reached. Once another layer is added, each neuron will act as a standard perceptron for the output of the neurons. A multilayer network does not provide an increase in computing power compared with networks with a single layer regardless of the activation function of the neuron. MLPs with one hidden layer are capable of approximating any continuous function and are often applied to supervised learning problems. In MLPs, training involves harmonizing the parameters, weights, or biases to minimize error. Back propagation is utilized to make the weight and bias fitting comparative with the error. In the next section a back propagation neural network (BPNN) and its applications are presented.

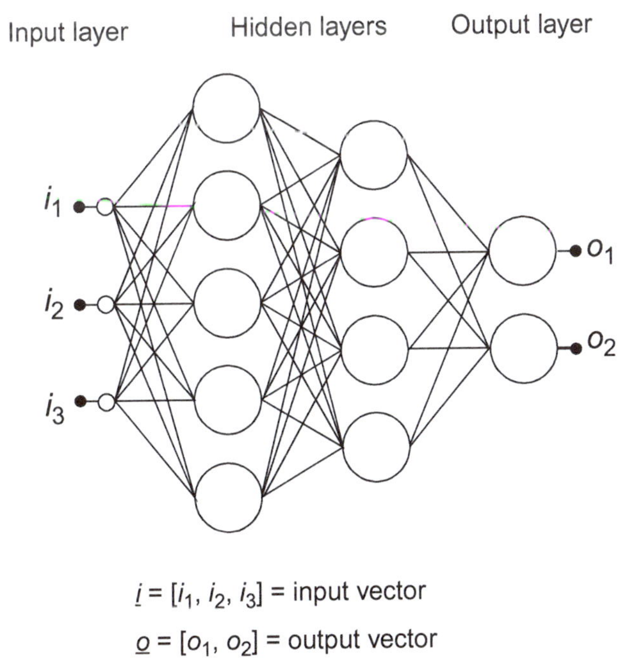

FIG. 7.1

A multilayer perceptron with two hidden layers.

Courtesy of M.W. Gardner, S. Dorling, Artificial neural networks (the multilayer perceptron) a review of applications in the atmospheric sciences, Atmos. Environ. 32 (14–15) (1998) 2627–2636.

7.1.1.2 Back propagation neural network

The BPNN algorithm is one of the most commonly used supervised algorithms in shallow neural networks, which was developed by Rumelhart et al. [1]. It is easy to implement and converges very fast and can therefore be used efficiently in classification and prediction studies. In the BPNN, input layers receive normalized values where these values are used to calculate the potential of each neuron in the next level (hidden layer) (Fig. 7.2). Then an activation function (ReLu, Tanh, Sigmoid, etc.) is used to calculate the output of each neuron. Afterward, in the output layer, these steps are repeated, and errors are propagated back to update biases and weights during the training process. Finally, root mean square error is used as stopping criteria for feedforward and feedback calculations are converged.

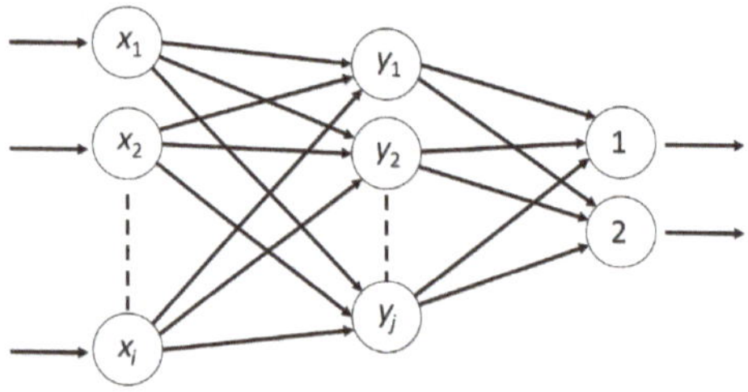

FIG. 7.2

General topology of a three-layered BPNN for *i* inputs, *j* hidden neurons, and two outputs.

7.1.1.3 Convolutional neural networks

A convolutional neural network (CNN) [2] is a neural network with a convolution operation instead of matrix multiplication in at least one of the layers. CNNs contain one or more of each of the following layers: convolution layer, rectified linear unit layer, pooling layer, fully connected layer, and loss layer (during the training process) (Fig. 7.3). CNNs are inspired by natural perception mechanisms of humans. It is a class of deep feedforward artificial neural networks that is applied to analyzing visual images. A CNN takes 2-D or 3-D images as the input while utilizing spatial and configuration information. CNNs utilize three mechanisms of receptive field, weights sharing, and subsampling, which help to reduce the freedom of the model. CNNs are primarily used in the field of pattern recognition within images. With this, image-specific features can be encoded into the architecture, thereby making the network more suited for image-focused tasks while further reducing the parameters required to set up the model. CNN applications include image classification, object detection, object tracking, pose estimation, text detection and recognition, end-to-end text test spotting, visual saliency detection, action recognition, and action recognition.

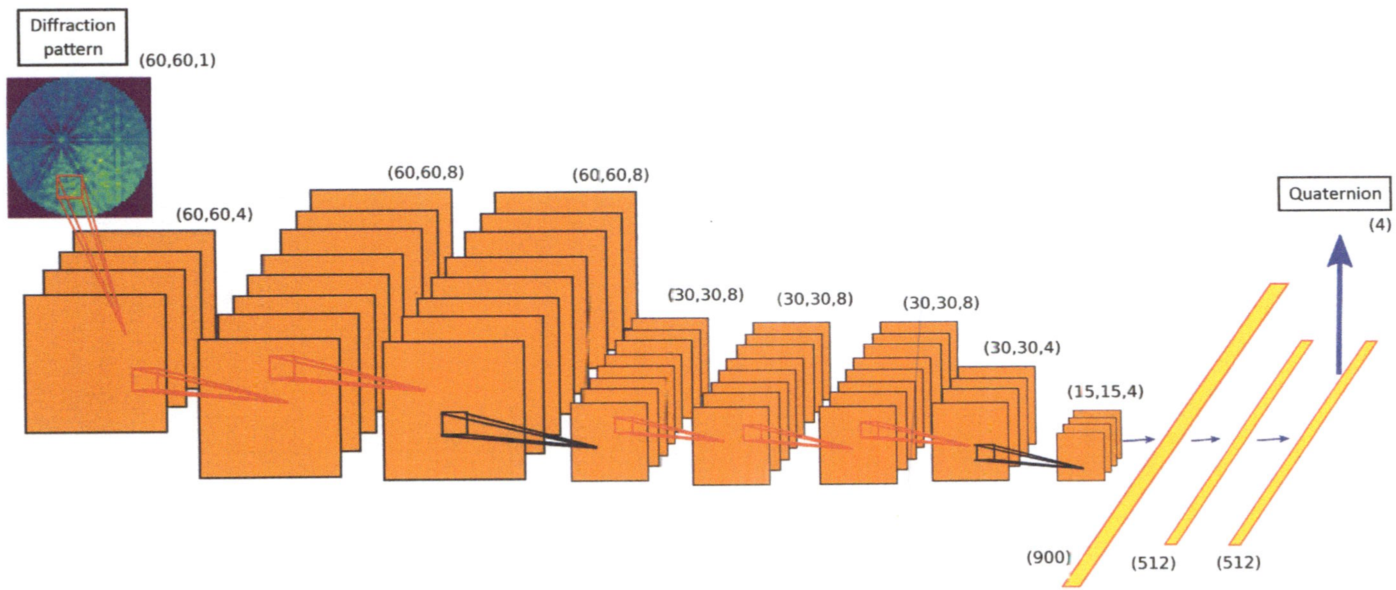

FIG. 7.3

Convolutional neural network architecture. The input is a diffraction pattern, which goes through several convolutional layers and then the fully connected layers. The output is four real-valued numbers corresponding to quaternion components that represent a crystal orientation. Numbers in the parentheses show the dimensions of each step. The convolutional operations are shown in *red*, max pooling operations are shown in *black*, and full connections are shown in *blue*.

Courtesy of Y.F. Shen, R. Pokharel, T.J. Nizolek, A. Kumar, T. Lookman, Convolutional neural network-based method for real-time orientation indexing of measured electron backscatter diffraction patterns, Acta Mater. 170 (2019) 118–131.

7.2 Applications on neurological and neuropsychiatric diseases

Neurological and neuropsychiatric diseases are disorders that arise from the damage and degeneration of the central nervous system. Examples of these disorders include Alzheimer's disease (AD), Parkinson's disease (PD), Huntington's disease, schizophrenia, Tourette syndrome, autism spectrum disorder (ASD), and attention-deficit/hyperactivity disorder (ADHD). The causes are associated with genetic, environmental factors, and injuries to the nervous system or other parts of the brain. This damage affects the communication of neurons giving rise to symptoms such as memory loss, mood swings, loss of bodily control, and behavioral changes. These symptoms can be neutralized with the help of various treatments in the early stages of the diseases, but diagnosis of the diseases in its earlier stages is inaccurate and challenging using current imaging techniques and variable human input; hence the disease can be misdiagnosed and progresses undetected. Neural networks, which are a form of artificial intelligence, can be applied in these cases to provide early and more accurate diagnosis of these diseases allowing for better and more effective treatment of affected patients and differentiating them from patients who may have other disorders or those who are healthy. These neural networks can learn from input data to create an improved output each time based on experience and can evolve without the need for human input, which improves accuracy as it removes human error and varied knowledge.

Artificial neural networks (ANNs) are types of machine learning algorithms that allow systems to learn from data and improve from experience without any human intervention by using training sets of real-world data to deduce models with a greater accuracy than human intervened models by stimulating the neural structure of the brain. They are proven to perform better in extracting the biomarkers of heterogeneous data sets, as in AD where the data volume and variety are great [3]. Hence, it is of great importance to use automated detection methods for precise detection and classification approaches. In the following sections, ANN applications on classification of AD, PD, ADHD, and ASD are presented.

7.2.1 Alzheimer's disease

AD is the most common type of neurodegenerative disease, which accounts for approximately 60%–80% of dementias [4], leading to an irreversible and gradual mental deterioration as a result of neuronal death in the brain, eventually leading to death. According to the Diagnostic and Statistical Manual of Mental Disorders IV (DSM-IV), AD is characterized by (1) new onset memory impairment; (2) another cognitive disturbance, for example, aphasia, agnosia, apraxia, or executive functioning; (3) a gradual and progressive course resulting in a significant amount of functional impairment [5]. Statistics show that there are approximately 47 million people on a global scale living with AD [6] with the number expected to double to about 100 million by 2050 [7]. There are currently no clinically proven treatments to avoid or stop the progression of the disease because the damage to the brain cells cannot be reversed and cannot be stopped. However, the symptoms of the disease can be targeted rather than its cause [8] using various therapeutic approaches such as drug therapy. It is reported that between 1998 and 2011, around 100 therapeutic drugs were tested and failed [9]. It was later found that the major reason for this series of failed clinical trials was the late intervention when brain damage had reached an advanced and irreversible stage with the current time-consuming diagnostic methods playing a major role in this factor [10]. This stresses the need to develop early and effective detection methods which are key for increasing the effectiveness of the current clinical therapies, thereby arresting symptoms of AD before significant damage has been done to the brain.

AD is neuropathologically characterized by the presence of amyloid plaques (caused by the aggregation of amyloid beta (Aβ) protein) and neurofibrillary tangles (NFTs) (caused by the aggregation of hyperphosphorylated tau protein), along with deficits in certain neurotransmitter systems [11]. The gradual neurodegenerative process, also referred to as "amyloid cascade hypothesis," begins when there is accumulation of Aβ either because of the failure to dispose of the protein or its overproduction, which leads to plaque deposits in the brain and NFT production and eventually neuronal necrosis, which gives rise to the symptoms of AD [12]. Aβ protein can thereby be used as a biomarker for AD diagnosis, and this can help in earlier diagnosis of the disease in its earlier stages before the first symptoms start to show [13].

Structural magnetic resonance imaging (sMRI) is one of the most frequently used imaging techniques in AD clinical assessment. sMRI is a stable biomarker that is essential in studying AD progression and intensity from the mild cognitive impairment (MCI) stages. The sMRI shows the relationship between neurodegeneration and cognitive decline, leading to its efficiency as an AD biomarker. When there is neuronal damage, it also leads to cerebral atrophy [14]. The disadvantages of using sMRI are that it cannot show AD behavior at a cellular level and may also give results that are inaccurate, as some atrophy patterns are the same as some other neurodegenerative diseases.

Functional magnetic resonance imaging (fMRI) has in recent years been used as functional neuroimaging and can detect changes in brain function in the earlier stages of the disease and track the progression of atrophy. Medial temporal lobe (MTL) memory structures are the source of neuropathological changes in AD. There is hypoconnectivity of the MTL versus healthy control of elderly patients [15], but it has recently been observed that there may be a phase of increased MTL activity, which indicates compensatory neural mechanisms with the aim of maintaining the healthy memory performance of the brain. When MCI converts to AD, this compensation is lost.

Positron emission tomography (PET) imaging is a functional imaging technique that provides unique information and has shown great sensitivity in tracking brain alterations over time. This has therefore led to PET imaging being considered the forerunner in in vivo assessment of amyloid load [16] with the overall goal being to achieve preclinical or early diagnosis of the disease [11]. ^{18}F-Florbetapir, also known as ^{18}F-AV45, is the preferred radiotracer because it boasts optimum kinetics and selectivity features, which bind specifically to amyloid plaques [17]. Therefore the prospects of PET AV45 (18F-florbetapir) being the preferred method of early diagnosis are increasing.

AD is a heterogeneous and multivariate disease that further complicates the extraction and classification of clinical data [10]. To this end, machine learning techniques can be employed with the aim of achieving early and accurate prediction of the disease. Machine learning techniques will also be able to differentiate healthy individuals and individuals suffering from AD and those who are just suffering from MCI (both in the early (EMCI) and late (LMCI) stages) and significant memory concern (SMC). MCI, also referred to as the AD predementia stage, is the prodromal stage of AD that may lead to AD or may remain stable in this stage without further progression [18], while SMC individuals are cognitively normal with slight memory concerns [19]. It is therefore of interest of researchers to be able to distinguish the presymptomatic stages of the disease that have not been well studied [20], allowing for a revised diagnosis criterion and the application of early intervention methods.

The Alzheimer's Disease Neuroimaging Initiative (ADNI) is a public-private partnership, led by Principal Investigator Michael W. Weiner, MD, and was launched in 2003. The goal of ADNI is to test whether serial magnetic resonance imaging (MRI), positron emission tomography (PET), other biological markers, and clinical and neuropsychological assessment can be combined to measure the progression of MCI and AD in its early stages by providing very large clinical and imaging data sets. Some examples of PET images with different radiotracers and MRI images from ADNI database are shown in Fig. 7.4.

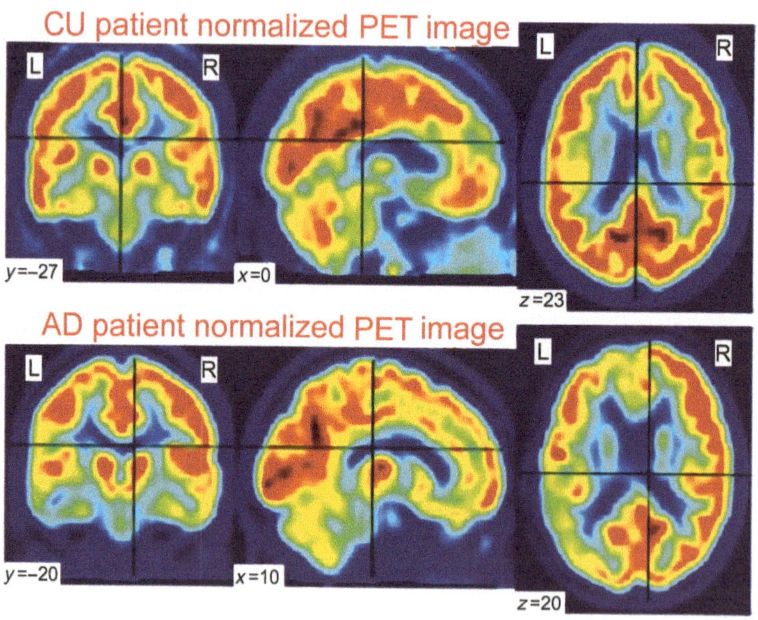

FIG. 7.4

Sample PET image slice for cognitively unimpaired (CU) and AD patients.

Courtesy of S. Singh, et al., Deep learning based classification of FDG-PET data for Alzheimers disease categories, in: Proceedings of SPIE-the International Society for Optical Engineering.

Many studies have used the ADNI database for the classification and detection of AD. Table 7.1 summarizes the results of different reports on the classification of AD with different neural network algorithms on the PET and MRI data sets and the use of biological, genetic, and cognitive measurements as supportive inputs.

Table 7.1 AD/NC classification accuracy results from different research groups.

Accuracy (%)	Method	Data set	References
94.0	SVM based	sMRI	[21]
98.3	DemNet	sMRI	[4]
94.7	STL based	sMRI	[22]
89.1	SVM	FDG-PET+MRI	[23]
95.4	SVM	FDG-PET+MRI	[24]
96.9	SVM	FDG-PET	[25]
98.1	MLP	FDG-PET	[16]
91.2	RBF-SVM	FDG-PET+MRI	[26]
87.9	RF	Florbetapir-PET+MRI	[26]
90.7	SVM	FDG-PET+MRI+CSF	[27]
92.4	MKL	FDG-PET+MRI++CSF+APOE+CS	[28]
91.8	OPLS	MRI+CSF	[29]
93.3	M3T	FDG-PET+MRI+CSF	[30]
89.0	RF	FDG-PET+MRI+CSF+genotype	[31]

CS, *cognitive score;* CSF, *cerebrospinal fluid;* IFAST, *implicit function as squashing time;* M3T, *multimodal multitask;* MKL, *multi kernel learning;* NIB, *natural image bases;* OPLS, *orthogonal partial least squares to latent structures;* STL, *self-taught learning.*

7.2.2 Parkinson's disease

Parkinson's disease (PD) is known to be a progressive disease with neurodegenerative effects on a person. It causes effects to the brain, muscles, coordination, and movement. PD has affected millions of people throughout the world from different cultures and races. This disorder was named after the doctor James Parkinson, who first described it in 1817. PD usually starts around the age of 60, but it can be detected 20 years earlier. Early onset of the disorder is when it begins before the age of 50, and this accounts for 5%–10% PD cases. These forms of PD are often inherited, even though they are not related to genetic mutations. The disease affects more men than women; however, younger people can also be diagnosed with PD. This is referred to as Young-Onset Parkinson's disease and is also known as juvenile parkinsonism. It runs in families and is related to genetic mutation.

The diagnosis of PD can be performed by physical examinations and imaging methods using the biomarkers in the brain to see the areas that are affected.

This diagnosis, which involves imaging, thereby using the biomarkers of the disease, has led to imaging procedures and clinical laboratory-based assays. Brain imaging studies using PET and single-photon emission computed tomography (SPECT) are the most commonly used methods to differentiate PD patients from normal healthy groups, but the similarities of PD with other neurodegenerative diseases and their respective indicators such as those of multiple system atrophy and supranuclear atrophy have made diagnosis more difficult and less accurate [32]. Early detection of the disease has also proven to be nonviable until certain low levels of dopamine neurons have been reached, and this may lead to the misdiagnosis of affected patients as healthy while the disease still progresses. This has left researchers with the objective of finding ways of detecting the disease in its early stages and with improved diagnostic accuracy, hence the application of ANN.

ANN is a computational algorithm that can model biological structures and systems using real-world data sets and can thereby learn and improve these data with great accuracy with little or no room for human variability. ANN is better suited for classifying nonlinear clinical data [33] such as that of PD because of its heterogeneous nature.

Many studies conducted on PD classification (Fig. 7.5) have used DaTscan (which gives functional information on dopamine transporters in striatal region) images from the Parkinson's Progression Markers Initiative (PPMI) database (www.ppmi-info.org/data). PPMI is an observational clinical study to verify progression markers in Parkinson's disease.

Table 7.2 summarizes the results of different studies on the classification of PD with different methods on the SPECT data set.

7.2.3 Attention-deficit/hyperactivity disorder

Attention-deficit hyperactivity disorder (ADHD) is a disorder that is prevalent with psychiatric symptoms affecting 39 million people as of 2013 [40]. Childhood and adolescence stages are characterized by various prevalent behavioral disorders, and among these disorders, ADHD affects approximately 10% of school-aged children in the United States [41]. ADHD-associated symptoms manifest in 2%–4% of adults when diagnosed [42]. The diagnosis of this disorder is made based on some symptoms that are manifested behaviorally, namely, impaired executive function, inattention, impulsivity, and hyperactivity. There is no known method or a diagnostic standard test for this disorder because most of them have low efficiency, which have long testing times, long interview time, and other inefficiencies that often result in misdiagnosis. There are several physiological tests carried out to test for this disorder, including the ADHD rating scale (ADHD-RS), Conners parent rating scale (CBRS), and Brown attention-deficit disorder scale (BADDS) [43, 44]. There is a significant need for an accurate and precise diagnostic method for detecting ADHD and also a need for defining experimental differences between subjects who have ADHD and normal subjects [45–49]. A further step in the study of this disorder has been since explored, which is the technique of using machine language with

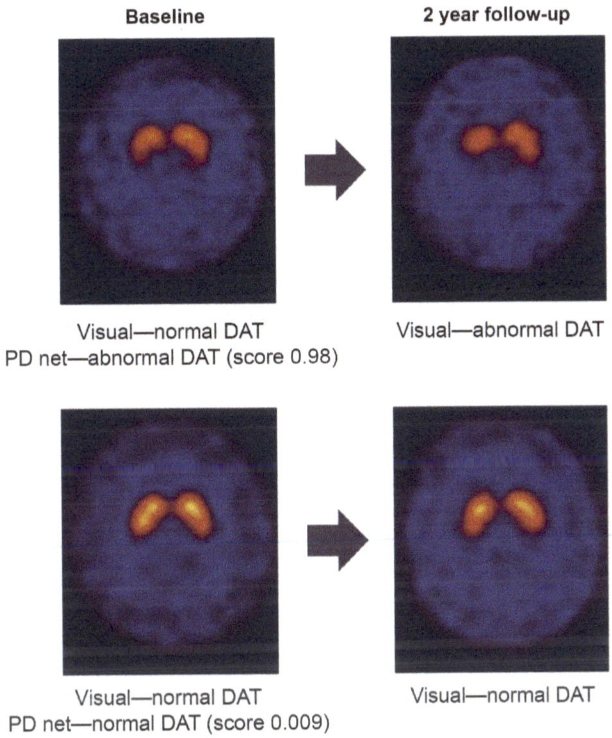

FIG. 7.5

Refining SWEDD classification using PD Net analysis. The representative two cases show different image diagnoses analyzed by PD Net. Two subjects had normal DAT according to the visual interpretation consensus, while PD Net revealed that one subject (in the preceding text) had reduced DAT in the striatum. The 2-year follow-up SPECT of the subject was abnormal according to the visual interpretation consensus. However, a SWEDD subject (in the succeeding text) who also showed normal DAT in PD Net persistently had normal DAT in the follow-up scan.

Courtesy of H. Choi, S. Ha, H.J. Im, S.H. Paek, D.S. Lee, Refining diagnosis of Parkinson's disease with deep learning-based interpretation of dopamine transporter imaging. Neuroimage Clin. 10(16) (2017) 586–594.

Table 7.2 Results of different studies on the classification of PD versus NC.

Accuracy (%)	Sensitivity (%)	Specificity (%)	Method	References
96.8	89.0	93.2	SVM	[34]
96	94.2	100	DCNN	[17]
97.9	97.8	98.1	SVM	[35]
94.8	93.7	97.3	SVD-NB	[36]
94.7	93.7	95.7	PLS-SVM	[37]
96.1	95.0	96.6	SVM	[38]
99.6	99.7	99.2	BPNN	[39]

DCNN, *deep convolutional neural network;* NB, *naive Bayes;* PLS, *partial least squares;* SVD, *singular value decomposition.*

pattern recognition based on structural MRI data used for both the diagnosis of this and other disorders like Alzheimer's disease using SVM to detect the early stages of the disorder. These traditional machine learning techniques are utilized to distinguish MRI data of subjects with such diagnosed defects. It involves different training sessions of data sets, which are classified and then their accuracy is tested [50–56].

The ADHD-200 consortium released a large data set of results from resting state fMRI (rs-fMRI) scans and from the personal characteristics of the subjects and they also supported the findings with another data set for testing, which was used for the 2011 ADHD-200 competition [57]. In studies from the past to the present, electroencephalography and magnetoencephalography have been used for recording brain activities, and they are often impacted by interferences that can affect the signals recorded [58–61]. Other imaging methods have also been employed in the studies of this disorder, including MRI [62] and fMRI [63] (Fig. 7.6), which are used to study

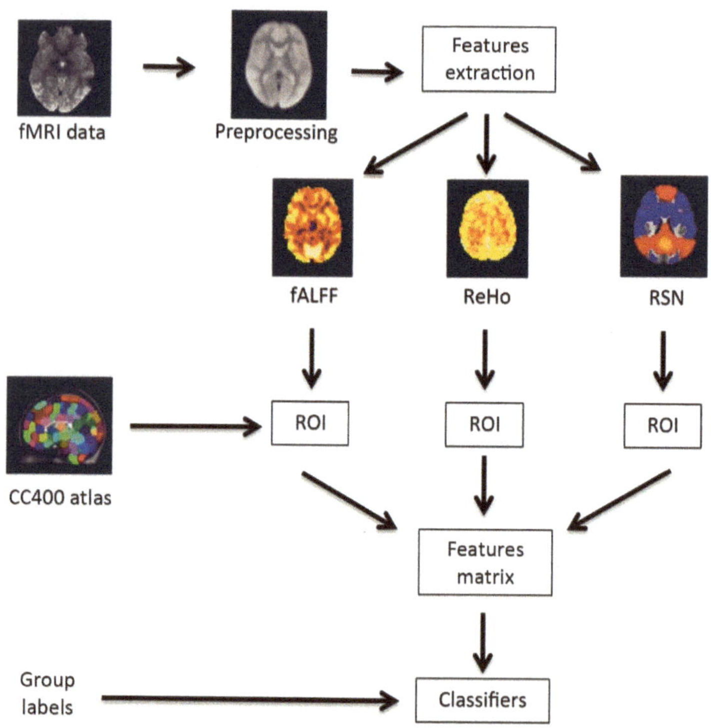

FIG. 7.6

Flow of data processing. The raw fMRI data are preprocessed; the feature maps for fALFF, ReHo, and RSN are obtained; the average coefficient of these maps within each ROI are calculated using the CC400 atlas; the data are then organized in a feature matrix that is then input to the classifiers.

Courtesy of J.R. Sato, M.Q. Hoexter, A. Fujita, L.A. Rohde, Evaluation of pattern recognition and feature extraction methods in ADHD prediction. Front. Syst. Neurosci. 6 (2012) 68.

the anatomy of brain disorders and the various differences between normal subjects and subjects with ADHD.

The development of an accurate, precise, effective, and automatic method of diagnosing ADHD to overcome all the deficiencies encountered when using the traditional clinical methods has been studied during the last decade. Kuang et al. used deep learning methods and were able to extract frequency domain features from each brain region, and they utilized a deep belief network with three hidden layers to discriminate ADHD [64]. The CNN is used to learn patterns from the inputted images [65]. Ji et al. used the 2-D CNN for 2-D images and performed 3-D convolutions in both space and time [66]. Li et al. later developed a 3-D CNN model, which was used for completing and integrating PET and MRI data [67]. A summary of the results on ADHD classification is presented in Table 7.3.

Table 7.3 ADHD versus NC classification results.

Accuracy (%)	Sensitivity (%)	Specificity (%)	Method	Cross validation	References
95.1	94.4	95.7	SVM	LOOCV	[68]
78.75	76.00	80.71	SVM	LOOCV	[69]
75.54	70.50	77.44	SVM	10-Folds CV	[69]
85	78	91	PCA-FDA	LOOCV	[70]
80	87	74	SVM	LOOCV	[71]
66	23	90	VM	10-Folds CV	[72]
55	33	80	VM	10-Folds CV	[73]
76	63	85	VM	LOOCV	[74]
90	N/A	N/A	ELM	LOOCV	[75]
61	N/A	N/A	H-ELM	10-Folds CV	[76]
83	84	82	SVM	LOOCV	[77]

CV, *cross validation;* LOOCV, *leave-one-out cross validation.*

7.2.4 Autism spectrum disorder

Autism spectrum disorder (ASD) is a severe neurodevelopmental condition characterized by a lifelong "triad" of impairments including repetitive behavior and deficits in social interactions and communication [78] that manifests in early childhood. It is estimated that about 1 in 68 children (1 in 42 boys and 1 in 189 girls) is suffering from ASD worldwide according to estimates from the Centers for Disease Control and Prevention (CDC) and Autism and Developmental Disabilities Monitoring (ADDM) Network [79]. ASD has severe consequences that affect not only the lives of patients but also their families with a variety of impacts on health, social integration, and quality of life along with an emotional and economic burden [80]. The CDC has estimated the total costs per year for children suffering from ASD in the United States alone to be between $11.5 and $60.9 billion (2011 US dollars) and ASD costs a family about $60,000 a year including medical care and special education. According to Statista (https://www.statista.com), the estimated total cost of ASD in the United States was $268 billion in 2015 and will reach $461 billion in 2025. The World Health Organization [81] states that there has been a global increase in the prevalence of the disorder, which will cause a further increase in the annual cost of ASD.

Affected individuals exhibit deficits in understanding how to behave and interact with others along with being unable to communicate with other people effectively, which is the first behavioral disturbance typically noted during the first 18–30 months. This is followed by the later development of imagination impairments including deficits in flexible thinking and stereotypical repetitive behaviors and limited interests when compared with typically developing children [82]. Nevertheless, the severity of the disease may show variations with the population, making the disease highly heterogeneous. Currently, ASD is diagnosed by carrying out behavioral and intellectual measurements. Such methods, however, can be subjective due to being entirely based on professional expertise and patient cooperation [83]. Additionally, they fail to provide an insight into the etiology of the disease along with being time consuming and requiring a long period to detect any abnormalities that are present [84]. It is known that early detection of ASD has a significant impact on the prognosis of the disease, and thus behavioral diagnostics are not suitable for early detection, as they only allow disease diagnosis after the manifestation of behavioral impairments has already taken place.

fMRI plays an important role in characterizing the pathophysiology of the disease and is considered as a promising candidate for producing objective biomarkers with the purpose of gaining a greater insight into the underlying causes of ASD [85]. fMRI is one of the most employed neuroimaging methods to search for novel biomarkers in brain function, by observing functional variations in brain activity to reveal regional associations during the performance of a task by detecting changes associated with blood flow [86]. The discovery that various areas of the brain still actively interact with each other and there is an intrinsic synchronous activity even when at rest (not actively participating in any task) corresponding to a functional network has prompted improvement in the resting state functional connectivity research in ASD [87]. Since then the use of resting state fMRI (rs-fMRI) is considered as a key imaging technique in examining brain networks [88], leading to many significant insights involved with the disease. Thus functional connectivity measures can be used as predictors in the identification of ASD.

However, as mentioned previously, ASD is a highly heterogeneous disease, leading to heterogeneous data sets. To this end, machine learning techniques can be employed to create an fMRI data-driven model to extract novel biomarkers of the disease and differentiate accurately ASD patients from healthy individuals to make an early and proper diagnosis. The importance of early diagnosis has previously been implicated in the literature [89], which allows for the application of early intervention methods. This is of great importance, as early intervention can significantly improve the quality of life of ASD patients [90] and disease prognosis, leading to improvements in cognition, language, and adaptive behavior [91] along with major reductions in the economic costs related to ASD.

Since an ANN allows systems to learn from data and improve from experience without any human intervention by using training sets of real-world data to deduce models with a greater accuracy than human intervened models, it simulates the neural structure of the brain and is significantly beneficial in situations where the data volume and variety are great. Hence, ANNs can perform better in extracting the novel biomarkers of heterogeneous data sets as in ASD [3]. Thus they have potential for gaining a greater understanding of the disorder and help to develop early diagnostic and therapeutic approaches. To this end, it is essential to focus on automated diagnosis

The multifaceted nature and heterogeneity of ASD make it necessary to conduct substantial scale tests that are hard to achieve in any individual lab. Accordingly the Autism Brain Imaging Data Exchange (ABIDE) provides previously gathered functional magnetic resonance imaging (rs-fMRI) data sets from over 500 people with ASD and nearly 600 typical controls (TCs). This grassroots activity included 16 international sites, yielding 1112 data sets comprising both MRI information and a broad cluster of phenotypic data. In compliance with 1000 Functional Connectomes Project/INDI protocols and Health Insurance Portability and Accountability Act rules, all data sets are anonymous, with no protected health information included. The ABIDE data set was obtained from 16 different imaging centers. For each patient, in addition to rs-fMRI data sets, phenotypic information and T1 structural brain images are provided, which is publicly available at http://preprocessed-connectomes-project.org/ [92]. The access information details were given by Di Martino et al. [93]. Studies using the fMRI data set for ASD classification are summarized in Table 7.4, and sample images for analyzing the images can be seen in Fig. 7.7.

Table 7.4 Classification accuracy results.

Accuracy (%)	Sensitivity (%)	Specificity (%)	Method	References
95.9	96.9	94.8	RCE-based SVM	[94]
65	68	62	SVM	[95]
63	60	58	RF	[95]
70	74	63	DNN	[95]
86	N/A	N/A	DNN	[83]
67	61	72	SVC	[96]
91	89	93	RF	[97]
90	92	87	PNN	[98]

PNN, *probabilistic neural network;* RCE, *recursive cluster elimination;* SVC, *support vector classification.*

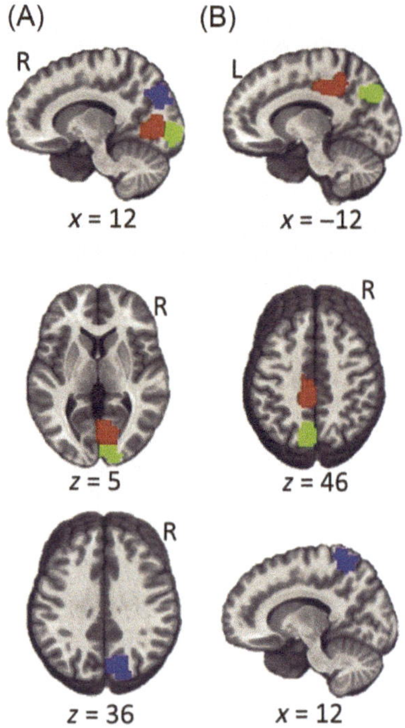

FIG. 7.7

Highly correlated (connected) areas for ASD subjects. (A) *Green* represents the source area: occipital pole. *Red areas* show the intracalcarine cortex. *Blue areas* show the lateral occipital cortex; superior division. (B) *Green* represents the source area: lateral occipital cortex; superior division. *Red areas* show the cingulate gyrus; posterior division. *Blue area* shows the postcentral gyrus.

Courtesy of A.S. Heinsfeld, A.R. Franco, R.C. Craddock, A. Buchweitz,F. Meneguzzi, Identification of autism spectrum disorder using deep learning and the ABIDE dataset. Neuroimage Clin. 17 (2018) 16–23.

7.3 Challenges and opportunities

ANN has proven to be a promising approach for the classification of medical imaging data. Unfortunately, several challenges remain [99]. The first challenge is the robustness of the data used. When classifying medical images, ANN requires a hugely insane amount of data for the best result during training. The performance of ANN is largely impacted by the quantity and quality of data [100]. However, unavailability of data set is one of the biggest barriers in the success of ANN in medical imaging classification [101]. Also, developing substantial medical imaging data can be demanding because annotation needs considerable time from medical imaging expert if expert opinion is desired to overcome human error [102].

The second challenge is that there is a black box character [103]. Even though a neural network performs excellently well after training, no one really understands how it works. This implies that the algorithms and mathematics used by the system are not explained. There is also an issue of reliability since it does not show how reliable the result is. Because of this the application of neural networks in medical imaging classification is limited.

The third challenge of ANN in medical image classification is that of the system's inability to explicit expert's opinion, knowledge, and experiences [104]. Also the real meaning of its joint weight is not clear. These challenges can be solved by combining neural networks with fuzzy logic and processing fuzzy information with neural networks. This enables the neural network to explicit network topological structure and qualitative knowledge and provides a clear physical meaning to the joint weight [105].

The fourth challenge is choosing which neural network model and architecture to use. Although there have been studies on model selection, however, there have not been an appropriate data in literature specifying the type of network to design for specific work and no generic exist to certify the most appropriate trade-off between variance for a particular size of the training set and model bias. Hence, networks are designed by trial and error, and this is difficult to surpass.

With the challenges come opportunities. First, numerous analysis methods for ANN is applicable to biological system modification; for example, the Canonical Correlation Analysis (CCA) only need access to activity recordings. CCA could be utilized to examine flexibility in activity pattern in similar neurons over time, across various layers, regions, or animal or to examine the correlation of depiction across subjects [106].

The second opportunity is that there is huge potential to overcome constraints that restrict the use of the analysis method in medical image classification. Black box variants are currently being developed. which will not require access to gradient [107]. It will be interesting for future studies to modify such methods to medical image classification.

Thirdly, ANNs can further enable researchers to quickly develop, test, and apply new data analysis techniques on models that can tackle complex sensory processing tasks.

Fourthly the neural network provides the possibility of modifying the environment for a range of mathematical systems. Medical processing with neural network also allows transferability of certain classifiers, which makes training difficult; however, it would produce high performance. On-the-job training would hence be a very valuable improvement for different medical image patterns.

Lastly the ANNs can be in the form of intelligent agents and a combination of neural networks. Also, neural networks and a combination of genetic algorithms with fuzzy fitness would provide a means for ANN advancement and effectiveness for medical image processing.

7.4 Future directions

Due to ANN complexity, understanding the mechanisms associated with the use of ANN would be a huge step toward developing better performing ANNs. To do this a sequence of processes should be considered such that major factors that out rightly affect the engineering problem are addressed, for example, adequate model input determination, division of data, selection of capable network architecture, selection of suitable internal parameters for optimization purposes, stopping criteria, and model validation. The data division method provides a systematic approach to improve the performance of ANNs in terms of trial and error with independent data sets, self-organization of maps, including fuzzy clustering [108], which can be applied to medical images. The models developed should be predictive to allow the generalization of similar data types to adequately train the network to be at their full potential. The model can be determined by checking the agreement of the prediction with the physical process and weight under observation [109].

Transparency of the model and knowledge extraction entails the ability of the user of an ANN model to interpret the model along with the effects of input model on the output model [110]. Model classification techniques are done according to colors such that the physical interpretation of the model phenomenon increases with respect to the physical knowledge used in model development. A color coding to represent mathematical models such as a white box for physical laws with known variables and parameters, a black box model for data or regressive processes where variable are either unknown or estimated, and a gray box model where the systems to be examined are conceptual and continue to derive more mathematical models. The black box model describes the ANNs and does not show transparency, hence hindering the ability to explain the physical process properly [110].

7.5 Summary

In this chapter the application of ANNs on neurological diseases such as AD, PD, ASD, and ADHD has been discussed. Classification performances of different methods on these diseases have been presented. Several challenges such as the robustness of the data, the system's inability to explicit expert's opinion still remain. Therefore, developing better performing ANNs requires deeper understanding of the models. Nevertheless, in its current stage, applications of ANNs have been shown to have very high performance in extracting the biomarkers of heterogeneous data sets where the data volume and variety are large.

Acknowledgments

We would like to thank Mubarak Mustapha, Kevin Meck, and Sunsley Tanaka Halimani from the Department of Biomedical Engineering at Near East University for their contributions.

References

[1] D.E. Rumelhart, G.E. Hinton, R.J. Williams, Learning representations by back-propagating errors, Nature 323 (1986) 533–536.

[2] K. Fukushima, Neocognitron: a self-organizing neural net-work for a mechanism of pattern recognition unaffected by shift in position, Biol. Cybern. 36 (4) (1980) 193–202.

[3] F. Pereira, T. Mitchell, M. Botvinick, Machine learning classifiers and fMRI: a tutorial overview, NeuroImage 45 (1) (2009) 199–209.

[4] C.D. Billones, et al., DemNet: a convolutional neural network for the detection of Alzheimer's disease and mild cognitive impairment, in: Region 10 Conference (TENCON), IEEE, 2016, pp. 3724–3727.

[5] S.W. Judith Neugroschl, Alzheimer's disease: diagnosis and treatment across the spectrum of disease severity, Mt Sinai J. Med. 78 (4) (2011) 596–612.

[6] S. Luo, et al., Automatic Alzheimer's disease recognition from MRI data using deep learning method, J. Appl. Math. Phys. 5 (2017) 1892–1898.

[7] R. Brookmeyer, et al., Forecasting the global burden of Alzheimer's disease, Alzheimers Dement. 3 (3) (2007) 186–191.

[8] M.A. Busquets, et al., Potential applications of magnetic particles to detect and treat Alzheimer's disease, Nanoscale Res. Lett. 9 (1) (2014) 538.

[9] K. Mullane, M. Williams, Alzheimer's therapeutics: continued clinical failures question the validity of the amyloid hypothesis-but what lies beyond? Biochem. Pharmacol. 85 (2013) 289–305.

[10] G.T. Saman Sarraf, Classification of Alzheimer's Disease Structural MRI Data by Deep Learning Convolutional Neural Networks, 2016. Computer Vision and Pattern Recognition.

[11] A.D. Cohen, W.E. Klunk, Early detection of Alzheimer's disease using PiB and FDG PET, Neurobiol. Disease 72 (2014) 117–122.

[12] J. Hardy, et al., Genetic dissection of Alzheimer's disease and related dementias: amyloid and its relationship to tau, Nat. Neurosci. 1 (1998) 355–358.

[13] A. Delacourte, et al., The biochemical pathway of neurofibrillary degeneration in aging and Alzheimer's disease, Neurology 52 (1999) 1158–1165.

[14] K.A. Johnson, et al., Brain imaging in Alzheimer disease, Cold Spring Harb. Perspect. Med. 2 (4) (2012). a006213.

[15] P. Vemuri, D.T. Jones, C.R. Jack, Resting state functional MRI in Alzheimer's disease, Alzheimers Res. Ther. 4 (2012) 2.

[16] S. Singh, et al., Deep learning based classification of FDG-PET data for Alzheimers disease categories, in: Proceedings of SPIE-the International Society for Optical Engineering, 2017.

[17] S.R. Choi, et al., Preclinical properties of 18F-AV-45: a PET imaging agent for Abeta plaques in the brain, J. Nucl. Med. 50 (11) (2009) 1887–1894.

[18] A. Khvostikov, et al., 3D CNN-based classification using sMRI and MD-DTI images for Alzheimer disease studies, 2018. Computer Vision and Pattern Recognition.

[19] S.L. Risacher, et al., APOE effect on Alzheimer's biomarkers in older adults with significant memory concern, Alzheimer's Dement. 11 (12) (2015) 1417–1429.

[20] V.K. Ithapu, et al., Imaging based enrichment criteria using deep learning algorithms for efficient clinical trials in MCI, Alzheimers Dement. 11 (12) (2015) 1489–1499.

[21] E. Gerardin, G. Chételat, M. Chupin, et al., Multidimensional classification of hippocampal shape features discriminates Alzheimer's disease and mild cognitive impairment from normal aging, NeuroImage 47 (4) (2009) 1476–1486.
[22] A. Gupta, et al., Natural image bases to represent neuroimaging data, in: Proc. of the 30th International Conf. on Machine Learning, pages 987-994, Atlanta, GA, 2013.
[23] M. Liu, D. Zhang, D. Shen, Hierarchical fusion of features and classifier decisions for Alzheimer's disease diagnosis, Hum. Brain Mapp. 35 (2013) 1305–1319.
[24] H. Suk, S. Lee, D. Shen, Hierarchical feature representation and multimodal fusion with deep learning for AD/MCI diagnosis, NeuroImage 101 (2014) 569–582.
[25] B. Lei, S. Chen, D. Ni, T. Wang, Discriminative learning for Alzheimer's disease diagnosis via canonical correlation analysis and multimodal fusion, Front. Aging Neurosci. 8 (2016).
[26] S. Nozadi, S. Kadoury, Classification of Alzheimer's and MCI patients from semantically parcelled PET images: a comparison between AV45 and FDG-PET, Int. J. Biomed. Imaging 2018 (2018) 1–13.
[27] O. Kohannim, X. Hua, D.P. Hibar, S. Lee, Y.-Y. Chou, A.W. Toga, C.R. Jack Jr., M. W. Weiner, P.M. Thompson, Boosting power for clinical trials using classifiers based on multiple biomarkers, Neurobiol. Aging 31 (8) (2010) 1429–1442.
[28] C. Hinrichs, V. Singh, G. Xu, S.C. Johnson, Predictive markers for AD in a multi-modality framework: an analysis of MCI progression in the ADNI population, NeuroImage 55 (2) (2011) 574–589.
[29] E. Westman, J.-S. Muehlboeck, A. Simmons, Combining MRI and CSF measures for classification of Alzheimer's disease and prediction of mild cognitive impairment conversion, NeuroImage 62 (1) (2012) 229–238.
[30] D. Zhang, D. Shen, Multi-modal multi-task learning for joint prediction of multiple regression and classification variables in Alzheimer's disease, NeuroImage 59 (2) (2012) 895–907.
[31] K.R. Gray, P. Aljabar, R.A. Heckemann, A. Hammers, D. Rueckert, Alzheimer's disease neuroimaging initiative. random forest-based similarity measures for multi-modal classification of Alzheimer's disease, Neuroimage 65 (2013) 167–175.
[32] S.S. Ahmed, W. Santosh, S. Kumar, H.T. Christlet, Metabolic profiling of Parkinson's disease: evidence of biomarker from gene expression analysis and rapid neural network detection, J. Biomed. Sci. 16 (2009) 63.
[33] R. Das, A comparison of multiple classification methods for diagnosis of Parkinson disease, Expert Syst. Appl. 37 (2010) 1568–1572.
[34] I.A. Illan, J.M. Gorrz, J. Ramirez, F. Segovia, J.M. Jimenez-Hoyuela, S.J. Ortega Lozano, Automatic assistance to Parkinson's disease diagnosis in DaTSCAN SPECT imaging, Med. Phys. 39 (10) (2012) 5971–5980.
[35] F.P. Olivera, M. Castelo-Branco, Computer-aided diagnosis of Parkinson's disease based on [123I] FP-CIT SPECT binding potential images, using the voxels-as-features approach and support vector machines, J. Neural Eng. 12 (2) (2015) 026008.
[36] D.J. Towey, P.G. Bain, K.S. Nijran, Automatic classification of 123I-FP-CIT (DaTSCAN) SPECT images, Nucl. Med. Commun. 32 (8) (2011) 699–707.
[37] F. Segovia, J.M. Gorriz, J. Ramirez, I. Alvarez, J.M. Jimenez-Hoyuela, S.J. Ortega, Improved Parkinsonism diagnosis using a partial least squares based approach, Med. Phys. 39 (7) (2012) 4395–4403.

[38] R. Prashanth, S. Dutta Roy, P.K. Mandal, S. Ghosh, Automatic classification and prediction models for early Parkinson's disease diagnosis from SPECT imaging, Expert Syst. Appl. 41 (7) (2014) 3333–3342.

[39] I. Ozsahin, B. Sekeroglu, P.C. Pwavodi, M. GSP, High-Accuracy Automated Diagnosis of Parkinson's Disease, Curr. Med. Imaging 15 (1) (2019) https://doi.org/10.2174/1573405615666190620113607.

[40] T. Vos, R.M. Barber, B. Bell, A. Bertozzi-Villa, S. Biryukov, I.B.F. Charlson, A. Davis, L. Degenhardt, D. Dicker, et al., Global, regional, and national incidence, prevalence, and years lived with disability for 301 acute and chronic diseases and injuries in 188 countries, 1990-2013: a systematic analysis for the global burden of disease study 2013, Lancet 386 (9995) (2015) 743.

[41] NIMH, https://www.nimh.nih.gov/health/statistics/attention-deficit-hyperactivity-disorder-adhd.shtml, 2017.

[42] G. Polanczyk, P. Jensen, Epidemiologic considerations in attention deficit hyperactivity disorder: a review and update, Child Adolesc. Psychiatr. Clin. N. Am. 17 (2008) 245.

[43] V. Simon, P. Czobor, S. Balint, A. Meszaros, Z. Murai, et al., Detailed review of epidemiologic studies on adult attention deficit/hyperactivity disorder (ADHD), Psychiatr. Hung. 22 (2007) 4–19.

[44] E. Willcutt, The prevalence of DSM-IV attention-deficit/hyperactivity disorder: a meta-analytic review, Neurotherapeutics 9 (2012) 490–499.

[45] I. Berger, Diagnosis of attention deficit hyperactivity disorder: much ado about something, Isr. Med. Assoc. J. 13 (2011) 571–574.

[46] T.E. Elder, The importance of relative standards in ADHD diagnoses: evidence based on exact birth dates, J. Health Econ. 29 (2010) 641–656.

[47] Y. He, Z.J. Chen, A.C. Evans, Small-world anatomical networks in the human brain revealed by cortical thickness from MRI, Cereb. Cortex 17 (2007) 2407–2419.

[48] R. Rader, L. McCauley, E.C. Callen, Current strategies in the diagnosis and treatment of childhood attention-deficit/hyperactivity disorder, Am. Fam. Physician 79 (2009) 657–665.

[49] T.W. Wilson, J.D. Franzen, E. Heinrichs-Graham, M.L. White, N.L. Knott, et al., Broadband neurophysiological abnormalities in the medial prefrontal region of the default-mode network in adults with ADHD, Hum. Brain Mapp. 34 (2013) 566–574.

[50] N.E. Adleman, S.J. Fromm, V. Razdan, R. Kayser, D.P. Dickstein, et al., Cross-sectional and longitudinal abnormalities in brain structure in children with severe mood dysregulation or bipolar disorder, J. Child Psychol. Psychiatry 53 (2012) 1149–1156.

[51] J.E. Brown, N. Chatterjee, J. Younger, S. Mackey, Towards a physiology based measure of pain: patterns of human brain activity distinguish painful from non-painful thermal stimulation, PLoS One 6 (2011).

[52] J. Dukart, K. Mueller, H. Barthel, A. Villringer, O. Sabri, et al., Meta-analysis based SVM classification enables accurate detection of Alzheimer's disease across different clinical centers using FDG-PET and MRI, Psychiatry Res. 212 (2013) 230–236.

[53] B. Magnin, L. Mesrob, S. Kinkingnéhun, M. Pélégrini-Issac, O. Colliot, et al., Support vector machine-based classification of Alzheimer's disease from whole-brain anatomical MRI, Neuroradiology 51 (2009) 73–83.

[54] L. O'Dwyer, F. Lamberton, A.L.W. Bokde, M. Ewers, Y.O. Faluyi, et al., Using support vector machines with multiple indices of diffusion for automated classification of mild cognitive impairment, PLoS One 7 (2012).

[55] M.G. Qiu, Z. Ye, Q.Y. Li, G.J. Liu, B. Xie, et al., Changes of brain structure and function in ADHD children, Brain Topogr. 24 (2011) 243–252.
[56] P. Shaw, M. Gilliam, M. Liverpool, C. Weddle, M. Malek, et al., Cortical development in typically developing children with symptoms of hyperactivity and impulsivity: support for a dimensional view of attention deficit hyperactivity disorder, Am. J. Psychiatr. 168 (2011) 143–151.
[57] M.R. Brown, G.S. Sidhu, R. Greiner, N. Asgarian, M. Bastani, P.H. Silverstone, A. J. Greenshaw, S.M. Dursun, ADHD-200 global competition: diagnosing ADHD using personal characteristic data can outperform resting state fMRI measurements, Front. Syst. Neurosci. 6 (2012) 69.
[58] H. Heinrich, H. Dickhaus, A. Rothenberger, V. Heinrich, G.H. Moll, Singles weep analysis of event-related potentials by wavelet networks—methodological basis and clinical application, IEEE Trans. Biomed. Eng. 46 (1999) 867–879.
[59] P. Missonnier, R. Hasler, N. Perroud, F.R. Herrmann, P. Millet, et al., EEG anomalies in adult ADHD subjects performing a working memory task, Neuroscience 241 (2013) 135–146.
[60] J.R. Sato, D.Y. Takahashi, M.Q. Hoexter, K.B. Massirer, A. Fujita, Measuring network's entropy in ADHD: a new approach to investigate neuropsychiatric disorders, NeuroImage 77 (2013) 44–51.
[61] L.Q. Uddin, A.M.C. Kelly, B.B. Biswal, D.S. Margulies, Z. Shehzad, et al., Network homogeneity reveals decreased integrity of default-mode network in ADHD, J. Neurosci. Methods 169 (2008) 249–254.
[62] C.-W. Chang, C.-C. Ho, J.-H. Chen, ADHD classification by a texture analysis of anatomical brain MRI data, Front. Syst. Neurosci. 6 (2012) 66.
[63] J.R. Sato, M.Q. Hoexter, A. Fujita, L.A. Rohde, Evaluation of pattern recognition and feature extraction methods in ADHD prediction, Front. Syst. Neurosci. 6 (2012) 68.
[64] D. Kuang, X. Guo, X. An, Y. Zhao, L. He, Discrimination of ADHD based on fMRI data with deep belief network, in: International Conference on Intelligent Computing, 2014, pp. 225–232.
[65] J. Kleesiek, G. Urban, A. Hubert, D. Schwarz, K. Maier-Hein, M. Bendszus, A. Biller, Deep MRI brain extraction: a 3D convolutional neural network for skull stripping, NeuroImage 129 (2016) 460–469.
[66] S. Ji, W. Xu, M. Yang, K. Yu, 3D convolutional neural networks for human action recognition, IEEE Trans. Pattern Anal. Mach. Intell. 35 (1) (2013) 221–231.
[67] R. Li, W. Zhang, H.-I. Suk, L. Wang, J. Li, D. Shen, S. Ji, Deep learning based imaging data completion for improved brain disease diagnosis, in: International Conference on Medical Image Computing and Computer Assisted Intervention, Springer, 2014, pp. 305–312.
[68] N. O'Mahony, B. Florentino-Liano, J.J. Carballo, E. Baca-García, A.A. Rodríguez, Objective diagnosis of ADHD using IMUs, Med. Eng. Phys. 36 (7) (2014) 922–926.
[69] X.H. Wang, Y. Jiao, L. Li, Identifying individuals with attention deficit hyperactivity disorder based on temporal variability of dynamic functional connectivity, Sci. Rep. 8 (2018) 11789.
[70] C.-Z. Zhu, et al., Fisher discriminative analysis of resting-state brain function for attention-deficit/hyperactivity disorder, NeuroImage 40 (2008) 110–120.
[71] X. Wang, Y. Jiao, T. Tang, H. Wang, Z. Lu, Altered regional homogeneity patterns in adults with attention-deficit hyperactivity disorder, Eur. J. Radiol. 82 (2013) 1552–1557.

[72] D. Dai, J. Wang, J. Hua, H. He, Classification of ADHD children through multimodal magnetic resonance imaging, Front. Syst. Neurosci. 6 (2012) 1–8.
[73] J.B. Colby, et al., Insights into multimodal imaging classification of ADHD, Front. Syst. Neurosci. 6 (2012) 59.
[74] W. Cheng, X. Ji, J. Zhang, J. Feng, Individual classification of ADHD patients by integrating multiscale neuroimaging markers and advanced pattern recognition techniques, Front. Syst. Neurosci. 6 (2012) 58.
[75] X. Peng, P. Lin, T. Zhang, J. Wang, Extreme learning machine-based classification of ADHD using brain structural MRI data, PLoS One 8 (2013) e79476.
[76] M.N. Qureshi, B. Min, H.J. Jo, B. Lee, Multiclass classification for the differential diagnosis on the ADHD subtypes using recursive feature elimination and hierarchical extreme learning machine: structural MRI study, PLoS One 11 (2016) e0160697.
[77] B. Jie, C.Y. Wee, D. Shen, D. Zhang, Hyper-connectivity of functional networks for brain disease diagnosis, Med. Image Anal. 32 (2016) 84–100.
[78] American Psychiatric Association, Diagnostic and Statistical Manual of Mental Disorders (DSM-5), American Psychiatric Association Publishing, Arlington, VA, 2013.
[79] CDC Reports, Centers for Disease Control and Prevention (CDC) Report, Available at: http://www.cdc.gov/media/releases/2014/p0327-autism-spectrum-disorder.html, 2014.
[80] M. Knapp, R. Romeo, J. Beecham, Economic cost of autism in the UK, Autism 13 (3) (2009) 317–336.
[81] WHO: World Health Organization, Autism Spectrum Disorder, Available at:http://www.who.int/mediacentre/factsheets/autism-spectrum-disorders/en/, 2017.
[82] I.L. Cohen, A neural network model of autism: implications for theory and treatment, in: Neuroconstructivism Vol 2: Perspectives and Prospects, Oxford University Press, 2006, pp. 231–264.
[83] X. Guo, et al., Diagnosing Autism spectrum disorder from brain resting-state functional connectivity patterns using a deep neural network with a novel feature selection method, Front. Neurosci. 11 (2017) 460.
[84] L. Nylander, et al., Attention- deficit/hyperactivity disorder (ADHD) and autism spectrum disorder (ASD) in adult psychiatry. A 20 year register study, Nord. J. Psychiatry 67 (5) (2013) 344–350.
[85] N.C. Dvornek, et al., Identifying Autism from resting-state fMRI using long short-term memory networks, Mac. Learn. Med. Imaging (2017) 362–370.
[86] N.J. Minshew, T.A. Keller, The nature of brain dysfunction in autism: functional brain imaging studies, Curr. Opin. Neurol. 23 (2) (2010) 124–130.
[87] M.E. Raichle, et al., A default mode of brain function, Proc. Natl. Acad. Sci. U. S. A. 98 (2) (2001) 676–682.
[88] C.S. Monk, et al., Abnormalities of intrinsic functional connectivity in autism spectrum disorders, NeuroImage 47 (2) (2009) 764–772.
[89] J.H. Elder, C.M. Kreider, S.N. Brasher, M. Ansell, Clinical impact of early diagnosis of autism on the prognosis and parent–child relationships, Psychol. Res. Behav. Manag. 10 (2017) 283–292.
[90] A. Pickles, A. Le Couteur, K. Leadbitter, E. Salomone, R. Cole-Fletcher, H. Tobin, I. Gammer, J. Lowry, G. Vamvakas, S. Byford, C. Aldred, V. Slonims, H. McConachie, P. Howlin, J.R. Parr, T. Charman, J. Green, Parent-mediated social communication therapy for young children with autism (PACT): long-term follow-up of a randomised controlled trial, Lancet 388 (10059) (2016) 2501–2509.

[91] G. Dawson, S. Rogers, J. Munson, M. Smith, J. Winter, J. Greenson, A. Donaldson, J. Varley, Randomized, controlled trial of an intervention for toddlers with Autism: the early start Denver model, Pediatrics 125 (1) (2016) e17–e23.
[92] C. Craddock, et al., The neuro bureau preprocessing initiative: open sharing of preprocessed neuroimaging data and derivatives, in: Neuroinformatics, Stockholm, Sweden, 2013.
[93] D. Martino, et al., The autism brain imaging data exchange: towards a large-scale evaluation of the intrinsic brain architecture in autism, Mol. Psychiatry 19 (2014) 659–667.
[94] G. Deshpande, L.E. Libero, K.R. Sreenivasan, H.D. Deshpande, R.K. Kana, Identification of neural connectivity signatures of autism using machine learning, Front. Hum. Neurosci. 7 (2013) 670.
[95] A.S. Heinsfeld, A.R. Franco, R.C. Craddock, A. Buchweitz, F. Meneguzzi, Identification of autism spectrum disorder using deep learning and the ABIDE dataset, Neuroimage Clin. 17 (2018) 16–23.
[96] A. Abraham, et al., Deriving reproducible biomarkers from multi-site resting-state data: an Autism-based example, NeuroImage 147 (2016) 736–745.
[97] C.P. Chen, C.L. Keown, A. Jahedi, A. Nair, M.E. Pflieger, B.A. Bailey, R.-A. Müller, Diagnostic classification of intrinsic functional connectivity highlights somatosensory, default mode, and visual regions in autism, Neuroimage Clin.8 (2015) 238–245.
[98] T. Iidaka, Resting state functional magnetic resonance imaging and neural network classified autism and control, Cortex 63 (2015) 55–67.
[99] D. Barrett, A. Morcos, J. Macke, Analyzing biological and artificial neural networks: challenges with opportunities for synergy? Curr. Opin. Neurobiol. 55 (2019) 55–64.
[100] N.A. Halvaei, K.H. Rahimi, Sensorless Direct Power Control of Induction Motor Drive Using Artificial Neural Network, Adv. Artif. Neural Syst. 2015 (2015) 1–9.
[101] Y. Xu, M. He, Improved artificial neural network based on intelligent optimization algorithm, Neural Netw. World 28 (4) (2018) 345–360.
[102] H. Bhasin, E. Khanna, Neural network based black box testing, ACM SIGSOFT Software Eng. Notes 39 (2) (2014) 1–6.
[103] S. Alam, U. Bajwa, N. ul Haq, N. Ratyal, M. Anwar, Skin disease classification using neural network, Curr. Med. Imaging Rev. 15 (2019).
[104] I. Tsoulos, A. Tzallas, D. Tsalikakis, Evolutionary based weight decaying method for neural network training, Neural. Process. Lett. (2017).
[105] M. Shahin, M. Jaksa, H. Maier, Recent advances and future challenges for artificial neural systems in geotechnical engineering applications, Adv. Artif. Neural Syst. 2009 (2009) 1–9.
[106] Z. Shi, L. He, Current status and future potential of neural networks used for medical image processing, J. Multimed. 6 (3) (2011).
[107] Z. Latt, Application of feedforward artificial neural network in Muskingum flood routing: a black-box forecasting approach for a natural river system, Water Resour. Manag. 29 (14) (2015) 4995–5014.
[108] A. Malatras, State-of-the-art survey on P2P overlay networks in pervasive computing environments, J. Netw. Comput. Appl. 55 (2015) 1–23.
[109] H. Maier, G. Dandy, Neural networks for the prediction and forecasting of water resources variables: a review of modelling issues and applications, Environ. Model Softw. 15 (1) (2000) 101–124.
[110] R. Turkson, F. Yan, M. Ali, J. Hu, Artificial neural network applications in the calibration of spark-ignition engines: an overview, Int. J. Eng. Sci. Technol. 19 (3) (2016) 1346–1359.

CHAPTER

Analysis and management of sleep data

8

Christoph Janott

Munich School of BioEngineering, Technical University of Munich, Garching, Germany

Abbreviations

AASM	American Academy of Sleep Medicine
AHI	Apnea-hypopnea index
CAP	Cyclic alternating pattern
CSA	Central sleep apnea
dB	Decibel
DISE	Drug-induced sleep endoscopy
ECG	Electrocardiography
EEG	Electroencephalography
EMG	Electromyography
EOG	Electrooculography
Hz	Hertz
ICSD	International Classification of Sleep Disorders
kHz	Kilohertz
MFCC	Mel-frequency cepstral coefficients
MSE	Multiscale entropy
OSA	Obstructive sleep apnea
PLMI	Periodic limb movement index
PLMS	Periodic limb movement disorder
PLP	Perceptual linear prediction
PSG	Polysomnography
RASTA	Relative spectral transform
RCNN	Recurrent convolutional neural network
RDI	Respiratory disturbance index
REM	Rapid eye movements
RMS	Root mean square
SER	Spectral energy ratio
SPL	Sound pressure level
SWS	Slow-wave sleep

Biomedical Signal Processing and Artificial Intelligence in Healthcare. https://doi.org/10.1016/B978-0-12-818946-7.00008-1

8.1 Introduction

In ancient cultures, sleep was considered a state of unconsciousness that was closely related to darkness, death, and the mystic phenomenon of dreaming.

In the Roman mythology, Somnus, the god of sleep, resided in the underworld. His brother was the death, and his sons, the Somnia, appeared in dreams in various shapes and forms.

The Greek god of sleep, Hypnos, and his twin brother Thanatos, the god of a peaceful death, could relieve humans from suffering and help them to die a peaceful death during sleep. Of his four children, Morpheus shaped the dreams, Ikelos represented people in dreams, and Phantasus could transform into objects. Phobetor was responsible for nightmares by appearing in the shape of monsters and animals.

In ancient China, dreams were an important factor for the diagnosis of illnesses, whereas the Egyptians believed that dreams were predictors of the future.

The ancient myths live on in a number of ubiquitous English words. Somnus has lent his name to the field of sleep research, somnology. Hypnosis stems from Hypnos, and euthanasia is derived from Thanatos. Finally, morphine is fittingly named after Morpheus, who used to rest in his dark cave among poppy flowers.

Today, it is well known that sleep is composed of a series of active processes of the human brain, rather than being perceived as a passive state of the brain being shut down. Measuring these processes serves to detect abnormalities in the sleep structure, which can be telling symptoms of an underlying disease. On the other hand, disturbed sleep by itself can lead to a variety of serious health conditions [1].

This chapter gives an overview of the basics of sleep diagnosis, the physiological parameters and standards of their measurements, and the current use of signal processing methods for their evaluation. Extensive literature references are provided to facilitate further reading and research.

8.2 Evolution of sleep medicine

In the 19th century the phenomenon of sleep was the subject of extensive research, which leads to the understanding that the brain was not simply turned off during sleep. Ernst Kohlschuetter in 1863 considered that "Sleep and waking are two opposing states of mental life. The same is not completely extinguished in sleep, which is proved by dreams and the possibility of awakening a sleeper by a strong local stimulus" [2]. Kohlschuetter measured the awaking reaction of sleeping subjects at different times during the night by applying acoustic stimuli of defined strength. He found that the depth of sleep changes during the course of the night, being deeper in the beginning and becoming shallower toward the morning.

Several theories were debated about the physiological mechanisms inducing the state of sleep. A common misconception was that sleep was induced by a blood congestion in the head, with the increased pressure on the brain causing unconsciousness [3]. Others thought that sleep is caused by increased cerebral blood flow [4] or decreased cerebral blood supply. Durham in 1860 published his observations of the blood circulation in dog brains, the skull of which he had cut open and covered with a glass window [5]. He reported that the blood flow in the brain is reduced during sleep. Consequently, sleeplessness was treated by substances reducing the cerebral blood flow, such as potassium bromide.

The debate as to whether sleep disorders should be treated pharmacologically or psychologically was already in full progress. For centuries, wine and opium were used as effective sleeping aids. In stark contrast, Russell in 1861 had a strong opinion that sleeping problems have their cause in the mental state of the sufferers and stated that "the physician's attention must be directed to regulating and strengthening the mind. Even in cases of organic disease, the chances of recovery depend quite as much on the state of the patient's mind as on that of his body" [6]. Russell's opinion should prove quite visionary. Recent research shows that behavioral therapy is an effective means in the treatment of primary insomnia [7].

A milestone in the understanding of the structure of sleep was the invention of electroencephalography (EEG) and its use for measuring the activity of the human brain in the early 20th century [8]. For the first time the brain could be directly monitored during sleep by means of its electric emissions. Not long after this discovery, distinct sleep states were observed and defined based on their electroencephalographical wave properties. It was discovered that in frequent cases, body "movement was immediately followed by a change of state upward, occasionally downward, and occasionally a movement occurred just after a change of state. During sleep there was a continual shift in states upward and downward, sometimes associated with recognized stimuli, sometimes without any external stimulus but probably as a result of internal stimuli" [9]. The sleep states defined at that time are still the basis of today's definition of depth of sleep. The phenomenon of rapid eye movements (REM) during sleep and its relation to dreaming was discovered in the 1950s [10]. Eventually, in the 1960s, a consensus committee of sleep specialists and researchers under the chairmanship of Allan Rechtschaffen and Anthony Kales agreed on standardized criteria for sleep staging. With the so-called R&K manual, they have created a standard piece of work for an internationally accepted system of sleep scoring, which is, with slight adaptations, valid to date and a reference for sleep research and diagnosis [11].

For a comprehensive overview on the history of sleep diagnosis and therapy, see [12, 13].

8.3 Sleep disorders

Today's key reference for the description of sleep anomalies is the International Classification of Sleep Disorders (ICSD), which is issued and regularly updated by the American Academy of Sleep Medicine (AASM) [14]. Table 8.1 lists the conditions that are described in this classification and their prevalence in healthy adults [15–21].

Table 8.1 Sleep anomalies according to the International Classification of Sleep Disorders [14].

Major diagnostic section	Prevalence	Disorder
Insomnia	2%–10%	Chronic insomnia disorder
Central hypersomnolence	4%–6%	Narcolepsy
		Hypersomnia
		Insufficient sleep syndrome
Circadian rhythm sleep-wake disorders	1%–2%	Delayed sleep-wake phase disorder
		Advanced sleep-wake phase disorder
		Irregular sleep-wake rhythm disorder
		Non-24-h sleep-wake rhythm disorder
		Shift work disorder
		Jet lag disorder
Parasomnias	<1%	NREM-related parasomnias
		REM-related parasomnias
		Other parasomnias
Sleep-related movement disorders	5%–15%	Restless legs syndrome
		Periodic limb movement disorder
		Leg cramps
		Bruxism
		Rhythmic movement disorder
Sleep-related breathing disorders	6%–38%	Obstructive sleep apnea syndromes
		Central sleep apnea syndromes
		Sleep-related hypoventilation disorders
		Sleep-related hypoxemia disorder

- *Insomnia* is characterized by problems to initiate or maintain sleep and the lack of adequate circumstances or opportunities to sleep. It also comprises the daytime consequences of this disorder. Chronic insomnia, as opposed to short-term insomnia, occurs at least three times a week and lasts longer than 3 months [14].
- *Central hypersomnolence* is characterized by a subjective complaint of excessive daytime sleepiness. A central hypersomnolence is diagnosed if this symptom cannot be related to other types of sleep disorders. This section subsumes

narcolepsy, characterized by sudden episodes of muscle weakness or loss of muscle tone, which is often triggered by strong positive or negative emotions. Narcolepsy can also go along with hypnagogic hallucinations and sleep paralysis. It is relatively rare with a prevalence of 0.03%–0.05% [14, 22, 23]. Hypersomnia is defined as excessive duration of nighttime sleep in combination with daytime sleepiness [24], while the insufficient sleep syndrome is simply a consequence of regularly getting less sleep than the body needs.

- *Circadian rhythm sleep-wake disorders* are defined as recurrent disruptions of the sleep-wake rhythm by a mismatch of the endogenous circadian timing system (the inner clock) with external requirements or circumstances. Mild forms of the disorder include the typical "early birds" or "night owls," meaning people who tend to wake up early or go to sleep late. Non-24-h sleep-wake rhythm disorder often occurs in blind people, where the inner circadian timer is not triggered by the natural light and dark rhythm of day and night. By definition, circadian rhythm sleep-wake disorders must last more than 3 months to be clinically relevant. Shift work disorder and jet lag are diagnosed whenever the symptoms can be related to the respective cause.
- *Parasomnias* are disruptive sleep disorders that involve abnormal behavior or perceptions during sleep. They are subdivided by their occurrence during either non-REM or REM sleep. Non-REM parasomnias include sleep walking, confusional arousals, and night terrors. REM sleep parasomnias are often characterized by an absence of muscle atonia while dreaming. Consequently, patients can act out their dreams, with the risk of injuring themselves or others. In rarer cases muscle atonia is still retained while waking up, leading to the symptom of incubus, the inability to move or speak while being awake and conscious [14].
- *Sleep-related movement disorders* are abnormal movements related to sleep. The restless legs syndrome is characterized by the urge to move the legs during periods of physical inactivity primarily occurring at nighttime or in the evening. In contrast, periodic limb movements, rhythmic movements, or other movement disorders such as bruxism (teeth grinding) or myoclonus (brief, irregular jerks) occur involuntarily during sleep.
- *Sleep-related breathing disorders* are the most common sleep abnormalities. They are defined as abnormal breathing behaviors during sleep, which can have different causes and characteristics. Obstructive sleep apnea (OSA) is characterized by repeated episodes of reduced or completely interrupted airflow despite an active breathing effort. It can be associated with morning headache, diurnal microsleep attacks, and excessive fatigue, and it is an independent risk factor for cardiovascular diseases such as hypertension and myocardial infarction [25].

Central sleep apnea (CSA) also involves repeated nightly breathing cessations. In contrast to OSA, however, these are caused by a central disorder of the ventilatory control system. In many sleep apnea patients, both OSA and CSA episodes can be detected, a condition sometimes referred to as mixed apnea or complex sleep apnea.

The reported prevalence in the general population varies. A recent systematic review [21] reports a prevalence in the range of 9% and 38% for mild OSA and between 6% and 17% for moderate OSA. OSA prevalence is higher in men than in women and increases with age.

Sleep-related hypoventilation and hypoxemia disorders are diagnosed by decreased oxygen and raised carbon dioxide levels in the blood, and they usually occur in overweight patients. Charles Dickens pointedly described a typical phenotype of a person suffering from the obesity hypoventilation syndrome in the character of *Little Fat Joe* in the Pickwick Papers [26]. Originally, this condition was named the *Pickwickian syndrome* after this novel [27].

8.4 Structure of sleep

8.4.1 Macrostructure, sleep phases

The macrostructure of sleep has distinct characteristics that are similar across humans, with no major differences between genders. Major research on normative sleep data was carried out starting in the 1960s by systematically collecting and analyzing polysomnographic data from healthy individuals of all age groups, leading to a compilation of average sleep characteristics that are considered normal [28].

Sleep is scored by a set of different sleep stages. The transition from one sleep stage to another is a continuous process with gradual changes in the biomedical signals. To make the analysis of the physiological data comparable and standardizable, clear and strict rules have been developed to interpret sleep data. It should be emphasized that "the scoring rules were devised to allow uniformity between sleep laboratories and to offer a conceptual simplicity rather than a rigid framework" [29]. This is especially the case for automated analysis of sleep data and machine classification applications, which require the rigid framework as a basis for unequivocal data labeling and do not allow for intuitive or subjective interpretation of data.

The Rechtschaffen and Kales scoring system is composed of five sleep stages: one REM sleep and four non-REM stages. This scoring model was revised and updated in 2007 by the American Academy of Sleep Medicine, reducing the number of non-REM sleep stages to three [30].

- Phases of being awake are indicated by the letter *W*.
- REM sleep is commonly marked *R* or *REM*. It is signified by pronounced ocular movements and related to dreaming.

- The three non-REM stages are named *N1*, *N2*, and *N3*, relating to the respective sleep depth, defined as the strength of stimulus required to disturb sleep or create awakening. Stage N3 is also sometimes referred to as *deep sleep* or *slow-wave sleep* (SWS). In deep sleep an external stimulus usually leads to a shift to shallower sleep stages, while in N1 and REM sleep, a stimulus often induces arousal.

Fig. 8.1 shows an example of the course of sleep stages during the night of a healthy adult sleeper. After sleep onset, which normally occurs within 5–15 min, a first phase of deep sleep of approximately 60–90 min is followed by an episode of REM sleep, completing a so-called N-R cycle. During the course of the night, several N-R cycles occur, with phases of deep sleep becoming shorter, REM phases getting longer, and occasional awakening happening more frequent.

Sleep efficiency is defined as the ratio of total sleep time and time in bed. It is usually around 90% in healthy adults. The proportion of deep sleep of the total sleep time and sleep efficiency decreases with age, leading to reduced total sleep time in the elderly on average, which is thought to be related to changes in circadian rhythm coinciding with age.

Sleep stages are scored in nonoverlapping intervals of 30 s length, called *epochs*. In each epoch the predominantly occurring patterns are used to determine the sleep stage. For example, standard criterion for scoring an awaking from sleep requires alpha wave activity showing in the EEG for a minimum of 15 s.

Table 8.2 shows the principle relationship between sleep stage and EEG, electrooculography (EOG), and electromyography (EMG) properties in healthy adults, while Table 8.3 summarizes the typical spectral energy bands of EEG waveform types. These are simplified representations; for details, refer to [30] or [31].

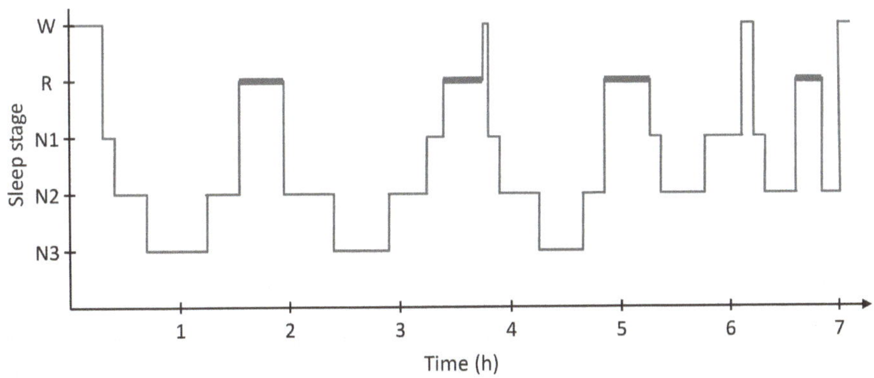

FIG. 8.1

Example of sleep macrostructure of a healthy adult.

Table 8.2 Simplified relationship between sleep stage, EEG, EOG, and EMG properties.

Stage	Waveform type	Phasic events	Eye movements	Muscle activity
W (active)	Beta	–	Eyes open	High
W (relaxed)	Alpha	–	Blinking, saccadic movements	Moderate
N1	Alpha, theta	–	Slow, rolling	Low
N2	Delta, theta	K-complexes, spindles	None	Low
N3	Delta, theta	Spindles (occasionally)	None	Low
REM	Theta, alpha, beta	–	Rapid	None

Table 8.3 Spectral energy bands of EEG waves.

Waveform type	Frequency range (Hz)
Delta	0.1–3.5
Theta	4–7
Alpha	8–13
Beta	14–30

8.4.2 Microstructure, cyclic alternating patterns

On a smaller time scale, a distinct microstructure of sleep exists, revealing *cyclic patterns* and *events*. The so-called *cyclic alternating pattern* (CAP) mainly occurs during N2 sleep and consists of an A and a B phase. Phase A is characterized by the presence of *phasic events*, such as *K-complexes* and *sleep spindles*. During phase A, responsiveness to external stimuli is increased. Phase B shows regular EEG activity without phasic events. One cycle of an A and B phase is usually between 10 s and 1 min in length, and to be scored as CAP sleep, several cycles must follow in sequence. A CAP episode often precedes a shift to lighter sleep or a phase of REM sleep [32, 33].

Depending on the amount of phasic events, phase A is subdivided into three subtypes, called A1, A2, and A3. While arousals normally do not occur in an A1 phase, they are more frequent in an A2 phase, whereas in an A3 phase, arousal occurs in more than 95% of cases [31].

8.4.3 Sleep-related events

- *Sleep spindles* are defined as a series of distinct waves with a frequency of 11–16 Hz, which mostly last between 0.5 and 1.5 s. They are generated in the thalamus and are considered to be important for consolidation of memory during sleep. Sleep spindles can also be named sigma waves or sigma bands.
- *K-complexes* are characterized by a clearly delineated initial negative sharp wave, which is followed by a positive component, lasting 0.5 s or more. Their function during sleep is still a matter of debate. Fig. 8.2 shows an EEG recording containing a short sleep spindle and a K-complex.
- *Arousals* are short awakenings of more than 3 but less than 15 s, followed by normal sleep. Arousals are normally not consciously recognized by the sleeper.

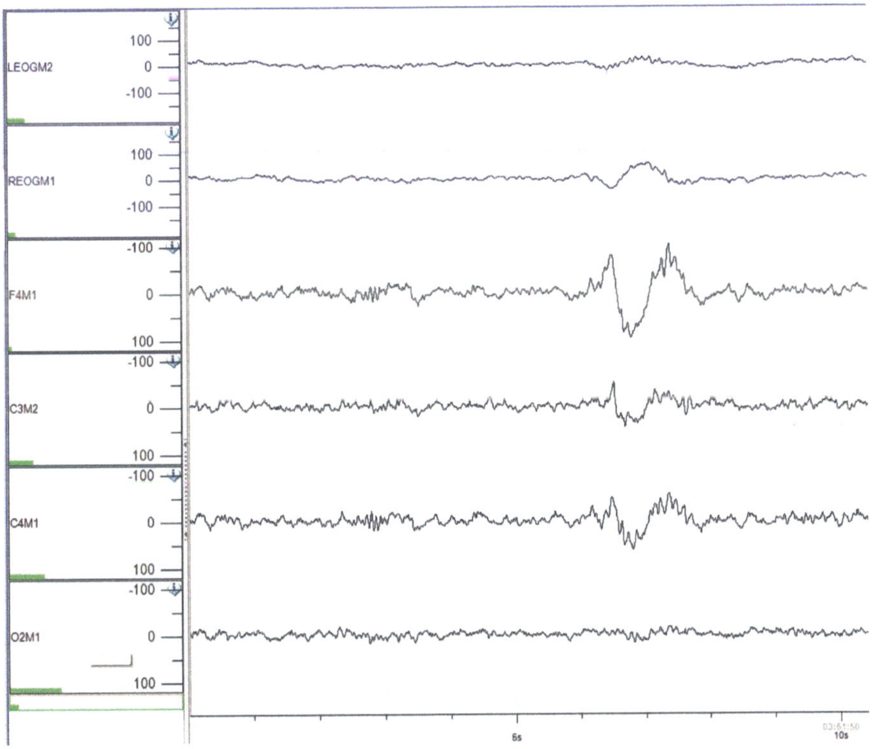

FIG. 8.2

Example EEG recording of N2 stage sleep during phase A of a CAP. A sleep spindle occurs at 2.5 s, while a K-complex can be seen from 6.5 s. All EEG derivations measured against reference electrodes at the mastoid. LEOGM2 = left EOG. REOGM1 = right EOG. F4M1 = frontal right derivation (right side on the forehead, F4). C3M2 and C4M1 = left and right central derivations (left and right side, approximately at the center of the head, C3 and C4). O2M1 = right occipital derivation (back of the head, O2).

- *Apneas* are complete cessations of airflow for at least 10 s. Stricter definitions require a drop in blood oxygen saturation by at least 3% as a result of the apneic event.
- *Hypopneas* are defined as a drop of 30% or more in peak airflow compared with the preevent baseline lasting for a minimum of 10 s and a drop in blood oxygen saturation by at least 3% or an arousal associated with the hypopneic event.

  The average number of apneas and hypopneas occurring per hour of sleep is measured by the apnea-hypopnea index (AHI). By common grading standards [30, 34], an AHI of 5 to less than 15 events per hour is considered mild OSA, between 15 and 30 is moderate, and more than 30 events per hour is defined as severe OSA. A similar measure is the respiratory disturbance index (RDI), which counts any respiratory event with a minimum of 10-s length if it is associated with an arousal, even if it does not meet the formal criteria of a hypopnea.
- *Periodic limb movements* (PLM) during sleep are regular, brief muscle activations of the arms or legs. A measure for the presence and severity of a sleep-related periodic limb movement disorder (PLMS) is the periodic limb movement index (PLMI), defined as the average number of limb movement events per hour of sleep. A PLMI below 5 is considered normal, between 5 and less than 25 is considered mild PLMS, and from 25 to 50 is moderate, while a value higher than 50 is defined as severe PLMS. Other definitions require a PLMI of 15 and related symptoms such as daytime sleepiness or disturbed sleep to qualify for a PLMS diagnosis.

Figs. 8.3–8.6 show example EEG recordings of different sleep stages.

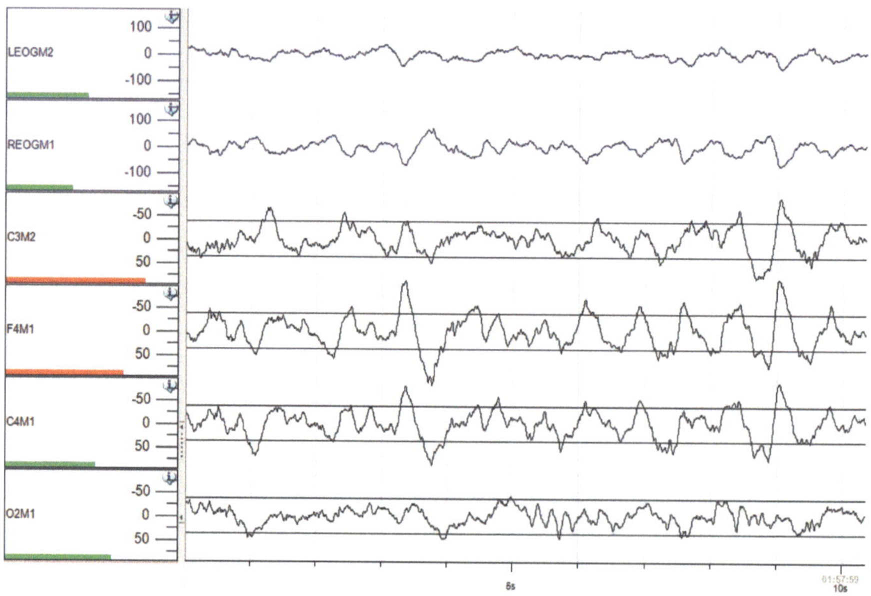

FIG. 8.3

Example EEG recording of N3 stage sleep. For description of derivations, please see Fig. 8.2.

8.5 Diagnostic standards for sleep data analysis

8.5.1 Polysomnography

Sleep structure and sleep events coincide with characteristic patterns of physiological activity that can be monitored through a variety of parameters. The most comprehensive method of sleep monitoring is polysomnography (PSG). PSG recordings were first documented in the 1960s and have become the gold standard for sleep diagnosis [35]. Full PSGs are carried out in sleep laboratories consisting of one or several bedrooms, fully equipped to record a patient's physiological parameters during sleep for a whole night. The definition of a whole night's sleep differs but is generally considered a minimum sleep time of 6 h. The physiological data are transferred to a central ward where the patients are monitored during the night, and the *somnogram* is recorded for subsequent evaluation.

Fig. 8.7 shows a typical bedroom in a sleep laboratory, while a central monitoring ward can be seen in Fig. 8.8.

8.5.1.1 Physiological parameters measured during polysomnography

A standardized measurement recommendation for polysomnography was developed in the 1950s and further refined in the following decades. The current recommended parameters are described as follows [36]:

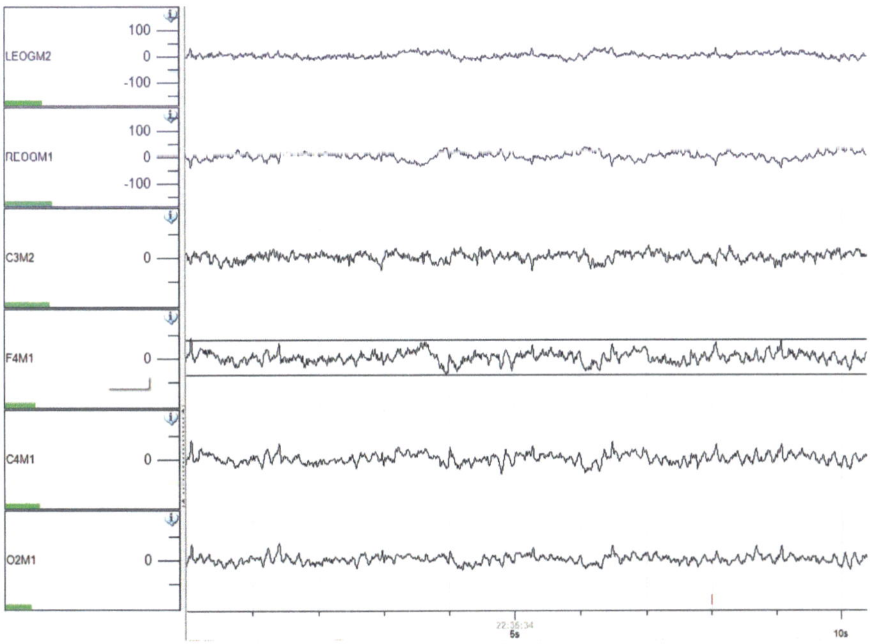

FIG. 8.4

Example EEG recording of N1 stage sleep. For description of derivations, please see Fig. 8.2.

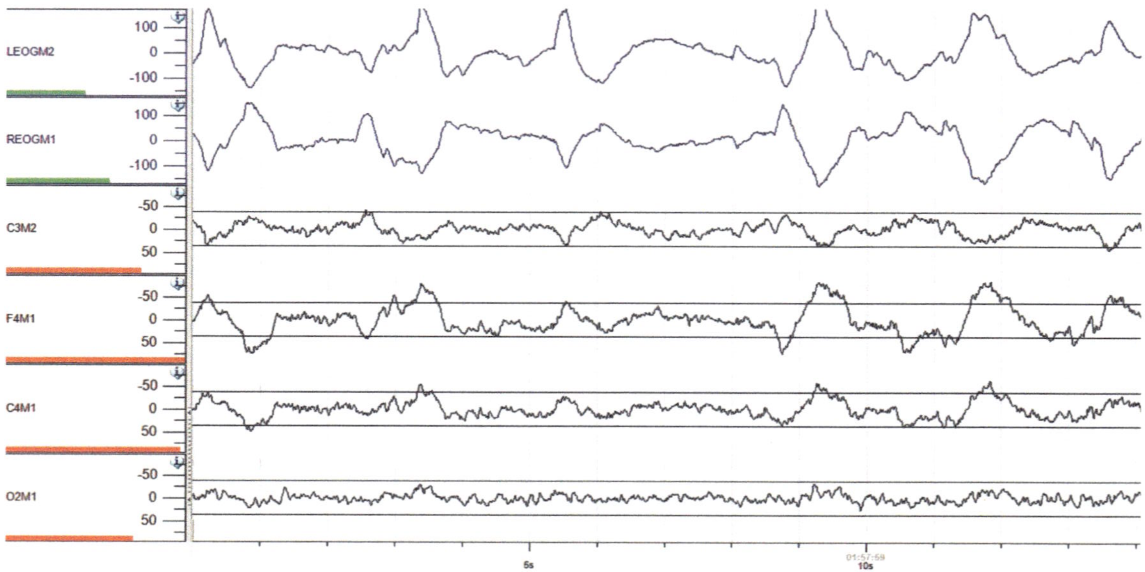

FIG. 8.5

Example EEG recording of a REM sleep phase. Rapid eye movements are clearly visible in the EOG derivations. For description of derivations, please see Fig. 8.2.

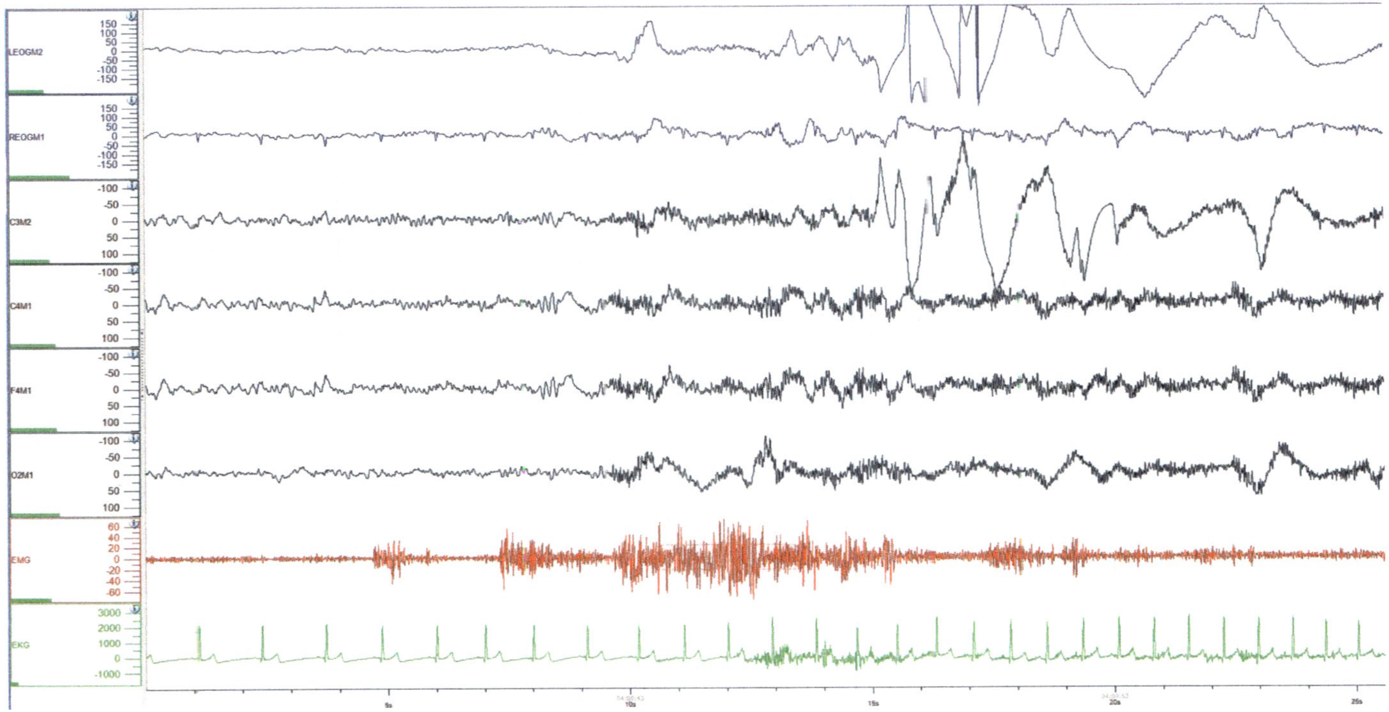

FIG. 8.6

Example EEG recording of an arousal (at 10 s) with subsequent wake stage. For description of derivations, please see Fig. 8.2.

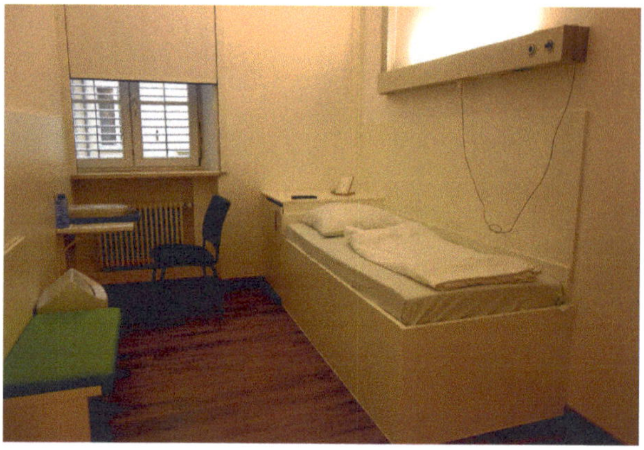

FIG. 8.7

Bedroom in a sleep laboratory.

Courtesy of Klinikum rechts der Isar, Munich, Germany.

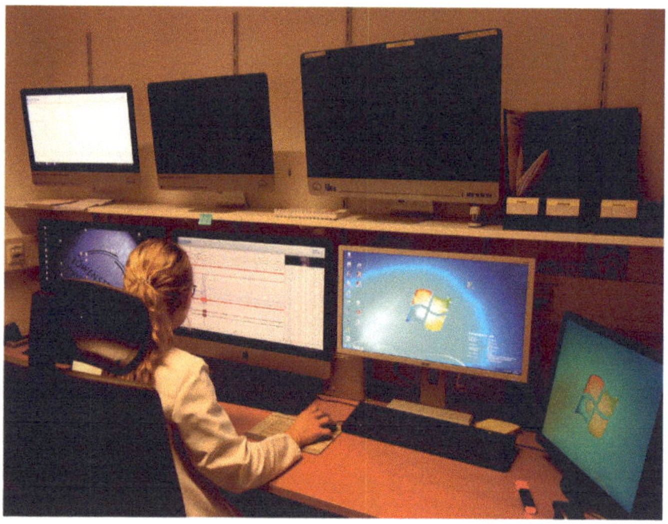

FIG. 8.8

Monitoring ward in a sleep laboratory.

Courtesy of Klinikum rechts der Isar, Munich, Germany.

- The brain activity measured through several EEG derivations is indispensable to detect sleep stages, which coincide with specific brain wave patterns. Derivations are unipolar against a central reference point, which is usually located at the ear lobe or mastoid bone.
- Eye movements are detected by electrooculography and are important indicators to detect REM sleep. Two electrodes attached to the right corner of the right

eye (right outer canthus), and the left outer canthus, respectively, record the muscle activity related to eye movements.
- Electromyograms are derived to aid in sleep phase estimation and to record limb movements. An electrode located above the chin is used to measure general muscle tone. Further the surface muscle tone of the right and left anterior tibial muscles are derived to detect leg movements.
- A one-channel electrocardiogram (ECG) is derived to measure heart rate and to detect tachycardia and cardiac arrhythmias.
- A finger or earlobe pulse oximetry sensor detects the course of oxygen saturation to determine apneic and hypopneic events.
- A contact microphone is attached to the neck in the tracheal region to detect snoring, coughing, and speaking activity.
- Nasal pressure sensors and oral airflow detectors record breathing by pressure changes and thermal differences between inspiration and expiration. The data are used to detect breathing irregularities during sleep.
- Chest and abdominal movements during inspiration and expiration are measured using two expansion belts applied above the bony thorax and above the umbilicus. Paradoxical thoracic and abdominal movements are a sign for breathing effort without airflow, signifying an obstructive apneic event, while simultaneous cessation of airflow and chest movements are a sign for a central apnea.
- A positional sensor is fixed to the thoracic belt to record the sleeping position.
- Optionally an infrared video recording of the sleeper is carried out to diagnose parasomnia and to allow for a differential diagnostic delimitation to certain forms of epilepsy [37].

Sample rates for EEG, EMG, ECG, and EOG data and the data from the microphone are recommended to be 500 Hz, while airflow, chest, and abdomen movements are sampled at 100 Hz. Oxygen saturation is sampled at 25 Hz, while the body position is recorded with a resolution of 1 Hz.

Fig 8.9 shows an example of a somnogram showing periodic limb movements. Fig. 8.10 illustrates an episode of subsequent obstructive apneic events, while Fig. 8.11 displays a series of central apneas, a condition also referred to as Cheyne-Stokes breathing. Finally, Fig. 8.12 contains an example of a primary snorer without any signs of respiratory disturbance.

8.5.1.2 Automated analysis of polysomnographic data

Until recently, sleep staging based on polysomnographic recordings, as well as the diagnosis of limb movement and sleep-related breathing disorders, is largely performed manually by sleep experts with the help of semiautomated PSG monitoring systems, providing assistance by suggesting sleep stages, movement, and respiratory events from the sleep recordings. However, the ultimate scoring is still made by a human expert.

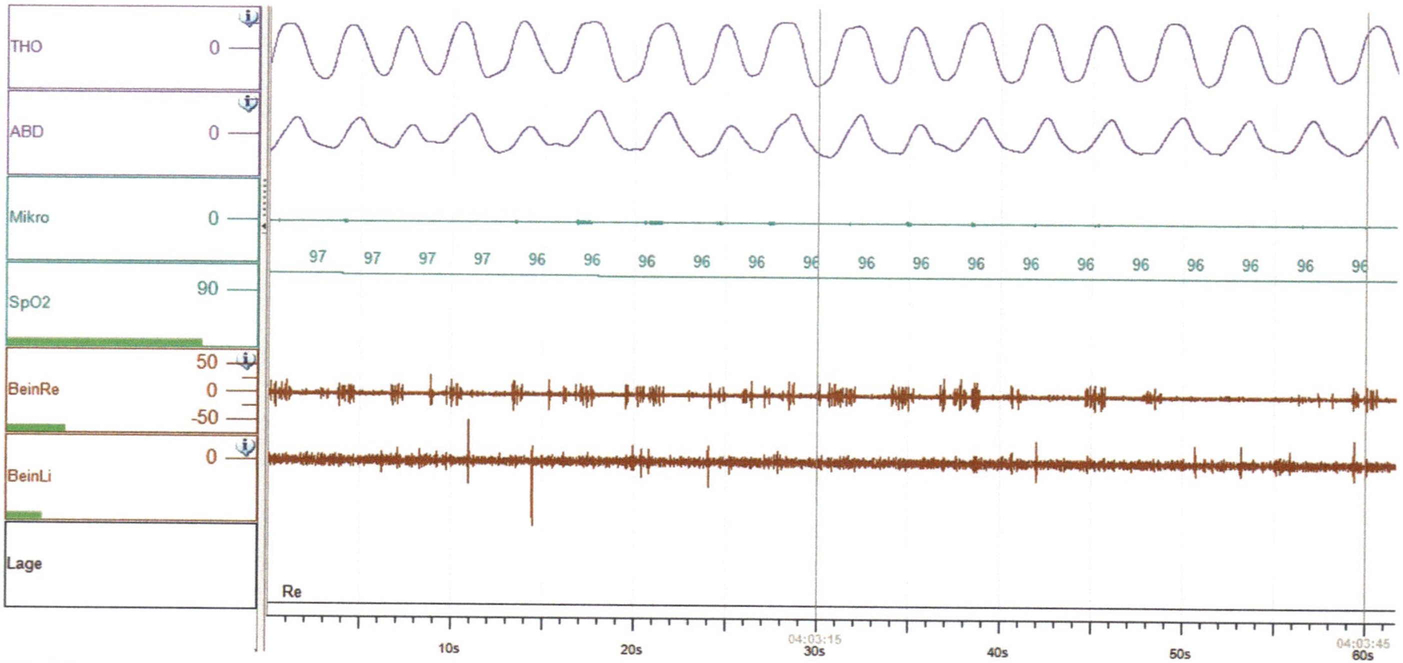

FIG. 8.9

Example of a somnogram of an episode of periodic limb movements. THO = thoracic movement and ABD = abdominal movement, showing regular respiratory activity. Mikro = contact microphone located on the neck, showing occasional snoring events. SpO2 = blood oxygen saturation. BeinRe and BeinLi = EMG derivations of right and left leg, showing periodic activity especially in the right leg. Lage = body position, lying on the right side.

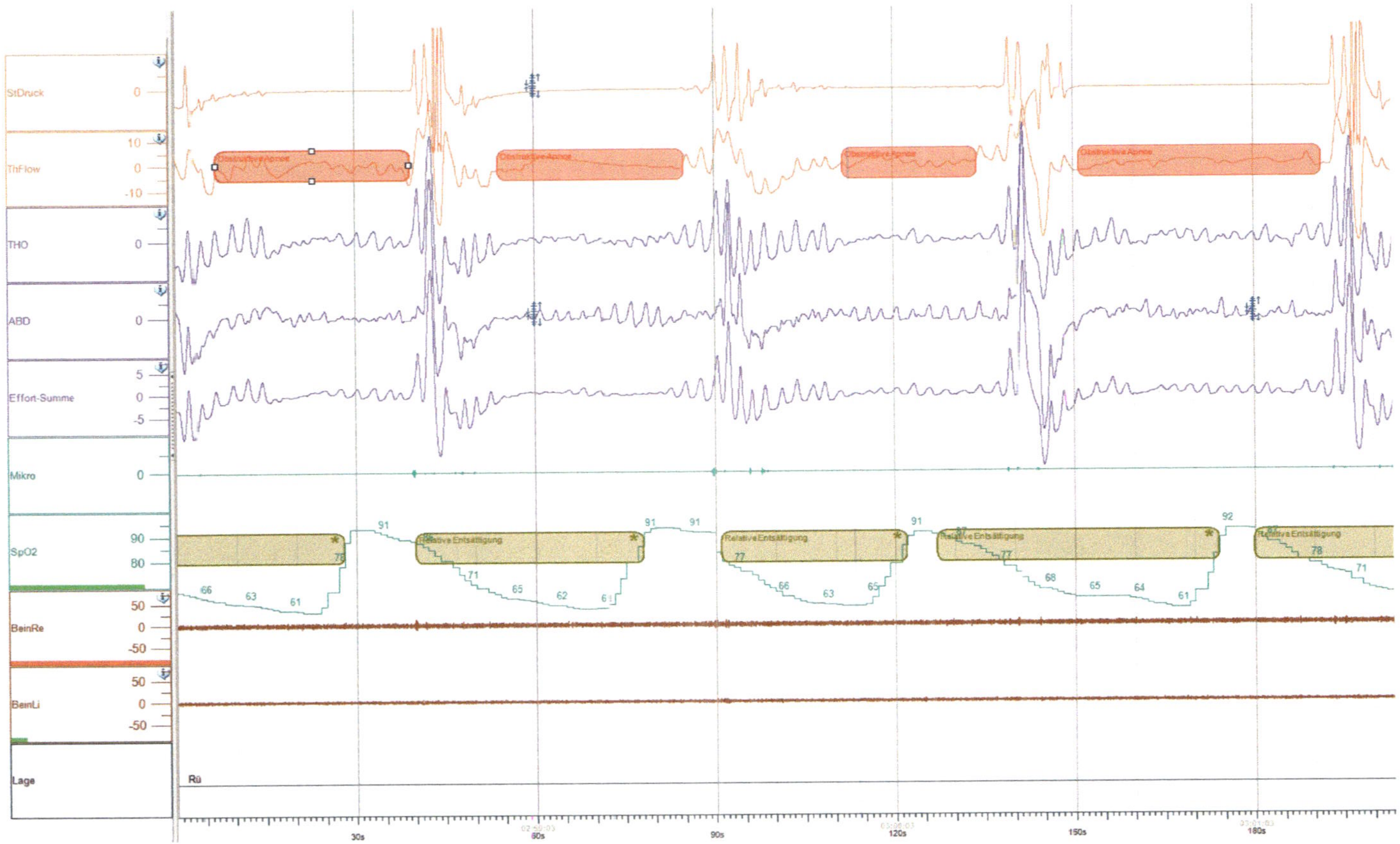

FIG. 8.10

Example of a somnogram of several subsequent obstructive events. StDruck = intranasal pressure. ThFlow = thermal airflow sensor, periods of airflow cessation are marked in *red* color. THO = thoracic movement. ABD = abdominal movement. Effort-Summe = combined thoracic and abdominal effort, showing a breathing effort (paradoxical movement of thorax and abdomen) during phases of apnea. Mikro = neck contact microphone, showing single snore events when breathing is restored. SpO2 = blood oxygen saturation, phases of severe desaturation are marked in *ochre* color. BeinRe and BeinLi = EMG derivations of right and left leg. Lage = body position, lying on the back.

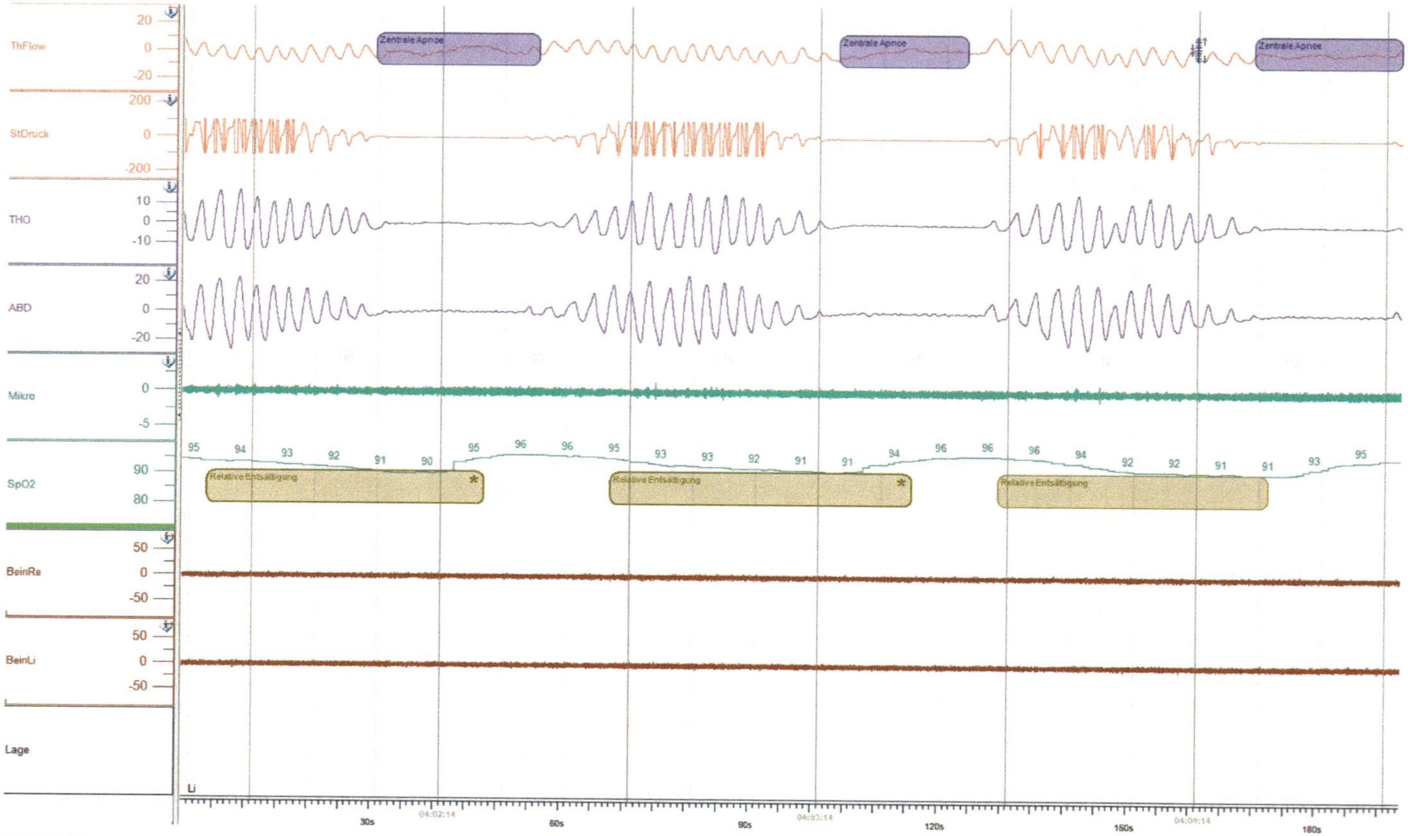

FIG. 8.11

Example of a somnogram of several subsequent central apneic events. StDruck = intranasal pressure. ThFlow = thermal airflow sensor, periods of airflow cessation are marked in *blue* color. THO = thoracic movement. ABD = abdominal movement, showing repeated cessations of breathing effort leading to apnea. Mikro = neck contact microphone. SpO2 = blood oxygen saturation, phases of desaturation are marked in *ochre* color. BeinRe and BeinLi = EMG derivations of right and left leg. Lage = body position, lying on the left side.

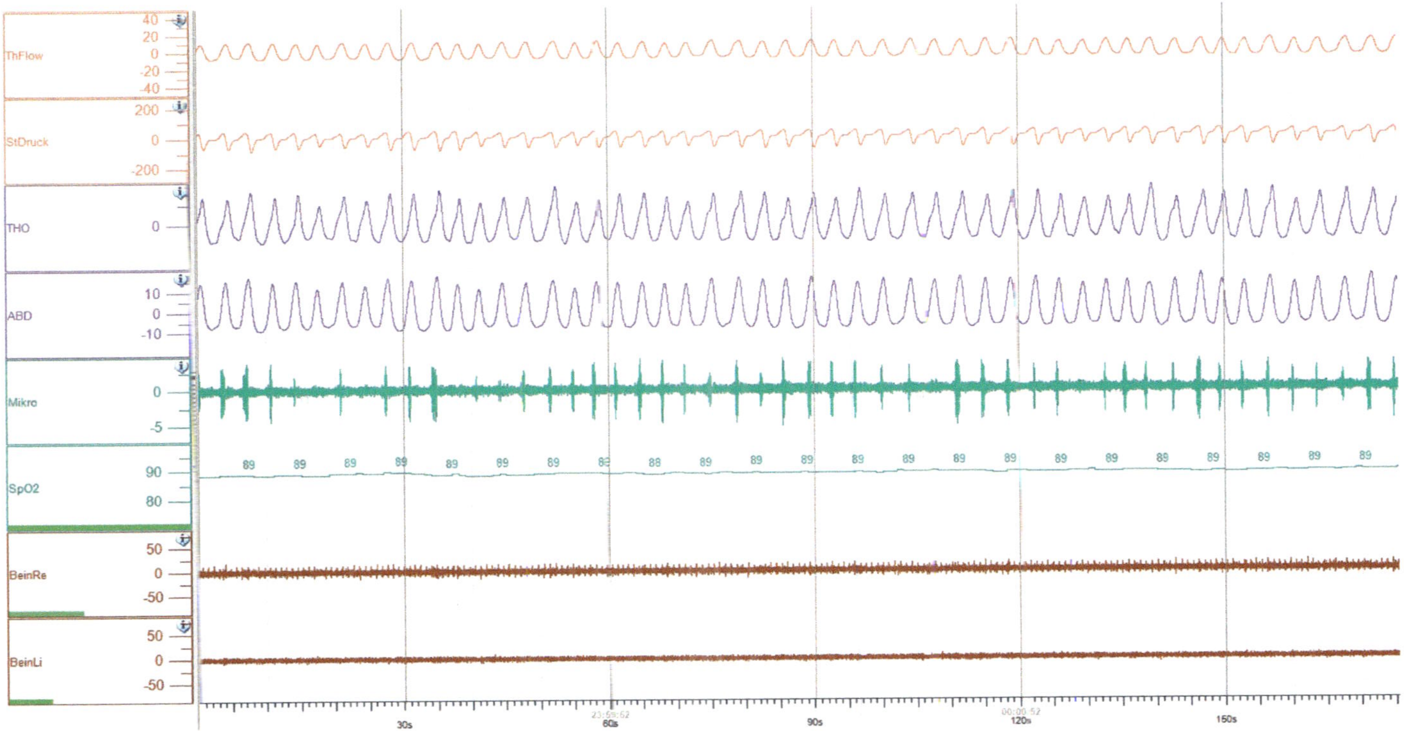

FIG. 8.12

Example of a somnogram of a primary snorer. StDruck = intranasal pressure. ThFlow = thermal airflow sensor. THO = thoracic movement. ABD = abdominal movement, showing regular breathing. Mikro = neck contact microphone, measuring regular snoring noise during inspiration. SpO2 showing normal blood oxygen saturation.

Recently, machine learning approaches have been evaluated for the automation of PSG analyses and data preprocessing, such as artifact detection [38]. Using combinations of different feature sets and classifiers, promising results could be achieved. Feature-based machine learning approaches often make use of the following temporal descriptions of the signal to be analyzed.

- *Line length* is the total length of the recorded graph from a derivation during a 30-s epoch. This temporal feature represents a mix of amplitude and frequency characteristics and can be used as part of a feature set for sleep phase classification.
- *Kurtosis* is a statistical parameter that can be useful to detect extreme value presence in a temporal signal representation to characterize signal properties as part of a feature set.
- *Sample entropy* is a temporal parameter to describe the unpredictability of a time series. In other words, sample entropy expresses the dependence of a data point on previous values in a given time period. It is a measure often applied to predict the existence of microevents in the background signal, such as spindles or K-complexes.
- *Multiscale entropy* (MSE) is another feature used for the analysis of complex physiological data in the time domain and has been applied for sleep staging. In short, MSE measures the structural complexity of a time series over multiple temporal scales [39].
- Complexity measures, in particular *fractal dimension* and *sample entropy*, of unipolar EEG derivations have been shown to be suitable predictors for the cycle type in a CAP. They can be applied for microsleep structure analysis and for the classification of sleep stages [40].

  For spectral analysis, short-term spectral transforms are usually deployed to capture temporal changes in the spectrum within an epoch. Frame lengths chosen are in the range of one to several seconds.
- *Relative spectral energy* or *power spectral density* and their statistical coefficients, such as different percentiles, minimum, mean, standard deviation, kurtosis, and derivations of successive frames, are used for classification of different types of brain waves to support sleep stage determination. Furthermore, complexity parameters and power spectral components have been tested to classify CAP A phases from EEG recordings with promising results [41, 42].
- *Wavelets* have been tested for the analysis of PSG data. Short-term time-spectrum transformations, such as Fourier transforms, generally result in a trade-off between temporal and spectral resolution. Often a detailed spectral resolution of the low-frequency range is desirable, whereas a fine resolution of the spectrum's temporal course is important for higher frequencies. Wavelet transformation allows both a fine low-frequency spectral and a detailed high-frequency temporal resolution and therefore provides useful information for analysis of nonstationary signals [43].

Wavelets are mathematical representations of oscillations that occur in a short period of time, and a wavelet transform represents the signal as a combination of scaled and translated wavelets that are defined in frequency and time.

A wavelet transform can be understood as a cascade of band-pass filters that decomposes the signal into a tree of orthogonal subspaces with an approximation part carrying the information of the low pass and a detail part that contains the high-pass information. A wavelet packet transform, in turn, decomposes both the approximation and the detail part of the original signal. Or to express it differently, while a WT employs only low-pass filters, a WPT uses both low-pass and high-pass filters.

Wavelet packet-based feature extraction algorithms have been tested successfully for the classification of EEG, EOG, and ECG signals [44]. Tunable Q-factor wavelet transform has been applied for the detection of sleep spindles and K-complexes with promising results [45].

- *Statistical inference*-based algorithms have been applied to assist human scorers in the detection of CAP phase borders [46].

Different advanced machine classifiers have been evaluated, such as extreme learning machines [47]. Deep learning methods have also been applied for PSG classification [48, 49], where an end-to-end approach was deployed to allow training of the classifier directly from the labeled raw signals without prior extraction of features.

Results show promising correlations with human expert scoring especially for deeper sleep (N2 and N3). Notably, classification of light sleep (N1) and REM sleep yields less accurate results in comparison with these stages tending to be confused with wake stages.

Most experiments are based on relatively small datasets. Using a large dataset of more than 10,000 nights of PSG recordings labeled by experts, Biswal et al. have trained a recurrent convolutional neural network (RCNN) in an end-to-end approach on EEG and EMG signals and signals from respiratory channels [48]. Labeling included sleep stages and limb movements and respiratory events. Good results were achieved in sleep stage classification (both non-REM and REM), limb movement detection, and in the measurement of OSA severity. Classification results were comparable with the interrater variations of human experts, except for light sleep (N1) and for existence of limb movements. Furthermore the model yielded promising results in the scoring of one of the most used parameters to score sleep-disordered breathing severity, the AHI index, although a finer distinction of types of breathing disorder has not been attempted.

8.5.2 Ambulatory cardiorespiratory screening

Full polysomnography has a number of disadvantages. It is expensive, limiting the number of nights that a subject can be investigated. Furthermore, it requires the subject to sleep in a dedicated sleep laboratory and therefore in an unfamiliar environment, which is likely to influence the sleep behavior, structure, and patterns. This effect is especially pronounced when the subject sleeps in a sleep laboratory for the first time, called the first-night effect.

To reduce the first-night effect and to allow for sleep monitoring over longer periods of several nights, ambulatory cardiorespiratory screening allows for the recording of a reduced number of parameters with a portable recording device that can be used in the home environment.

Often, these systems allow recording of oxygen saturation levels, airflow, breathing effort, heart rate, and body position. Since they do not record EEG data, their use is limited to the diagnosis of sleep-related breathing disorders.

8.5.3 Actigraphy

Introduced to clinical use in the 1990s, actigraphy plays an important role in the assessment of activity-rest patterns. Usually, actigraphy measurements are carried out over a longer period of time covering several days and nights.

The core of an actigraphy recorder is a set of motion sensors measuring acceleration in different axes to detect gross motor activity and to record the motions over the duration of the examination. Actigraphy recorders are small devices usually worn on the wrist.

In recent years, smartphone apps have been developed as an alternative for actigraphy recordings. While the built-in acceleration sensors of modern smartphones are sensitive and precise enough for the task at hand, none of the software solutions available are certified as medical devices to date (September 2019).

In addition to motor activity, some devices additionally measure further parameters, such as light intensity, skin temperature, or noise volume level. A comprehensive overview on the available technologies comprising medical grade and consumer products is given by Bianchi [50].

A recent review evaluates the use of actigraphy for the evaluation of mood disorders. The authors found that actigraphy can in principle distinguish between mood disorder patients and healthy controls [51].

Actigraphy in combination with the measurement of tracheal respiratory noise using a contact microphone has been investigated for the monitoring of sleep structure [52]. The authors found a moderate correlation of REM, non-REM, and awake stages with polysomnographic sleep staging, suggesting that actigraphy, especially in combination with other parameters, can be useful for sleep screening.

8.5.4 Body temperature

Skin temperature and core body temperature are related to sleep. More than an hour before sleep onset, peripheral vasodilatation leads to an increase of skin temperature, consequently increasing heat loss of the body to the environment and a fall in core body temperature. This effect is maintained during the early phases of sleep, and its strength is correlated with the duration of the first deep sleep phase [53].

Thermoregulation of the human body differs depending on the sleep stage; during REM sleep the thermoregulatory response to environmental temperature changes is reduced. However, the nightly course of body temperature and macrosleep rhythm is only partly correlated, since body temperature is not only a direct effect of the current stage of sleep but also controlled by the circadian rhythm [54].

Skin and core temperature measurement is a useful additional parameter to determine sleep onset in combination with other parameters [55, 56]. Furthermore, it has been shown that anomalies in skin temperature can be an indicator for impairment of the circadian rhythm [57].

8.5.5 Multichannel pressure measurement

Polysomnography and cardiorespiratory screening are valuable tools to identify the existence and severity of a sleep-related breathing disorder. However, they do not reveal information about the actual mechanisms that lead to the breathing difficulties. Multichannel pressure measurement helps to identify the locations within the upper airways in which narrowing or obstructions occur [58–60]. A thin tube with multiple pressure sensors is introduced into the upper airway. The pattern of pressure changes during breathing of the different sensors allows for a determination of the obstruction location during an apneic or hypopneic event. This method can in principle be used in natural sleep. However, the tube within the upper airway is not tolerated by every patient.

Fig. 8.13 shows the principle of multichannel pressure measurement in the upper airways.

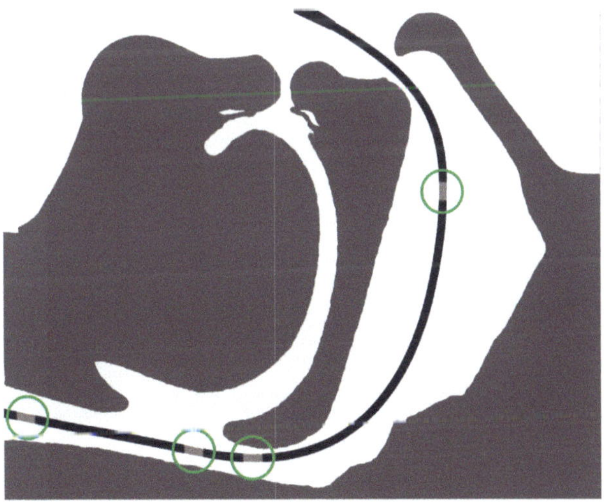

FIG. 8.13

Principle of multichannel pressure measurement. A thin tube with multiple pressure sensors is introduced intranasally into the upper airways.

8.5.6 Drug-induced sleep endoscopy

Another method to identify obstruction mechanisms in the upper airways is drug-induced sleep endoscopy (DISE). Invented in the late 1980s and first described by Croft and Pringle [61], it is increasingly used by surgical sleep specialists as a diagnostic tool in addition to PSG, especially in the therapy planning for sleep-disordered breathing patients [62].

For a DISE examination a state of artificial sleep is induced using titrated doses of narcotic agents, such as propofol or midazolam. Being in a state of unconsciousness that resembles sleep, the upper airways are intranasally inspected using a flexible nasopharyngoscope. Sleep experts evaluate the video image for the location and mechanism of airway narrowing or obstruction. Snoring activity provides additional information for diagnosis and therapy planning [63].

DISE comes with certain disadvantages. It is costly and requires the availability of qualified medical personnel and sophisticated endoscopic equipment. Furthermore a DISE investigation often takes more than 20 min overall. Also a subject would not remain asleep undisturbed through the introduction and movement of the endoscope during the procedure, so DISE cannot be performed in natural sleep.

Fig. 8.14 shows the principle setting of a DISE evaluation.

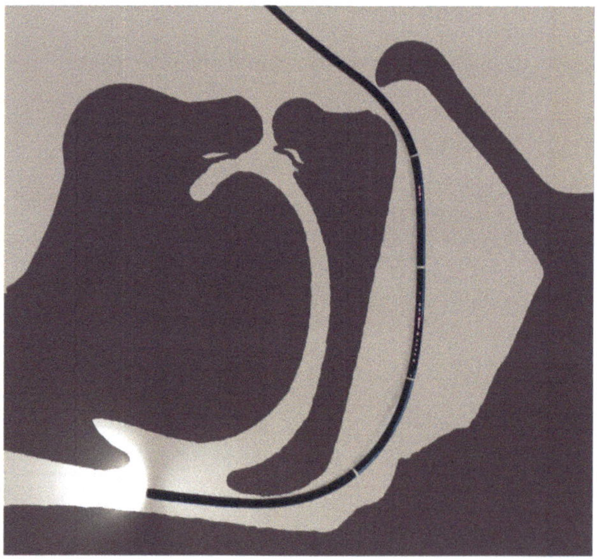

FIG. 8.14

Principle of a drug-induced sleep endoscopy procedure. A flexible nasopharyngoscope is introduced intranasally into the upper airways. By moving the tip of the endoscope back and forth, different planes of the pharynx can be observed during sleep to identify the vibration and obstruction mechanisms.

8.5.7 Acoustic analysis of breathing-related noise

Acoustic breathing and snoring noise analysis, applying machine learning methods, has become a popular field of scientific research in recent years. A large part of published research deals with OSA diagnosis. Herein, two main objectives can be distinguished:

1. Differentiation between nonobstructive (primary) snoring and obstructive sleep apnea or classification of OSA severity. The validation of the data is usually based on polysomnographic results, using the AHI or RDI as an objective reference (ground truth).
2. Detection of apneic events. Using expert-labeled polysomnographic evaluations as objective reference, a direct identification of false-positive and false-negative event detection is possible and in turn allows qualifying the sensitivity and specificity of the method.

A number of features have been investigated for use in acoustic OSA analysis with different kinds of machine classifiers.

- *Periodicity*

  Instead of analyzing the actual acoustic properties of individual acoustic events, the temporal relationship of successive events within a snoring episode can provide valuable information on the type of snoring. Primary snoring is considered to have a higher periodicity than snoring in OSA. Also a certain level of periodicity can be used in the detection of snoring and its elimination from nonsnoring acoustic events. Figs. 8.15 and 8.16 show examples of snoring episodes with high and low periodicity.
- *Fundamental frequency and harmonics*

  A sound consists of a fundamental frequency and a series of harmonics. The fundamental frequency determines the perceived pitch, while the structure of the

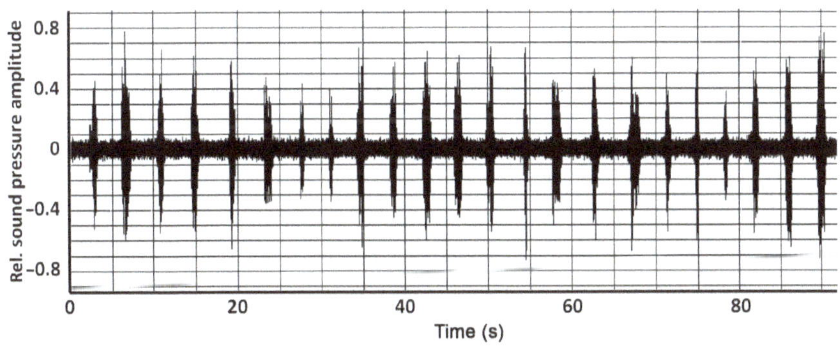

FIG. 8.15

Snoring episode of a primary snorer, showing a high periodicity.

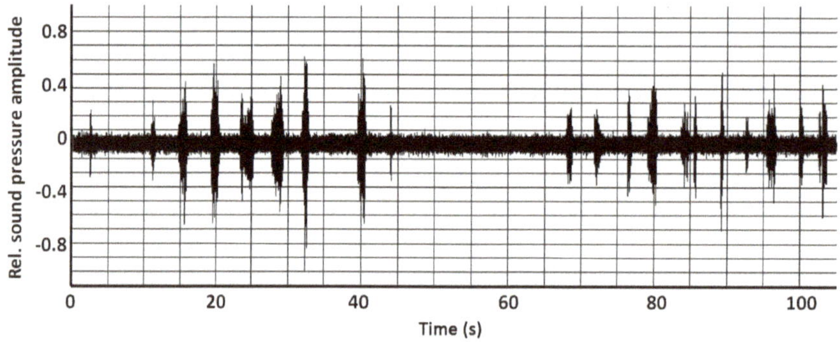

FIG. 8.16

Snoring episode of a snorer with obstructive sleep apnea.

harmonics determines the timbre. For example, the chamber note *A*, played on a piano and a guitar, has the same fundamental frequency but a different harmonic spectrum, which characterizes the sound of the instrument. In contrast, noise contains no tonal components and therefore has no distinctive harmonic structure [64].

Several studies conclude that primary snoring has more pronounced tonal components compared with snoring of OSA patients, assuming that primary snoring is generated on the velopharyngeal level, while OSA-related snoring is excited in the retrolingual or hypopharyngeal level. In some studies a lower fundamental frequency was found in velum snorers compared with lingual snorers [65, 66]. Sleep endoscopic pilot studies revealed a direct correlation between acoustic properties and the location of sound generation [67]. Notably, these results could not be reproduced in the natural sleep of the same volunteers, and further conclusions should be drawn with caution.

– *Crest factor*

The crest factor is used to quantify the tonal fraction of a snoring sound. It describes the ratio of peak value to root mean square (RMS) or effective value of a signal amplitude. High crest factors not only signify a high fraction of harmonics but also can be caused by strong impulses in a signal [68].

Pilot studies with small sample sizes conclude that the crest factors of palate snorers are significantly higher compared with the nonsoft palate snorers [69]. In natural sleep the crest factor can vary overtime, suggesting that the type of snoring may change during the night and that sleep video endoscopy may not be representative of snoring behavior during natural sleep [70].

– *Spectral energy ratio*

A long-standing approach is to differentiate between primary and OSA-related snoring by the ratio of energy content in the snoring noise signal below and above a certain cutoff frequency. The exact definition of the cutoff frequency varies but is usually in the order of 1 kHz. An alternative approach is to determine the frequency above and below of which the energy content of the sound signal is equal.

Several studies show that primary snoring contains higher low-frequency energy components than OSA-related snoring [71–73]. It is found that the soft palate vibrates with a fundamental frequency well below 1 kHz and the harmonic's energy decreases with increasing frequency. Consequently the main energy content of the signal is in the low-frequency range. Snoring at tongue base level, as it often occurs in OSA-related snoring, generates a higher portion of nonperiodic, noise-like signals caused by turbulent airflow in the constricted areas. Hence the energy spectrum of the resulting noisy signal contains a larger ratio of high-frequency energy components.

However, the results are based on statistical evaluation of the relationship between spectral energy ratio and AHI, assuming that a high AHI is related to tongue base snoring. A direct distinction of velar and nonvelar snoring based on the spectral energy ratio has not yet been demonstrated.

- *Pitch*

  In speech signal analysis, pitch refers to the course of the fundamental frequency of speech over time [74]. Accordingly, pitch can be used to describe the course of the fundamental frequency over the duration of a snoring event, see Fig. 8.17.

  Pitch analysis, to distinguish between primary and OSA-related snoring, has been described in several publications. A distinction between snorers with and without OSA was demonstrated based on the stability of the fundamental frequency of snoring sounds [75]. Pitch discontinuities (jumps in the fundamental frequency within a snoring event) also indicate OSA-related snoring [76].

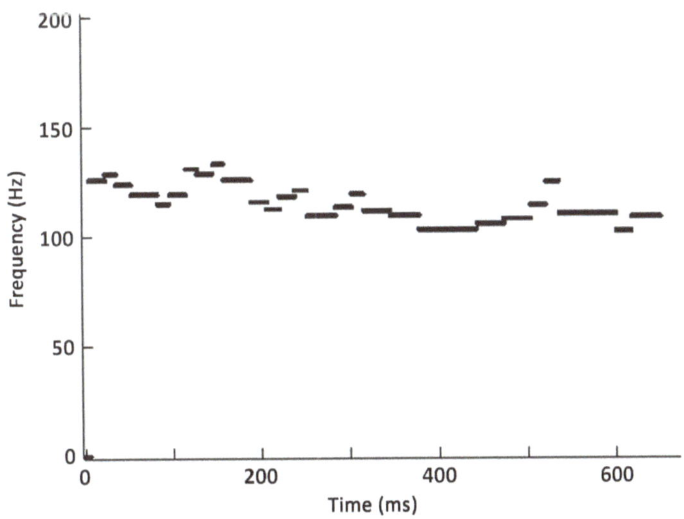

FIG. 8.17

Pitch diagram of a velum snore event.

– *Sound pressure level*

The sound pressure level (SPL) has been used in numerous studies to quantify snoring. For example, a relationship between SPL and RDI was shown in a large cohort of more than 1000 subjects [77].

It should be noted that the measurement of the absolute SPL in snorers can be very error prone. The SPL of a point source (e.g., a snorer) decreases with the square of the distance from the source. Consequently the distance between recording microphone and mouth and nose of the snorer has a considerable influence on the measured value. Additional potential error factors are the room acoustics (reverberation of the room) and the sleeping position. Especially in an environment that is not completely controllable over the course of the recording process, analyzing absolute SPL values involves a high risk of uncertainty.

– *Formants*

In speech analysis the resonance frequencies of the respiratory tract's transfer function are called *formants*. These are essentially influenced by the position of tongue, soft palate, and lips. Formants are independent of the stimulating signal. For example, they remain constant with changing pitch. It is reasonable to assume that different types of snoring have characteristic resonance frequencies determined by the typical positions of the tongue and soft palate and the different overall length of the acoustically active part of the upper respiratory tract, which could be referred to as *snoring formants*. See Fig. 8.18 for an example of a typical velum-snoring spectrum.

While contact microphones attached to the neck at tracheal level are routinely used in PSG to detect snoring, an airborne sound microphone is required to

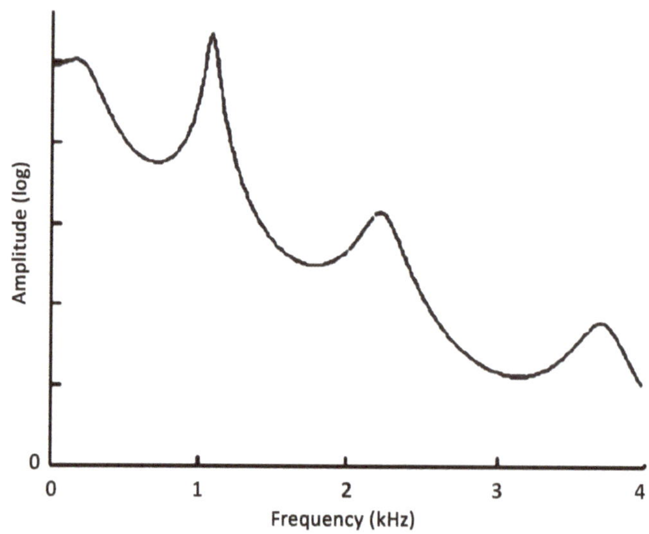

FIG. 8.18

Snoring formants of a velum snore event.

measure snoring formants, since the spectrum shaped by the upper respiratory tract becomes audible only when the sound exits the nose and mouth.

Snoring formant characteristics for the classification of OSA severity have been investigated in several studies [78, 79], reporting statistical correlations between the first snoring formant and the severity of OSA.

- *Mel-frequency cepstral coefficients (MFCC)*

  Calculated from a psychoacoustically warped power spectrum of a discretely Fourier-transformed short-term segment of a signal, MFCCs are a compact representation of a signal's spectral properties. They are regularly used in speech recognition applications because they allow for a separation of the properties of excitation signal and transfer function.

  In sleep laboratory studies of test subjects, the stability of MFCCs over the entire night was used to distinguish between primary and OSA snorers [75], finding that MFCCs were more stable in primary snorers. It is assumed that OSA is associated with an unstable muscular balance in the upper respiratory tract, which is acoustically expressed in a variability of its transfer function overtime.
- *Perceptual linear prediction (PLP) and relative spectral transform perceptual linear prediction (RASTA-PLP)*

  PLP is a psychoacoustically adjusted approximation of the vocal tract's spectral transfer function [80], and RASTA-PLP adds a step of linear band-pass filtering to each energy band after the spectral transformation, to reduce the impact of slowly varying and constant signal components. RASTA filtering especially provides superior results over PLP for signals overlaid with static background noise [81]. PLP and RASTA-PLP features have been tested in the classification of the excitation locations of snoring sounds with promising results [82, 83].
- *Wavelets*

  The usefulness of wavelets has been explored for the identification of obstructive events in OSA patients [84]. Using a continuous wavelet transform, higher fractions of high-frequency energy components in the snoring event, directly following the apneic event, were found. Wavelet transforms and wavelet packet transforms were applied as features to classify the excitation location of snoring sounds, achieving comparable results with large feature space extraction approaches [85, 86].

8.6 Conclusion

In the handbook of clinical neurology, issued in 2011 [31], it was stated that "the great expectation from computerization was to provide reliable automatic sleep stage scoring and to enhance our ability to understand physiologic information in new, clinically useful ways; however, we are still waiting for these hopes to be realized."

Research results from recent years show that machine learning methods for the interpretation and classification of sleep data have made a big leap forward toward reaching these goals. The results are promising to support clinical experts in the interpretation of sleep data and support diagnosis, freeing personnel from time-consuming manual routine work.

The development of sophisticated machine learning models for the interpretation of PSG data can also facilitate more accurate sleep monitoring with a reduced number of channels or novel combinations of sleep parameters. This will allow for a more cost-effective and mobile sleep monitoring that is more convenient for the sleeper. Also, there will be less sleep disturbance and longer-term sleep data recording.

With the availability of larger datasets of longer-term sleep data, new findings in the correlation of sleep structure and diseases will most likely be possible, deepening the understanding of the underlying properties of sleep and improving diagnoses.

Sleep research has been a fascinating field of research over the past centuries, and it is most likely to remain fascinating especially with the introduction of advanced methods of sleep signal processing and automated evaluation to support medical diagnosis and therapy decision-making.

Acknowledgments

The author holds a German patent on a method and system for the determination of anatomical causes of snoring noise (DE102012219128B4). The author would like to thank Katharina Eckbauer and Clemens Heiser from Klinikum rechts der Isar, Munich for providing example polysomnograms and making their sleep laboratory available for photos.

References

[1] T. Young, M. Palta, J. Dempsey, J. Skatrud, S. Weber, S. Badr, The occurrence of sleep-disordered breathing among middle-aged adults, N. Engl. J. Med. 328 (1993) 1230–1235.

[2] E. Kohlschuetter, Messungen zur Festigkeit des Schlafes, Z Rat Med. 17 (1863) 209–253.

[3] R. MacNish, The Philosophy of Sleep, WR M'Phun, Glasgow, 1830.

[4] R. Wittern, Sleep theories in the antiquity and in the Renaissance, in: J.A. Horne (Ed.), Sleep 88, Fischer Verlag, Stuttgart, 1989, pp. 11–22.

[5] A.E. Durham, The Physiology of Sleep, Guy's Hospital Reports, Vol. 6, 1860, pp. 149–173.

[6] J. Russell, On sleepiness, Br. Med. J. 2 (1861) 488–490.

[7] C.M. Morin, P.J. Hauri, C.A. Espie, Nonpharmacologic treatment of chronic insomnia. An American Academy of Sleep Medicine review, Sleep 22 (1999) 1134–1156.

[8] H. Berger, Ueber das Elektrenkephalogramm des Menschen, Archiv Psychiatr. Nervenkr. 87 (1929) 527–570.

[9] A.L. Loomis, E.N. Harvey, G.A. Hobart, Cerebral states during sleep, as studied by human brain potentials, J. Exp. Psychol. 21 (1937) 127–144.

[10] E. Aserinsky, N. Kleitman, Regularly occurring periods of eye motility, and concomitant phenomena, during sleep, Science 118 (1953) 273–274.

[11] A. Rechtschaffen, A. Kales, A Manual of Standardised Terminology, Techniques and Scoring System for Sleep Stages of Human Subjects, Brain Information Service/Brain Research Institute, Los Angeles, 1968.
[12] M.J. Thorpy, History of sleep medicine, Handb. Clin. Neurol. 98 (2011) 3–25.
[13] H. Schulz, P. Salzarulo, The development of sleep medicine: a historical sketch, J. Clin. Sleep Med. 12 (7) (2016) 1041–1052.
[14] M.J. Sateia, International classification of sleep disorders-third edition, Chest 146 (5) (2014) 1387–1394.
[15] M. Partinen, Epidemiology of sleep disorders, Handb. Clin. Neurol. 98 (2011) 275–314.
[16] M. Partinen, C. Hublin, Epidemiology of sleep disorders, in: M.H. Kryger, T. Roth, W. Dement (Eds.), Principles and Practice of Sleep Medicine, third ed., WB Saunders Co, Philadelphia, PA, 2000, pp. 558–579.
[17] S. Ram, H. Seirawan, S.K.S. Kumar, G.T. Clark, Prevalence and impact of sleep disorders and sleep habits in the United States, Sleep Breath. 14 (1) (2010) 63–70.
[18] Y. Takaesu, Y. Inoue, A. Murakoshi, Y. Komada, A. Otsuka, K. Futenma, et al., Prevalence of circadian rhythm sleep-wake disorders and associated factors in euthymic patients with bipolar disorder, PLoS One 11 (7) (2016). e0159578.
[19] L. Zhu, P.C. Zee, Circadian rhythm sleep disorders, Neurol. Clin. 30 (4) (2012) 1167–1191.
[20] Y. Dauvilliers, A. Buguet, Hypersomnia, Dialogues Clin. Neurosci. 7 (4) (2005) 347–356.
[21] C.V. Senaratna, J.L. Perret, C.J. Lodge, A.J. Lowe, B.E. Campbell, M.C. Matheson, et al., Prevalence of obstructive sleep apnea in the general population: a systematic review, Sleep Med. Rev. 34 (2017) 70–81.
[22] M.W. Calik, Update on the treatment of narcolepsy: clinical efficacy of pitolisant, Nat. Sci. Sleep 9 (2017) 127–133.
[23] S.W. Black, A. Yamanaka, T.S. Kilduff, Challenges in the development of therapeutics for narcolepsy, Prog. Neurobiol. 152 (2017) 89–113.
[24] C.F. Reynolds, R. O'Hara, DSM-5 sleep-wake disorders classification: overview for use in clinical practice, Am. J. Psychiatry 170 (10) (2013) 1099–1101.
[25] C. Janott, M. Schmitt, Y. Zhang, K. Qian, V. Pandit, Z. Zhang, et al., Snoring classified: the Munich-Passau Snore Sound Corpus, Comput. Biol. Med. 94 (2018) 106–118.
[26] C. Dickens, The Posthumous Papers of the Pickwick Club, Chapman & Hall, England, 1837.
[27] A.G. Bickelmann, C.S. Burwell, E.D. Robin, R.D. Whaley, Extreme obesity associated with alveolar hypoventilation; a Pickwickian syndrome, Am. J. Med. 21 (5) (1956) 811–818.
[28] R.L. Williams, I. Karacan, C.J. Hursch, EEG of Human Sleep: Clinical Applications, Wiley, New York, 1974.
[29] R.K. Malhotra, A.Y. Avidan, Sleep stages and scoring technique, in: Atlas of Sleep Medicine, Elsevier Inc, 2014, pp. 77–99.
[30] C. Iber, S. Ancoli-Israel, A.L. Chesson, S.F. Quan, The AASM Manual for the Scoring of Sleep and Associated Events: Rules, Terminology and Technical Specifications, first ed., American Academy of Sleep Medicine, 2007.
[31] M. Hirshkowitz, A. Sharafkhaneh, Normal sleep-recording and scoring techniques, Handb. Clin. Neurol. 98 (2011) 29–43.
[32] M.G. Terzano, D. Mancia, M.R. Salati, G. Costani, A. Decembrino, L. Parrino, The cyclic alternating pattern as a physiologic component of normal NREM sleep, Sleep 8 (2) (1985) 137–145.

[33] L. Parrino, R. Ferri, O. Bruni, M.G. Terzano, Cyclic alternating pattern (CAP): the marker of sleep instability, Sleep Med. Rev. 16 (1) (2012) 27–45.
[34] B. Stuck, A. Dreher, C. Heiser, M. Herzog, T. Kühnel, J. Maurer, et al., Sk2 guidelines diagnosis and therapy of snoring in adults compiled by the sleep medicine working group of the German Society of Otorhinolaryngology, head and neck surgery, HNO 61 (2013) 944–957.
[35] H. Gastaut, C.A. Tassinari, B. Duron, Polygraphic study of the episodic diurnal and nocturnal (hypnic and respiratory) manifestations of the Pickwick syndrome, Brain Res. 1 (2) (1966) 167–186.
[36] G.M. Barthlen, Schlafdiagnostik (Polysomnographie), in: H. Matthys, W. Seeger (Eds.), Klinische Pneumologie, Springer Berlin Heidelberg, Berlin, 2002, pp. 103–111.
[37] G. Mayer, I. Fietze, J. Fischer, T. Penzel, D. Riemann, A. Rodenbeck, et al., S 3-Leitlinie. Nicht erholsamer Schlaf–Schlafstoerungen, Springer, 2011.
[38] E. Saifutdinova, D.U. Dudysova, L. Lhotska, V. Gerla, M. Macas, Artifact detection in multichannel sleep EEG using random forest classifier, in: 2018 IEEE International Conference on Bioinformatics and Biomedicine (BIBM); December, 2018, pp. 2803–2805.
[39] M. Costa, A.L. Goldberger, C.K. Peng, Multiscale entropy analysis of complex physiologic time series, Phys. Rev. Lett. 89 (6) (2002) 068102.
[40] I. Chouvarda, V. Rosso, M.O. Mendez, A.M. Bianchi, L. Parrino, A. Grassi, et al., EEG Complexity during Sleep: on the effect of micro and macro sleep structure, in: 2010 Annual International Conference of the IEEE Engineering in Medicine and Biology; August, 2010, pp. 5959–5962.
[41] R. Ferri, O. Bruni, S. Miano, G. Plazzi, M.G. Terzano, All-night EEG power spectral analysis of the cyclic alternating pattern components in young adult subjects, Clin. Neurophysiol. 116 (10) (2005) 2429–2440.
[42] S. Mariani, E. Manfredini, V. Rosso, A. Grassi, M.O. Mendez, A. Alba, et al., Efficient automatic classifiers for the detection of A phases of the cyclic alternating pattern in sleep, Med. Biol. Eng. Comput. 50 (4) (2012) 359–372.
[43] S. Mallat, A Wavelet Tour of Signal Processing, Academic Press, 1999.
[44] R.N. Khushaba, S. Kodagoda, S. Lal, G. Dissanayake, Driver drowsiness classification using fuzzy wavelet-packet-based feature-extraction algorithm, IEEE Trans. Biomed. Eng. 58 (2011) 121–131.
[45] A.R. Hassan, M.I.H. Bhuiyan, A decision support system for automatic sleep staging from EEG signals using tunable Q-factor wavelet transform and spectral features, J. Neurosci. Methods 271 (2016) 107–118.
[46] J.M. Tenorio, A. Alba, M.O. Mendez, A.M. Bianchi, A. Grassi, E. Arce-Santana, et al., A novel method to assist the detection of the cyclic alternating pattern (CAP), in: Annual International Conference of the IEEE Engineering in Medicine and Biology Society. IEEE Engineering in Medicine and Biology Society. Annual Conference 2012, 2012, pp. 3656–3659.
[47] H. Sun, J. Jia, B. Goparaju, G.B. Huang, O. Sourina, M.T. Bianchi, et al., Large-scale automated sleep staging, Sleep 40 (10) (2017).
[48] S. Biswal, H. Sun, B. Goparaju, M.B. Westover, J. Sun, M.T. Bianchi, Expert-level sleep scoring with deep neural networks, J. Am. Med. Inform. Assoc. 25 (12) (2018) 1643–1650.
[49] S. Chambon, V. Thorey, P.J. Arnal, E. Mignot, A. Gramfort, A deep learning architecture to detect events in EEG signals during sleep, in: 2018 IEEE 28th International Workshop on Machine Learning for Signal Processing (MLSP); September, 2018, pp. 1–6.

[50] M.T. Bianchi, Sleep devices: wearables and nearables, informational and interventional, consumer and clinical, Metab. Clin. Exp. 84 (2018) 99–108.

[51] Y. Tazawa, M. Wada, Y. Mitsukura, A. Takamiya, M. Kitazawa, M. Yoshimura, et al., Actigraphy for evaluation of mood disorders: a systematic review and meta-analysis, J. Affect. Disord. 253 (2019) 257–269.

[52] C. Kalkbrenner, R. Brucher, T. Kesztyus, M. Eichenlaub, W. Rottbauer, D. Scharnbeck, Automated sleep stage classification based on tracheal body sound and actigraphy, Ger. Med. Sci. 17 (2019). p. Doc02.

[53] I. Montgomery, J. Trinder, S. Paxton, Physical exercise and sleep: the effect of the age and sex of the subjects and type of exercise, Acta Physiol. Scand. 133 (1988) 36–40.

[54] L.C. Lack, K. Lushington, The rhythms of human sleep propensity and core body temperature, J. Sleep Res. 5 (1996) 1–11.

[55] E.H. Geschickter, P.A. Andrews, R.W. Bullard, Nocturnal body temperature regulation in man: a rationale for sweating in sleep, J. Appl. Physiol. 21 (2) (1966) 623–630.

[56] K. Krauchi, C. Cajochen, E. Werth, A. Wirz-Justice, Functional link between distal vasodilation and sleep-onset latency? Am. J. Physiol. Regul. Integr. Comp. Physiol. 278 (3) (2000) R741–R748.

[57] A. Martinez-Nicolas, M. Guaita, J. Santamaria, J.M. Montserrat, M.A. Rol, J.A. Madrid, Circadian impairment of distal skin temperature rhythm in patients with sleep-disordered breathing: the effect of CPAP, Sleep 40 (6) (2017).

[58] H. Demin, Y. Jingying, W.J.Y. Qingwen, L. Yuhua, W. Jiangyong, Determining the site of airway obstruction in obstructive sleep apnea with airway pressure measurements during sleep, Laryngoscope 112 (2002) 2081–2085.

[59] M. Reda, G.J. Gibson, J.A. Wilson, Pharyngoesophageal pressure monitoring in sleep apnea syndrome, Otolaryngol. Head Neck Surg. 125 (2001) 324–331.

[60] B.A. Stuck, J.T. Maurer, Airway evaluation in obstructive sleep apnea, Sleep Med. Rev. 12 (2008) 411–436.

[61] C.B. Croft, M. Pringle, Sleep nasendoscopy: a technique of assessment in snoring and obstructive sleep apnoea, Clin. Otolaryngol. Allied Sci. 16 (1991) 504–509.

[62] M.R. El Badawey, G. McKee, H. Marshall, N. Heggie, J.A. Wilson, Predictive value of sleep nasendoscopy in the management of habitual snorers, Ann. Otol. Rhinol. Laryngol. 112 (2003) 40–44.

[63] C. Janott, W. Pirsig, C. Heiser, Akustische Analyse von Schnarchgeräuschen, Somnologie-Schlafforschung und Schlafmedizin 18 (2014) 87–95.

[64] M. Cremer, Vorlesungen über Technische Akustik, Springer-Verlag, Berlin, 1990.

[65] J. Schafer, How can one recognize a velum snorer? Laryngorhinootologie. 68 (1989) 290–294.

[66] S.J. Quinn, L. Huang, P.D. Ellis, J.E. Williams, The differentiation of snoring mechanisms using sound analysis, Clin. Otolaryngol. Allied Sci. 21 (1996) 119–123.

[67] S. Agrawal, P. Stone, K. McGuinness, J. Morris, A.E. Camilleri, Sound frequency analysis and the site of snoring in natural and induced sleep, Clin. Otolaryngol. Allied Sci. 27 (2002) 162–166.

[68] R. Flosdorff, G. Hilgarth, Elektrische Energieverteilung, Vieweg+Teubner, Wiesbaden, 2005.

[69] P.D. Hill, B.W.V. Lee, J.E. Osborne, E.Z. Osman, Palatal snoring identified by acoustic crest factor analysis, Physiol. Meas. 20 (1999) 167–174.

[70] P.D. Hill, E.Z. Osman, J.E. Osborne, B.W.V. Lee, Changes in snoring during natural sleep identified by acoustic crest factor analysis at different times of night, Clin. Otolaryngol. Allied Sci. 25 (2000) 507–510.

[71] J.R. Perez-Padilla, E. Slawinski, L.M. Difrancesco, R.R. Feige, J.E. Remmers, W.A. Whitelaw, Characteristics of the snoring noise in patients with and without occlusive sleep apnea, Am. Rev. Respir. Dis. 147 (3) (1993) 635–644.
[72] M. Herzog, A. Schmidt, T. Bremert, B. Herzog, W. Hosemann, H. Kaftan, Analysed snoring sounds correlate to obstructive sleep disordered breathing, Eur. Arch. Otorhinolaryngol. 265 (1) (2008) 105–113.
[73] J.A. Fiz, J. Abad, R. Jane, M. Riera, M.A. Mananas, P. Caminal, et al., Acoustic analysis of snoring sound in patients with simple snoring and obstructive sleep apnoea, Eur. Respir. J. 9 (11) (1996) 2365–2370.
[74] M.H. Hayes, Statistical Digital Signal Processing and Modeling, Wiley, 1996.
[75] N. Ben-Israel, A. Tarasiuk, Y. Zigel, Nocturnal sound analysis for the diagnosis of obstructive sleep apnea, in: Annual International Conference of the IEEE Engineering in Medicine and Biology Society. IEEE Engineering in Medicine and Biology Society. Annual Conference 2010, 2010, pp. 6146–6149.
[76] U.R. Abeyratne, A.S. Wakwella, C. Hukins, Pitch jump probability measures for the analysis of snoring sounds in apnea, Physiol. Meas. 26 (2005) 779–798.
[77] K. Wilson, R.A. Stoohs, T.F. Mulrooney, L.J. Johnson, C. Guilleminault, Z. Huang, The snoring spectrum: acoustic assessment of snoring sound intensity in 1,139 individuals undergoing polysomnography, Chest 115 (1999) 762–770.
[78] A.K. Ng, T. San Koh, E. Baey, T.H. Lee, U.R. Abeyratne, K. Puvanendran, Could formant frequencies of snore signals be an alternative means for the diagnosis of obstructive sleep apnea? Sleep Med. 9 (2008) 894–898.
[79] E. Dafna, A. Tarasiuk, Y. Zigel, Automatic detection of whole night snoring events using non-contact microphone, PLoS One 8 (12) (2013). e84139.
[80] H. Hermansky, Perceptual linear predictive (PLP) analysis of speech, J. Acoust. Soc. Am. 87 (1990) 1738–1752.
[81] H. Hermansky, N. Morgan, RASTA processing of speech, IEEE Trans. Speech Audio Process. 2 (1994) 578–589.
[82] B. Schuller, S. Steidl, A. Batliner, E. Bergelson, J. Krajewski, C. Janott, et al., The INTERSPEECH 2017 computational paralinguistics challenge: addressee, cold & snoring, in: Proceedings of INTERSPEECH; Stockholm, 2017, pp. 20–24.
[83] K. Qian, C. Janott, V. Pandit, Z. Zhang, C. Heiser, W. Hohenhorst, et al., Classification of the excitation location of snore sounds in the upper airway by acoustic multi-feature analysis, IEEE Trans. Biomed. Eng. 64 (2017) 1731–1741.
[84] D. Matsiki, X. Deligianni, E. Vlachogianni-Daskalopoulou, L.J. Hadjileontiadis, Wavelet-based analysis of nocturnal snoring in apneic patients undergoing polysomnography, in: Proceedings of the IEEE EMBS 29th Annual International Conference, 2007, pp. 1912–1915.
[85] K. Qian, C. Janott, J. Deng, C. Heiser, W. Hohenhorst, M. Herzog, et al., Snore sound recognition: on wavelets and classifiers from deep nets to kernels, in: 39th Annual International Conference of the IEEE Engineering in Medicine and Biology Society (EMBC); Seogwipo, 2017, pp. 3737–3740.
[86] K. Qian, C. Janott, Z. Zhang, C. Heiser, et al., Wavelet features for classification of vote snore sounds, in: 2016 41st IEEE International Conference on Acoustics, Speech and Signal Processing (ICASSP), 2016, pp. 221–225.

Index

Note: Page numbers followed by *f* indicate figures and *t* indicate tables.

E

F

M

N

O

P

Kolibri 360 GmbH
Ferdinand-Jühlke-Straße 7
99095 Erfurt, Deutschland
produktsicherheit@kolibri360.de